Physical Fitness Digest

By
George B. Anderson
and
Pamela J. Johnson

DBI BOOKS, INC. / NORTHFIELD, ILLINOIS

STAFF

EDITORIAL CONSULTANT
Ron Wellman/Director Athletics, Elmhurst College

PHOTOGRAPHY
John Hanusin
Elmhurst College Photography Staff

COVER PHOTOGRAPHY
John Hanusin

MODELS
Linda Turney
William J. Factor
Rich Williams
George Dunne

ASSOCIATE PUBLISHER
Sheldon L. Factor

ISNB 0-695-81275-0
Library of Congress Catalog Card Number 79-50058

Acknowledgments

The authors of this book are indebted to the cooperation of and contributions from the following people and U.S. government publications: Robert C. Fellows, Linda Turney, William Factor, Ron Guenther, Iligene Anderson, *Adult Physical Fitness, Youth Physical Fitness, Fitness and Work Capacity, The Fitness Challenge in the Later Years* and *Aqua Dynamics*.

Contents

CHAPTER 4: ENDURANCE

CHAPTER 5: NUTRITION AND WEIGHT

CHAPTER 6: PROGRAMS

CHAPTER 7: NOW IT'S UP TO YOU

PHYSICAL FITNESS

Physical fitness is a quality of life. It is the condition that helps a person to look and feel well, to carry out his daily duties and responsibilities successfully, and yet have enough physical reserves to enjoy his other social, civic, cultural, and recreational interests. In addition, it enables him to meet unusual or emergency demands.

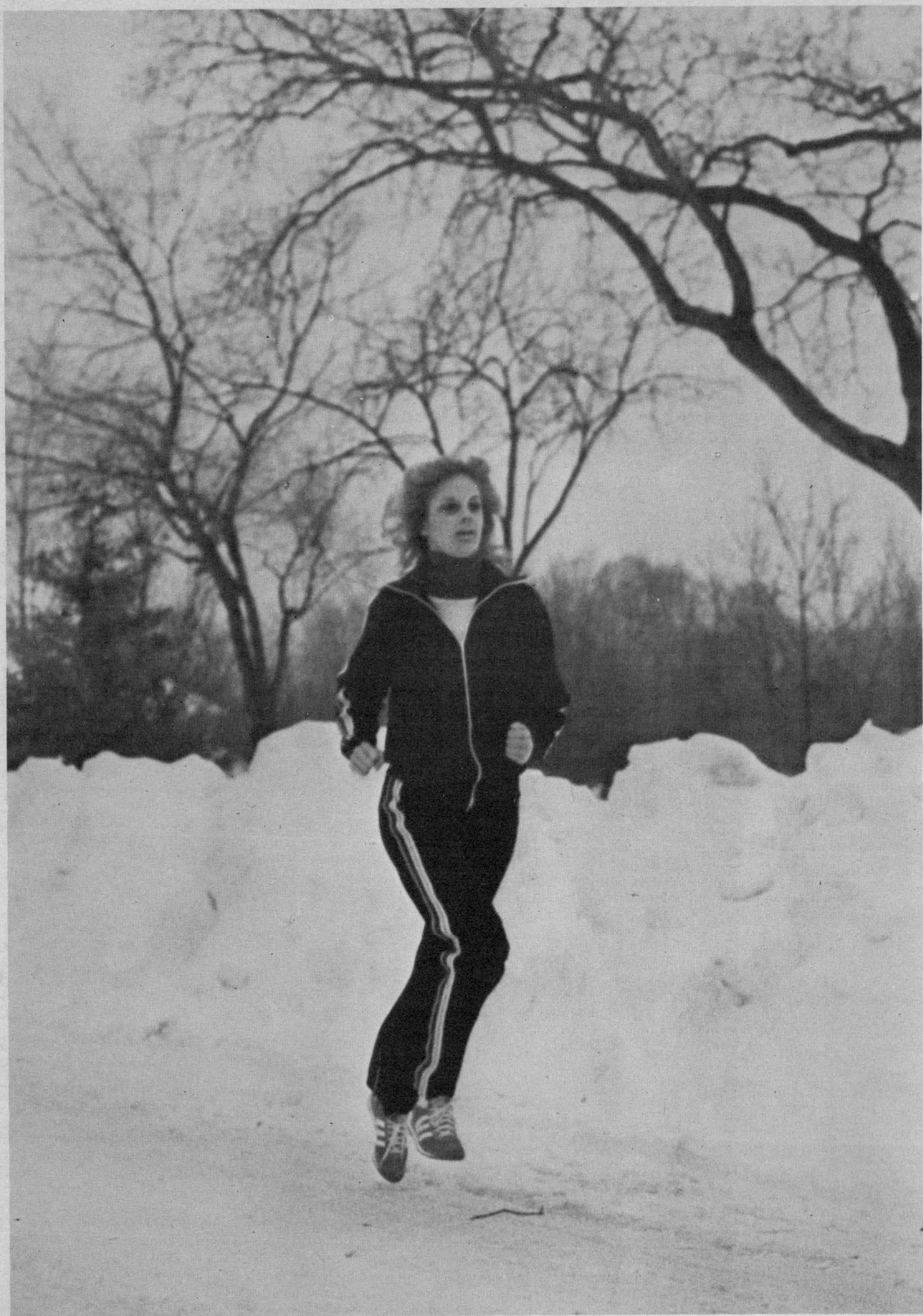

chapter 1

Physical Fitness

EVERYONE AGREES that physical fitness is a good thing. Argue *against* it, and you'll be a minority of one.

Nearly everyone also agrees that most of us don't get enough regular, healthful exercise. This same majority believes exercise is "good for you" and that they should get into better physical shape and then follow a regimen that will keep them physically fit.

So what? The same people unanimously agree that taxes are too high, that the price of gas is exorbitant, that the weather leaves a lot to be desired, and that there's too much red tape in government. Having agreed on all of these problems, having acknowledged that they exist, most of us do absolutely nothing to remedy the situation.

Yes, there are many perplexing problems—but the problem of physical fitness is a comparatively easy one to solve. However, to do it, every individual must take that first step—from awareness to action. Regular exercise is something that most of us agree we *should* do—and even *will* do—but not today, maybe tomorrow, or next week, or next month, or next year. Unfortunately many of us wait until we're faced with a life threatening situation. A doctor told a close friend of mine that he had to take off 80 pounds, repeating that warning every time my friend got a checkup. He once half-heartedly started a diet routine so unappetizing that I doubt I'd have stayed with it more than a couple of days. My

fitness in america:

These are highlights of the National Adult Physical Fitness Survey conducted by Opinion Research Corporation of Princeton, N.J., for the President's Council. Here are some specific findings:

• Forty-five percent of all adult Americans do not engage in physical activity for the purpose of exercise.

• Only 55% of American men and women do any exercise at all, but 57% say they believe they are as physically active as they should be.

• Persons who don't exercise are more inclined to say they get enough exercise than are those who do exercise. Sixty-three percent of the non-exercisers say they get enough exercise, while only 53% of the exercisers believe they are as physically active as they should be.

• Of the 60 million American men and women who engage in various forms of exercise, nearly 44 million walk for exercise. More than 18 million ride bicycles for exercise (as opposed to recreation), 14 million swim for exercise, and 14 million do calisthenics.

friend held firm for 5 days and then ate like a glutton when he was invited out to dinner. From that time on, the diet was forgotten—forgotten, that is, until he had a severe coronary.

He pulled through, but the doctor then told him that he'd have to follow a regular, vigorous exercise program and strict diet or he'd soon be dead. That was a choice my friend understood. He found exercise and diet much more attractive than dying. Today, he's a healthy man again, and looks 10 years younger than he did before his heart attack. He thoroughly enjoys his physical fitness program and tries to convert others.

But the point I'm making is that he did absolutely nothing to improve his health until he was forced to do it.

My son, an active sports participant in high school and college, entered the business world and was so successful that he soon found he didn't have time for sports. But he soon began putting on weight—too much weight—and decided he had to do something to get back into the kind of physical condition he'd previously enjoyed.

He discovered the president of the company liked to play tennis and got on a schedule of playing tennis at least two mornings a week before the business day began. Then he booked time at a tennis club two nights a week, where he plays tennis, racquetball and handball.

He and his family spend their summer weekends at a Wisconsin lake. One of the neighbors has a good tennis court which he uses every Saturday and Sunday. He also does a lot of swimming and water skiing. So far this summer, he's taken his family on three kayak trips on nearby rivers. In the winter, he and his family do a lot of both downhill and cross-country skiing.

He's physically hard as a rock, and he now says being "too busy" was nothing more than an excuse for not keeping fit. He has 10-speed bikes for his whole family, and they go on frequent bike-trail jaunts. As a result of his fitness program, he's much closer to his two young sons than most sedentary fathers are, and the boys are in fine physical condition, as is his wife.

Because he took that relatively easy first step—playing tennis with the boss—he soon got back into the swing and is now a confirmed exercise advocate.

My daughter and son-in-law, who live with their little son and daughter in Boulder, Colorado, follow the same kind of a routine, except that brisk jogging, both winter and summer in all kinds of weather is a part of their life-style. They also do a great deal of mountain hiking and bicycling.

My daughter and the children are on a brisk swimming program, and the children have regular classes in gymnastics. From an easy start,

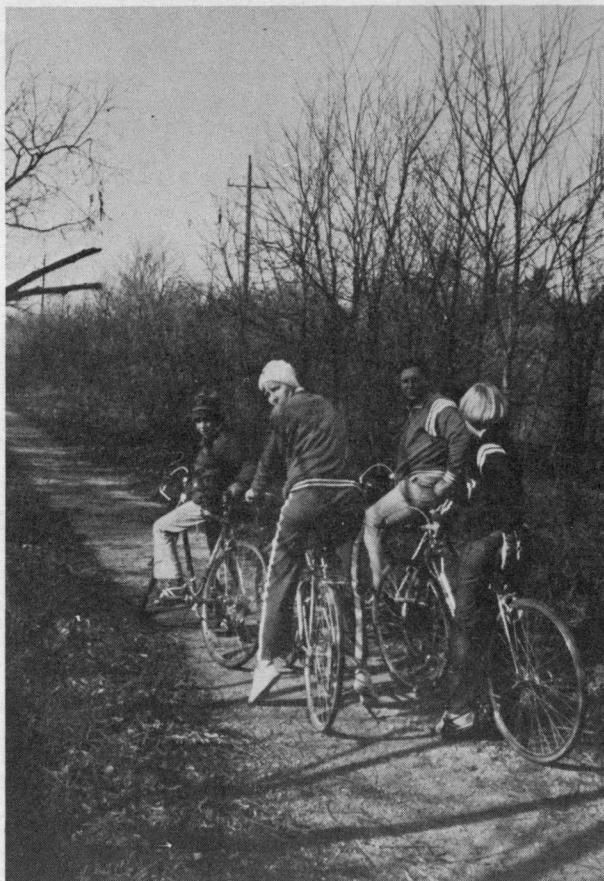

If there is a better cardiovascular pulmonary exercise for a family than bicycling, the authors haven't found it.

they've progressed to the point where they thoroughly enjoy the athletic life and wouldn't consider changing it.

Getting started is the important thing, and getting started requires that you first indoctrinate yourself with a health philosophy. First, you accept the fact that you need more exercise—a fact you quickly admit and can hardly avoid. But getting started is work—and *not* working is easier than working. It isn't as pleasant as loafing. For

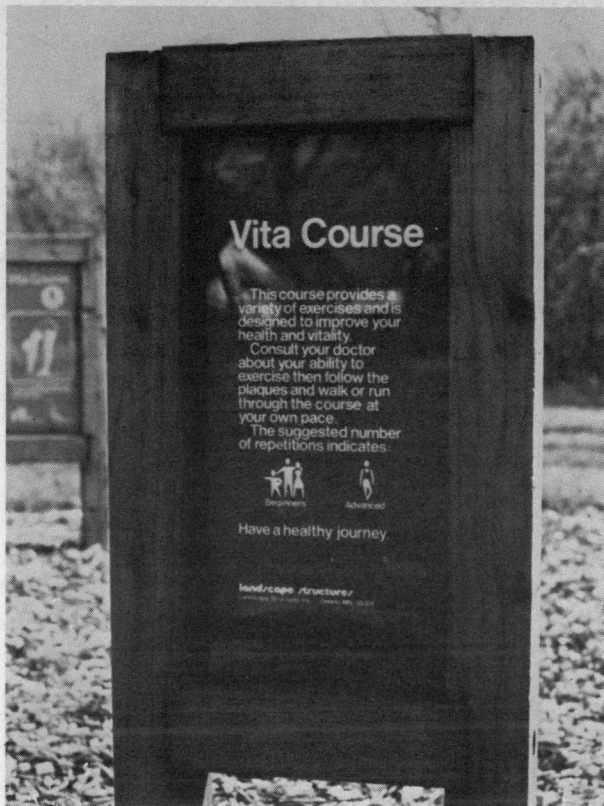

Community exercise programs are comparatively new, particularly programs that apply to a community's total citizenry—children, teenagers, adults and senior citizens. These new and popular programs provide carefully worked out routines that engage the participant in flexibility, strength and endurance exercises. The Elmhurst, Illinois Park District's "Vita Course" is an example of such a program. It is spread over a dozen exercise stations or stops, with an excellent sod running or jogging path to be traversed between stations. It is an excellent example of what is embodied in a proper physical fitness philosophy.

that reason, many of us have an anti-exercise prejudice. To overcome that prejudice, all we have to do is ask ourselves four questions.

1. **Would I rather be a physical mess than a healthy person?**
2. **Would I rather look trim and presentable or sloppy and run-down?**
3. **Do I want to take the high-risk gamble of cardiovascular disease, high blood pressure and hypertension that menace people who don't get sufficient exercise?**
4. **Do I want to be physically old at an early age?**

Experience has shown me that most people can read those four questions and not be bothered at all. It isn't *enough* just to read them. Right now, go back and ask yourself every one of the four questions and give your answer *out loud*. There's only one sane way anybody *can* answer them.

Of course, you don't always *know* when you need more exercise. Just yesterday, I learned that a successful stockbroker I greatly admire is in the cardiac care unit of a nearby hospital, after having suffered a serious heart attack that came without warning.

It was a shock, because this man had always *looked* healthy. He burned up a lot of energy on the job. But after he gets out of the hospital, which I certainly hope he does, he'll be faced with the vital necessity of a cardiovascular pulmonary rebuilding program that will call for regular, vigorous exercise. Because he's a smart man, he'll follow the doctor's advice. And that brings up an important thing about your physical fitness starting program. It must be one you can live with comfortably—one that's not downright unpleasant for you. For most of us, the *only* way we'll embrace a fitness program we don't like is to be scared into it.

Which brings up another important point in embracing a personal philosophy which establishes physical fitness as a way of life.

You pick types of exercise that are not only pleasant and stimulating but that also accomplish what you want exercise to do for you.

I don't think my son would ever stick with a program of calisthenics because the exercises wouldn't be fun for him. On the other hand, I have one friend who finds competitive sports distasteful. He thinks too much emphasis is put on winning, and he shrinks from violent body contact. He's a rope jumper, among other things, and he's become so proficient at it that his routines could well be exhibitions. He delights in learning and doing more and more intricate rope jumping routines. And while he doesn't like body contact, he's become a whiz with the punching bag, which he also enjoys.

Don't set your goals too high at the outset. A baby creeps before it can walk. There is no quick-easy exercise program that will make you a Charles Atlas or Lionel Strongfort or Arnold Schwartzenegger overnight. Indeed, people who've gotten into poor physical condition sometimes need a preliminary conditioning program to get them ready for the simplest beginning exercises. A man who gets out of breath and exhausted from walking up a short flight of steps isn't going to embark on an exercise program that will have him in competition for the Boston Marathon or Mr. America title in a month or two.

The exercise programs recommended in this book recognize that an exercise which is probably a little mild for one person may be too tough for another. Also, one particular exercise that looks good to you may be all wrong for a person in your particular physical condition. It may create stresses that you aren't presently able to take. Likewise, it may not be the kind of exercise you really need most.

Quite a few people badly need corrective exercises for physical ailments or defects, and in some instances, those corrective exercises must accomplish at least a part of their purpose before any real physical fitness program is started. You may have body malfunctions or weaknesses that make certain exercises, good for most people, downright destructive for you. Not all good exercises are good for all people.

It may be that proper diet should play an important part in your fitness program. Thirty-seven million women and 33 million men are at least 10 percent overweight. No two human bodies are *exactly* alike. That's why certain preliminary steps are tremendously important before you even begin your physical fitness program.

HOW PHYSICALLY FIT ARE YOU?

Physical Examination

The first step, an absolute must, is a consultation with your family doctor or a visit to a physical fitness evaluation center. If you're as lax about regular physical examinations as most people are, a complete physical would be in order. Most of us are unaware of our true physical conditions and therefore run the risk of injuring ourselves by embarking on an exercise program which may be too strenuous. If you are *under 30,* have had a physical exam in the past year and the doctor found nothing wrong with you, you can start exercising. If you are *30-59,* you should have a medical checkup at least 3-4 months prior to beginning an exercise program. In all cases, an EKG should be taken while you're exercising. *Over 59* have a checkup, including an EKG, immediately prior to embarking on an exercise program. In addition, for those who are overweight, have a history of high blood pressure or heart trouble, an exercise program should *never* be begun without your doctor's approval.

The physical exam should include examination of your blood pressure, cardiovascular system, condition of your muscles and joints and a blood test for cholesterol and triglycerides.

The doctor is all in favor of your starting and keeping with a physical fitness program. He's also in a position to know if any of the forms of exercise you have in mind would be unwise for you. You should also ask him if there's any particular kind of exercise he thinks you need to stress. Find out your major physical weaknesses and ask him if he'd suggest corrective exercises to alleviate them.

Unfortunately, some doctors are overworked and are much too busy to spend any length of time with their patients unless they feel it's absolutely necessary. For that reason, it's a good idea to have a written list of questions for the doctor to answer. By having such a list, you'll be able to confine your visit to the physician to the items which concern you.

You'll probably have specific questions in addition to these, but here's a basic list for a starter:

1. Do I have any physical condition for which any type of exercise could be dangerous? What is it? Do you know of any corrective exercises for it?

2. Do I need to lose any weight? How much? What kind of diet would you recommend to accomplish such a weight loss?

3. How are my heart and pulse? What's my blood pressure? What effect should these things have on an exercise program?

4. Is my back all right? How about my kidneys?

5. Do I have to worry about my legs, kneecaps or hip joints? What kind of exercise would be harmful for them?

6. Do I have any indication of diabetes? What effect should it have on my exercise program?

The medical doctor can definitely establish the

QUESTIONS TO ASK YOUR DOCTOR

1. Do I have any physical condition for which any type of exercise could be dangerous? What is it? Do you know of any corrective exercises for it?

2. Do I need to lose any weight? How much? What kind of diet would you recommend to accomplish such a weight loss?

3. How are my heart and pulse? What's my blood pressure? What effect should these things have on an exercise program?

4. Is my back all right? How about my kidneys?

5. Do I have to worry about my legs, kneecaps or hip joints? What kind of exercise would be harmful for them?

6. Do I have any indication of diabetes? What effect should it have on my exercise program?

strained? How does your heart react to this same exercise? Is the stress too much for your heart? How efficiently is your cardiovascular pulmonary system working? If you wish to embark on a strenuous fitness program, the answers to these questions could be *very* important.

Usually the stress test takes one of two forms—the individual pedals a stationary bicycle or walks and/or alternately runs on a motorized treadmill while being monitored by an EKG. By watching the EKG readings, blood pressure rate and respiration rate, the doctor can tell you the limits of your physical capacity and many times prescribe a program for you to increase your cardiovascular pulmonary endurance.

There are two major drawbacks to the stress test—lack of doctors and centers which perform these tests and the cost, which can run from $100 for the stress test to $250 for a complete fitness evaluation including strength, stamina and body composition. If you can afford such a fitness analysis, first try your local hospital and see if they have a cardiologist on staff who will conduct the test. If you live in a big city, try your local YMCA or YWCA. If you live in a university town, phone their medical school or physical education department and inquire about the stress test. In addition to these sources, there are four stress test centers in the United States:

Vital Fitness Evaluation Center
  1 Embarcadero Plaza
  San Francisco, Calif. 94111
  (415) 433-7286

Institute for Aerobics Research
  12100 Preston Road
  Dallas, Tex. 75230
  (214) 239-7223

George Sheehan
  Stress Testing Program
  Riverview Hospital
  Red Bank, N.J. 07701
  (201) 741-2700

Cardio-Metrics Institute
  295 Madison Avenue
  New York, NY 10017
  (212) 889-6123

state of your physical health. Then, to give you good advice, he must know the type of physical fitness program you want to start with, and whether it will have a light or strenuous start.

He can come close to estimating the physical tolerance of your body, but once he has done that, you, yourself, can be the best judge of when you're approaching the limit of your physical tolerance. That tolerance, of course, depends on your age as well as your physical condition.

The Stress Test

As mentioned above, your physical checkup should include an EKG while you are engaged in a physical activity. (An EKG taken while at rest really does not tell you how much stress your circulorespiratory system can handle.) Why is such a test important? A stress test evaluates and tests the fitness of your heart, lungs and circulatory system. How long can you walk at a steady pace before your breathing becomes

Stress Test/Fitness Evaluation Alternatives

Most of us can't afford to shell out $100 for a stress test, and if that were the criterion for starting a fitness program, most of us would not think twice about starting. Fortunately, there are much simpler ways to test your cardiovascular endurance, body composition (percentage of fat), and your strength, stamina and flexibility. However, you should have your doctor's okay before trying these tests.

The Step Test is one of a number of tests designed to measure your cardiovascular endurance. By putting you through 4 minutes of strenuous exercise, it will tell you how hard your

To take the Step Test you will need a bench and a stopwatch, wristwatch or clock with a second-hand.

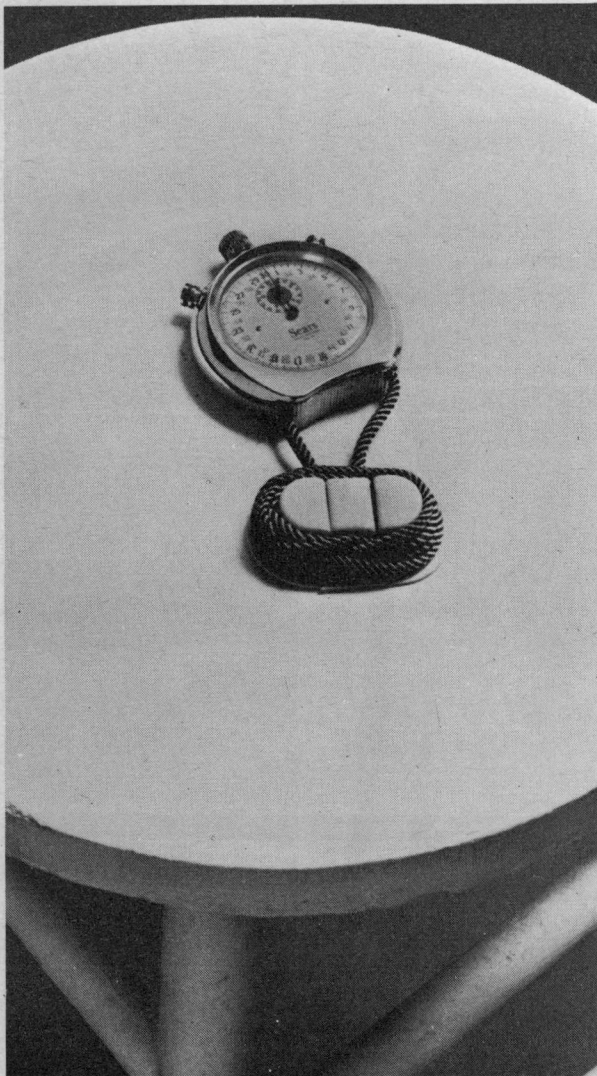

STEP TEST

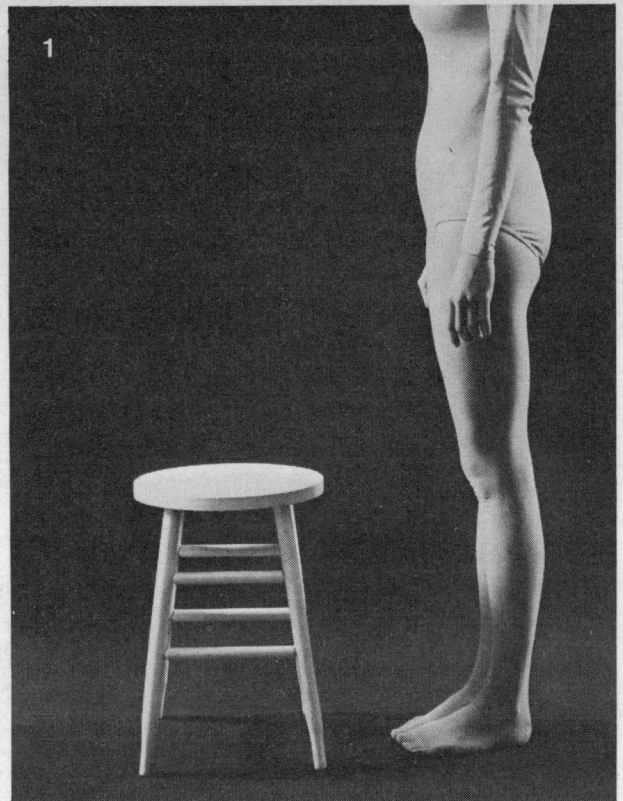

heart has to work, in order to move blood through your system during the exercise and how fast it recovers from that strain. *Do not smoke or engage in any physical activity 2 hours prior to taking this test.* You will need: a bench (see chart below for correct size), and a stopwatch, wristwatch or clock with a second hand. The bench can be a chair, two steps, an ottoman, etc.

If You Are	Bench Should Be
Under 5' tall	12" high
5'1" to 5'3" tall	14" high
5'3" to 5'9" tall	16" high
5'9" to 6' tall	18" high
Over 6' tall	20" high

The test consists of stepping up and down from bench to floor 30 times a minute for 4 minutes. To begin, stand facing the bench and, starting with either foot, place your foot on the bench and then step up so both feet are on the bench. Then immediately step down so both feet are on the floor. This test should be performed rhythmically

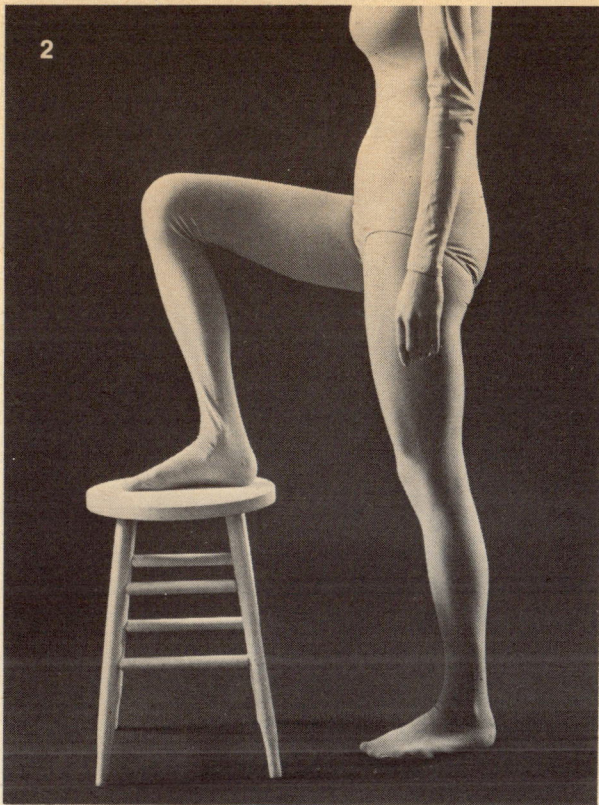

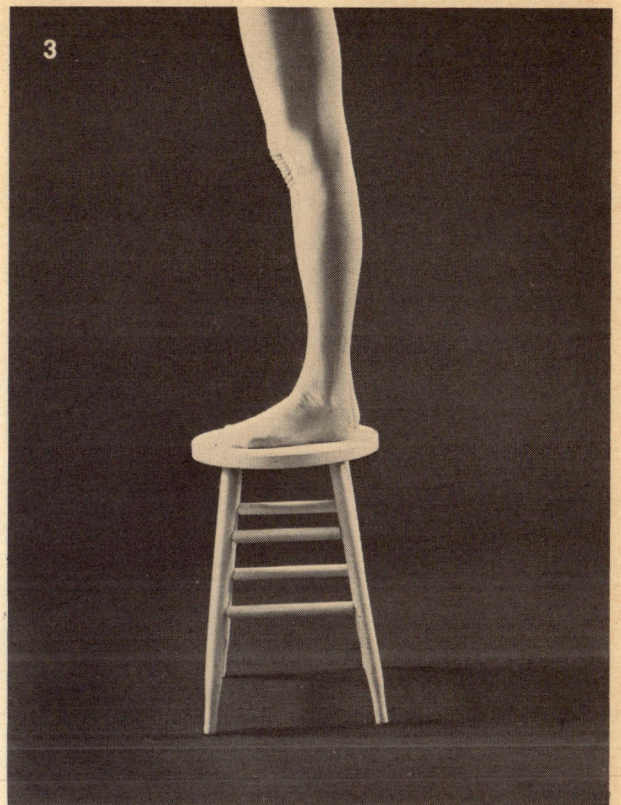

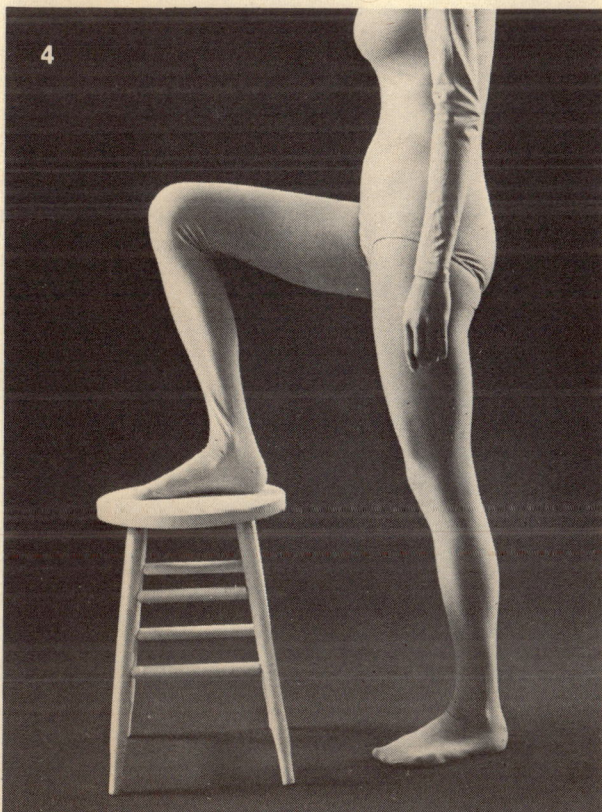

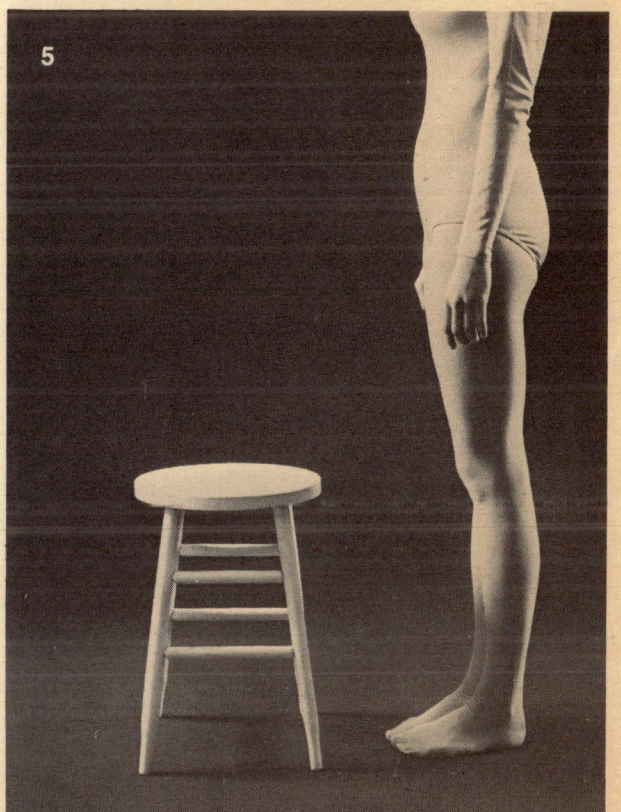

so that every 2 seconds you complete the up and down motion. After 4 minutes of continuous exercise, sit down and remain quiet for 1 minute. Take your pulse rates and record them as follows:

1. Pulse rate taken 1 minute after exercise—take for 30-second period.
2. Pulse rate taken 2 minutes after exercise—take for 30-second period.
3. Pulse rate taken 3 minutes after exercise—take for 30-second period.

To determine your cardiovascular fitness, add the three pulse counts and refer to the table below.

When the three 30-second pulse counts total:	**Recovery Index is:**	**Then the response to this test is:**
199 or more	60 or less	Poor
from 171-198	between 61-70	Average
from 150-170	between 71-80	Good
from 133-149	between 81-90	Very Good
132 or less	91 or more	Excellent

Determine your cardiovascular fitness rating by taking your pulse for 30 seconds each of 3 times — 1 minute, 2 minutes and 3 minutes after the Step Test. Record the counts. After the third count add up the pulse counts and consult the chart above.

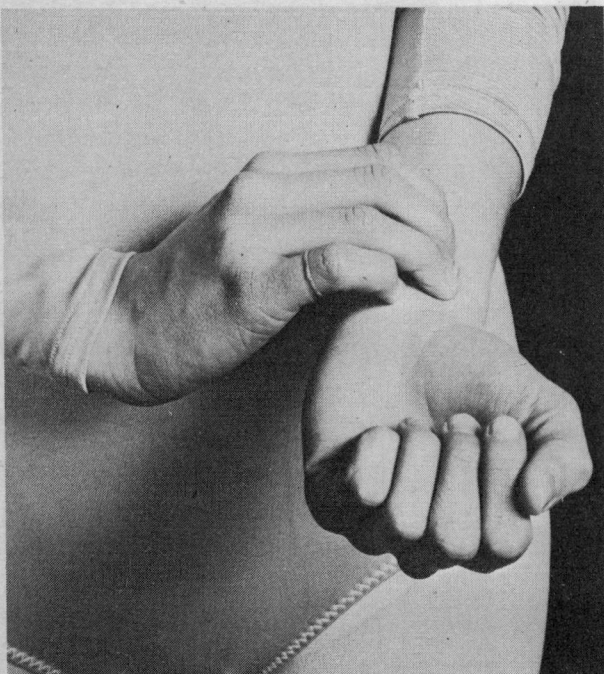

You may find that you can not complete this test. Don't get discouraged. Just rate your fitness "poor" and make up your mind to do something about it. However, if you could not complete the test and/or after the test any of these symptoms appear, it's advisable to see your doctor: excessive breathlessness long after exercise; bluing of the lips; pale or clammy skin or cold sweating; unusual fatigue; persistent shakiness or weakness 10 minutes after the exercise; muscle twitching following exercise.

Remember to record your rating for this test on the Personal Physical Fitness Evaluation Chart (page 21). Retake this test after 2 weeks on a fitness program to see how much you have improved.

Body Fat Measurement will tell you if you are carrying around too much body fat; in other words, it tells you if you are obese. Although obesity is usually evident from appearances alone, appearances may be deceiving. Most of us refer to the Department of Agriculture height/build/weight chart to determine whether we are overweight or whether we fall into the normal weight range. What that chart does not tell you is how much of your weight is body fat. In the average healthy man, the total body weight is 15 percent fat, 23 percent water, 58 percent muscle and organs and 4 percent bone mineral. The percentage of body fat for a woman will be slightly higher. In the obese person, the percentage of body fat far exceeds these average amounts, so that even though your total body weight may fall in the normal range for your height and build, your percentage of body fat may be too high.

Most of us are aware of the dangers we face if there is excess fat in the body—increased chance of heart disease, high blood pressure, diabetes, etc. How can you tell whether you are carrying around too much body fat?

Pinch Test: This test can be done by your doctor who will use a measuring device called a caliper to measure the thickness of a fold of skin on the back of your arm. However, you can get a rough idea at home by gently gripping with thumb and forefinger the skin behind your upper arm midway between elbow and shoulder. If the thickness is from ¼- to ½-inch, rate yourself excellent (¼-inch) or good (½-inch). If the thickness is more than that, you have some work to do and rate yourself poor.

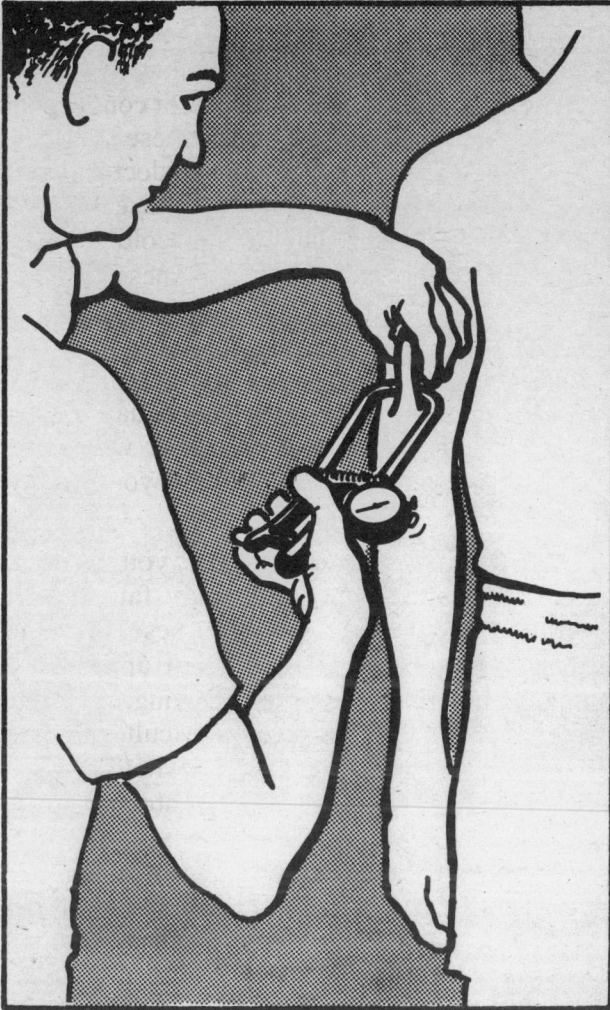

To determine if you are carrying around too much body fat, you can have your doctor measure the thickness of a fold of skin on the back of your arm with a measuring device called a caliper, or take the Pinch Test.

Weight Gain Test: Can you remember how much you weighed at the age of 25? How about at age 16? If you can, take the lower of the two weights. Your weight now if you are a light-boned person should only be 5-10 percent more, and if you are a muscular or heavyset person, your weight should be 5-10 percent less. Rate yourself exellent if you passed this test and poor if you did not.

The Flexibility Test will tell you the range of motion, or lack thereof, through which your limbs are able to move. Since there are many joints in our bodies, there is no one general test which will tell you your overall flexibility fitness. However, most of us tend to lose flexibility in the hamstring, low back and neck areas first. So these are the joints to be tested with the Sitting Stretch.

Sitting Stretch: Put two pieces of tape on the floor about 5 inches apart and align them horizontally. Next, sit down on the floor, legs stretched out straight, toes pointing upward. Place your heels on each piece of tape. You should have a marker of some sort—a checker, backgammon chip, etc. Now bend forward, slowly stretching as far as possible. Touch the finger tips to the floor, placing the outer edge of the marker at the forward tip of fingers. Now measure the distance between the tape and the outer edge of your marker. If you could reach 8 inches (men) or 12 inches (women) beyond the tape, your flexibility is excellent. From 5-6 inches (men) or 6-8 inches (women) is good. From 1-4 inches (men) or 1-5 inches (women) is average flexibility. Below that you need work—rate yourself poor.

Muscular Strength Test does as its name implies—it tests the strength of your muscles. As was true for the Flexibility Test, there is no one general test that can determine your overall muscular strength fitness. We will test the muscles, that, as we grow older, tend to lose strength first—the abdominal muscles, shoulder and arm muscles and upper and lower back muscles. You should be able to do all three of these tests. These are the very minimum tests for strength fitness. The failure to do even one test is an indication of very poor muscular strength. Score yourself for all three with either pass or fail.

Pushup (arm and shoulder strength): Lie face down on the floor, legs together, hands on floor palms down under shoulders with fingers pointing straight ahead. Extend arms, pushing body off the floor so that your weight rests on your hands and toes. Keeping your back straight lower your body until chest touches the floor.

Prone Arch (upper and lower back muscles): Lie face down, hands tucked under thighs. Arch back, raising legs and chest off the floor. Hold that position for a count of 10. *Caution:* If you have lower back problems, you should not try this test.

Situp (abdominal muscles): Lie on your back, legs slightly bent, feet about 1-inch apart. Tuck your toes under a sofa or have a partner hold your ankles—your heels must be in contact with the floor during the situp motion. Lace your fingers behind your neck. Curl up to the sitting position.

17

FLEXIBILITY TEST

Sitting Stretch: The sitting stretch is designed to test the flexibility of your back, hamstring and neck muscles. **(1)** Put two pieces of tape on the floor about 5 inches apart. **(2)** Sit down on the floor, legs stretched out straight, placing one heel on each piece of tape. Bend forward slowly, stretching as far as possible and place outer edge of marker at forward tip of fingers **(3)** Measure distance between the tape and outer edge of marker.

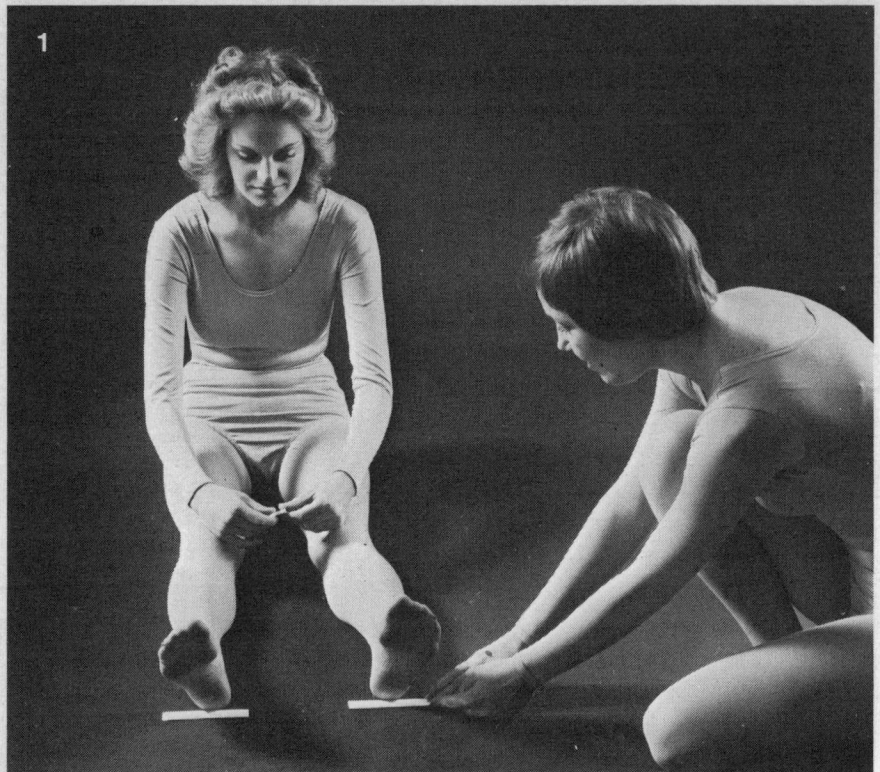

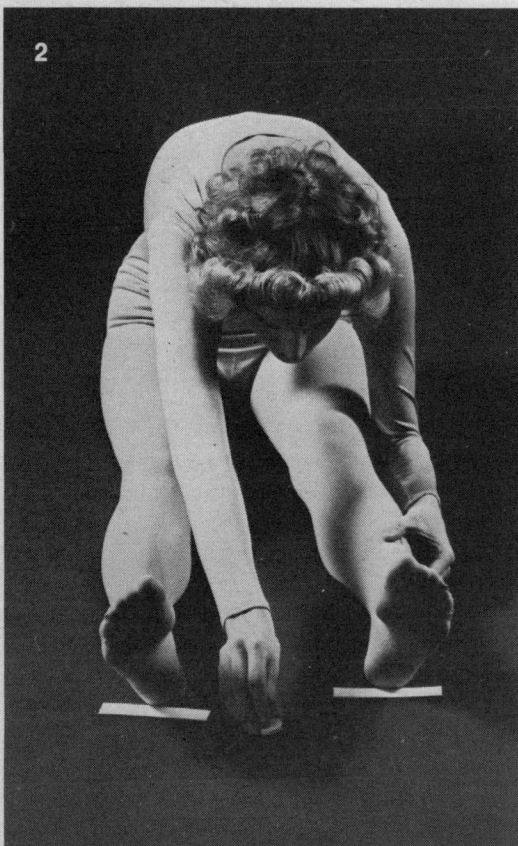

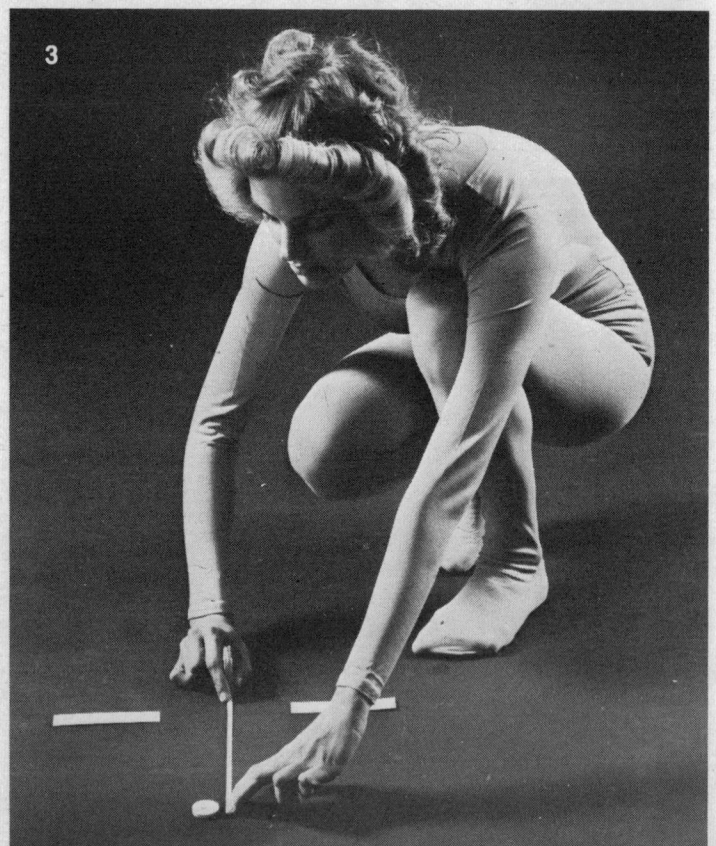

MUSCULAR STRENGTH TEST

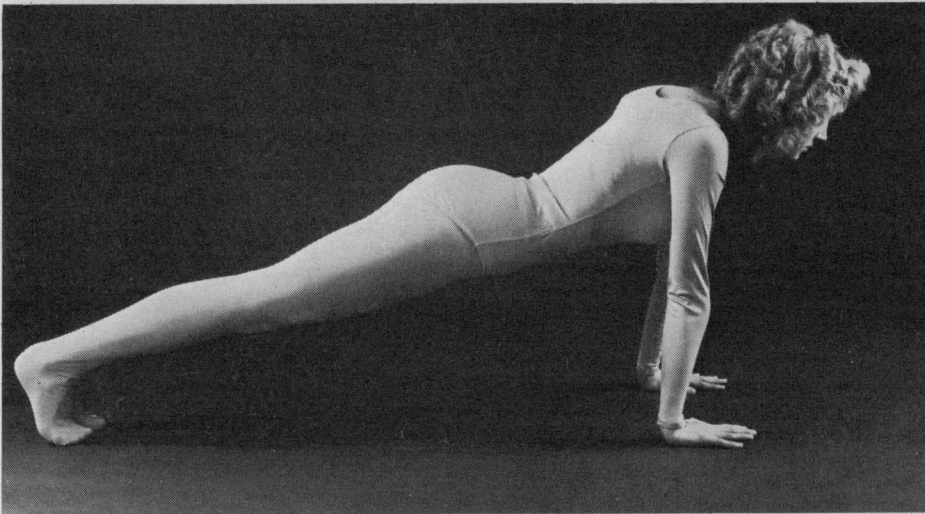

Pushup: The pushup is designed to test the muscular strength of your shoulder and arm muscles. Lying face down on the floor with palms on floor under shoulders you **(1)** extend arms pushing body off the floor. **(2)** Keeping your back straight, lower your body until your chest touches the floor.

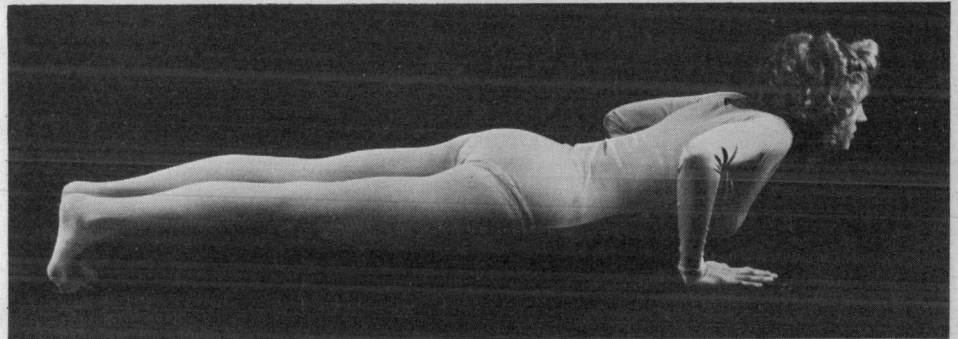

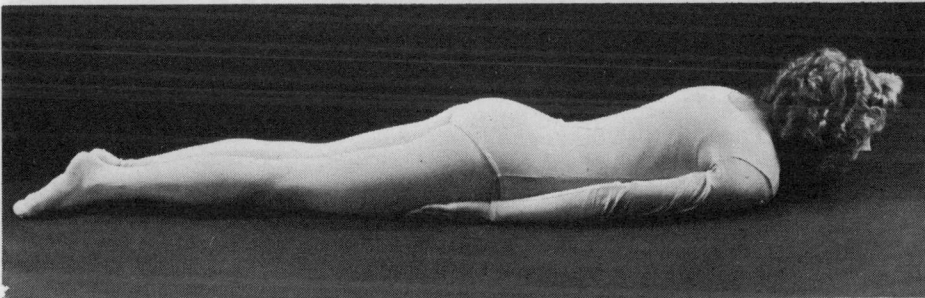

Prone Arch: The prone arch is designed to test the muscular strength of your lower back muscles. **(1)** Lie face down on the floor, hands tucked under thighs. **(2)** Arch back raising legs and chest off the floor and hold for a count of 10.

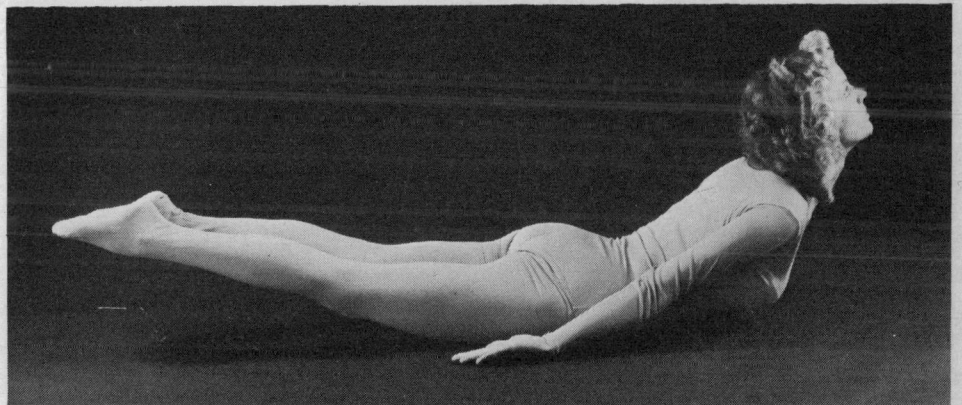

MUSCULAR STRENGTH AND ENDURANCE TEST

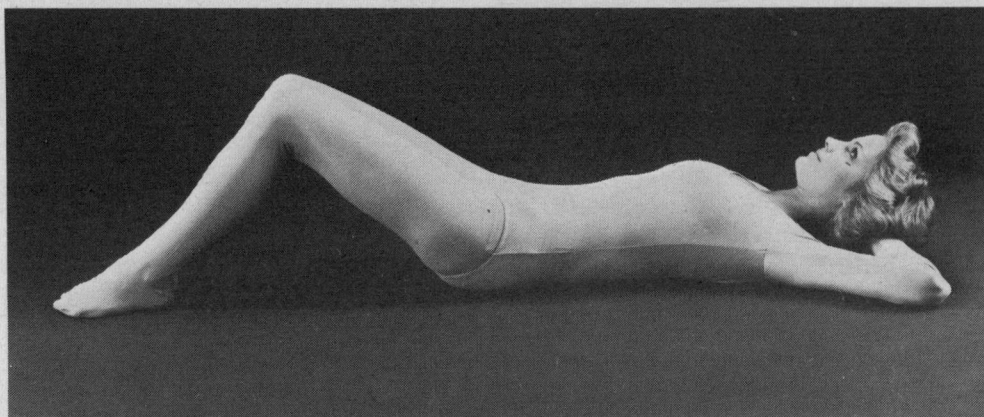

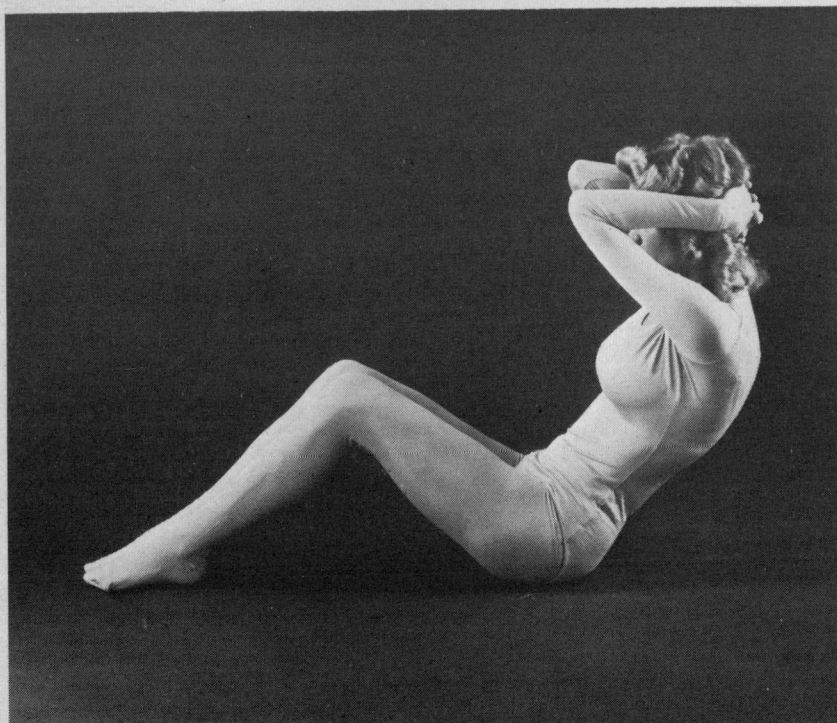

Situp: The situp is designed to test both the muscular strength and endurance of your abdominal muscles. The primary difference between testing for strength and endurance is the number of repetitions. Strength is the ability of a muscle to overcome a maximum resistance in *one* effort. Endurance, on the other hand, is the ability of a muscle to *sustain* an effort for a period of time. Thus to test for a minimum amount of strength in the abdominal muscles one situp must be completed. To test for the endurance capacity of your abdominal muscles you see how many situps you can complete. To do the situp you **(1)** lie on your back, legs slightly bent, feet about 1 inch apart with toes tucked under a sofa or with a partner holding your ankles. Your fingers should be laced behind your neck. **(2)** Curl up into the sitting position.

Muscular Endurance Test tests the ability of a muscle to perform a specific task for a length of time. Once again, there is no one test to determine the endurance of each of your muscles. The situp, however, is the most widely accepted and used test for muscular endurance.

Situp (abdominal muscle endurance): Perform the situp as described in the Muscular Strength Test. Do as many situps as you can.

For both men and women, a score of 50 or more situps is excellent. A score of 40-49 (men), 35-49 (women) is good and a score of 25-39 (men), 22-34 (women) is average. If you could not complete 25 (men) or 22 (women) situps, you scored below average. Rate yourself poor. You need work.

PERSONAL PHYSICAL FITNESS EVALUATION CHART

How physically fit are you? This chart will help you take an overall view of your present state of physical fitness. For each of the tests you just completed, put a check mark down by your rating. You can now easily see in which areas you need the most work.

TEST

Cardiovascular Endurance
Step Test

Body Fat Measurement
Pinch Test

Weight Gain Test

Flexibility
Sitting Stretch

Muscular Strength
Pushup
Prone Arch
Situp

Muscular Endurance
Situps

RATING

_____ Excellent
_____ Very Good
_____ Good
_____ Average
_____ Poor

_____ Excellent
_____ Good
_____ Poor

_____ Excellent
_____ Poor

_____ Excellent
_____ Good
_____ Average
_____ Poor

_____ Pass _____ Fail
_____ Pass _____ Fail
_____ Pass _____ Fail

_____ Excellent
_____ Good
_____ Average
_____ Poor

THE THREE BASIC BODY TYPES

Now that you have a pretty fair evaluation of your present physical fitness status, you have one more aspect to consider—your body type. People come in many shapes and sizes. Some are thin and wiry and others are muscular and heavy. In between is a myriad of combinations—top heavy with thin legs, bottom heavy with narrow chest and on and on. However, everyone falls into one of the three basic body types.

Why is it important to know your body type? First of all, you must face the fact that you can't do much to change your basic body type—no matter how much training or exercise you do. If you fall into the thin muscled and boned, slender body type, no amount of weight training is going to turn you into an Arnold Schwartzenegger. In fact, weight training for such a body type is usually very frustrating. There are other exercises for building strength that a person with such a body type would be much more successful with. The exercises listed under each of the three body types are all activities using large muscle groups. These are the types of exercises that are best suited for that particular body type. This doesn't mean that if your body type is Endomorphic, for example, you should not or cannot jog. It simply means your body type is best suited to other types of exercises, and you will be more successful in performing those than you will in attempting to jog.

Endomorph

The endomorph has noticeable soft musculature with a round face, short neck, double chin and wide hips. There is little muscle development and small bones.

Exercises: Exercises best suited to the endomorph are bowling, bicycling, swimming, tennis and badminton.

Mesomorph

The mesomorph is solid, muscular, big-boned and rugged. Generally of medium height with large chest, slender waist, long torso and short powerful legs.

Exercises: Exercises best suited to the mesomorph are bowling, bicycling, golf, handball, weight training, swimming, jogging and hiking.

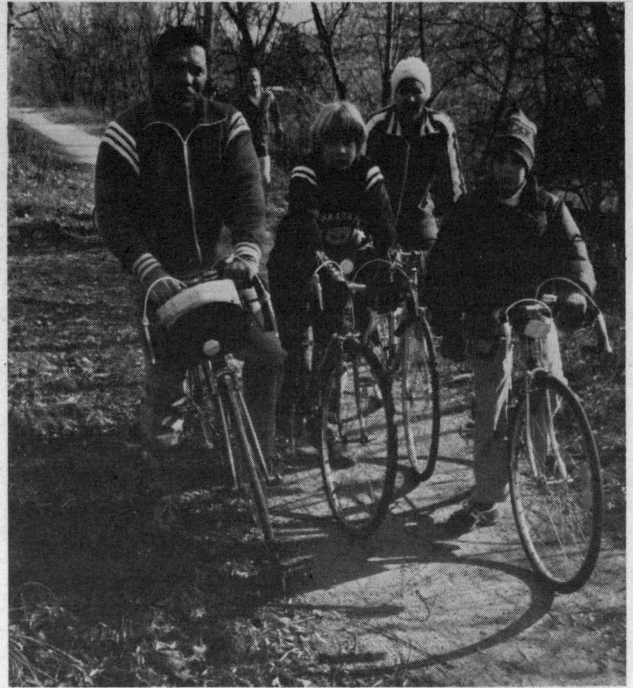

The author's son, daughter-in-law and two grandchildren on their 10-speed bikes taking one of their regular tours of the bike trails.

Ectomorph

The ectomorph has a slender body, is thin muscled and thin boned, has a long slender neck, narrow chest and has very little body fat.

Exercises: Exercises best suited to the ectomorph are badminton, basketball, bicycling, golf, hiking, jogging, tennis and running.

METHODS OF EXERCISE

Now that you know your present state of physical fitness and the types of large muscled activities best suited to your body type, let's look at the methods of exercise you will be using to improve your fitness. There are five basic methods of exercise—*aerobics, calisthenics, isometrics, isotonics* and *isokinetics*. Each method has its followers and its detractors. For the purposes of this book, we recognize that each of these exercise methods helps the individual build and improve one or more aspects of the total fitness spectrum—*flexibility, muscle strength, muscle endurance* and *cardiovascular pulmonary endurance*. However, no one method can be used as a total fitness program. No one method is best suited to improve all four aspects of the total fitness spectrum.

THE FOUR TOTAL PHYSICAL FITNESS ELEMENTS

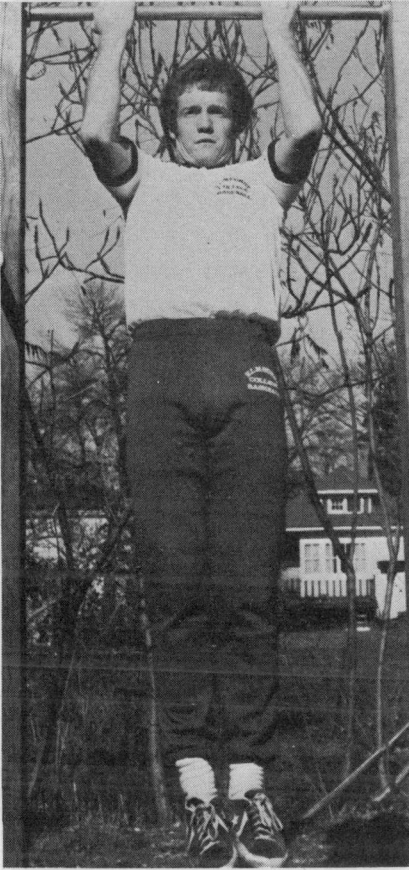

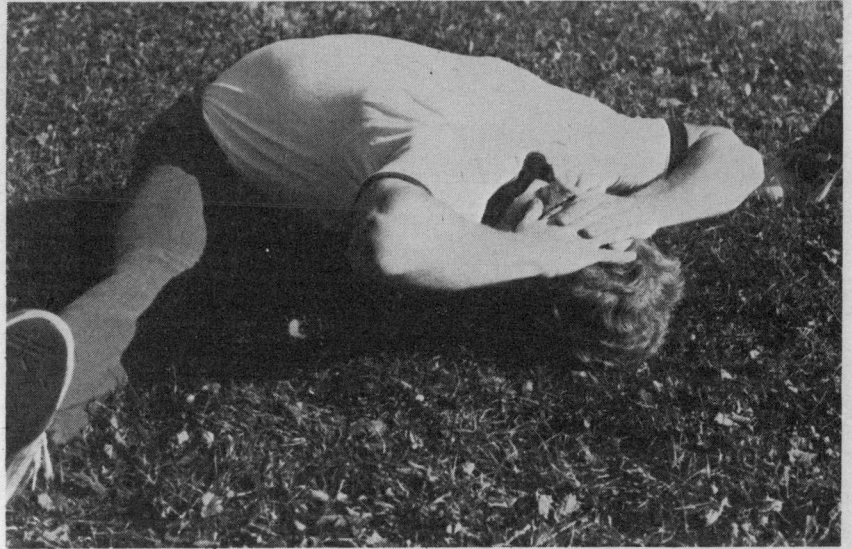

FLEXIBILITY

STRENGTH

CARDIOVASCULAR ENDURANCE

MUSCULAR ENDURANCE

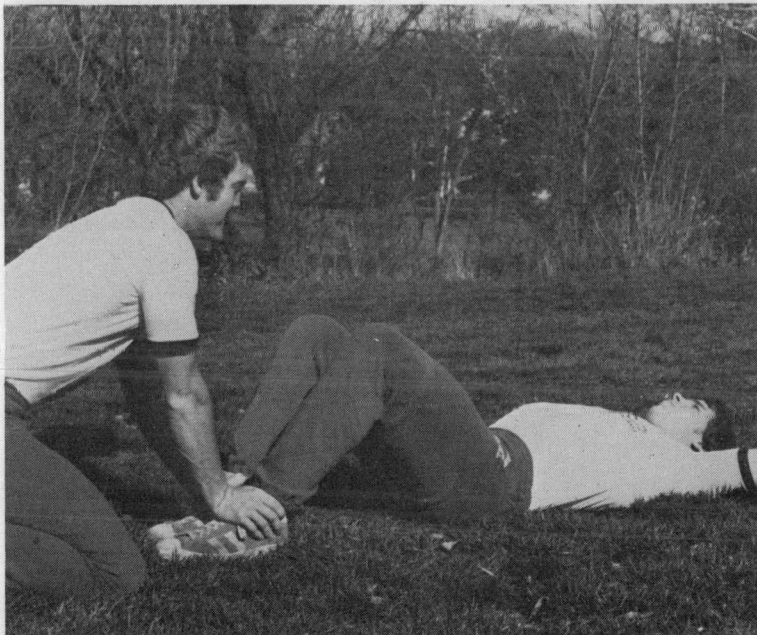

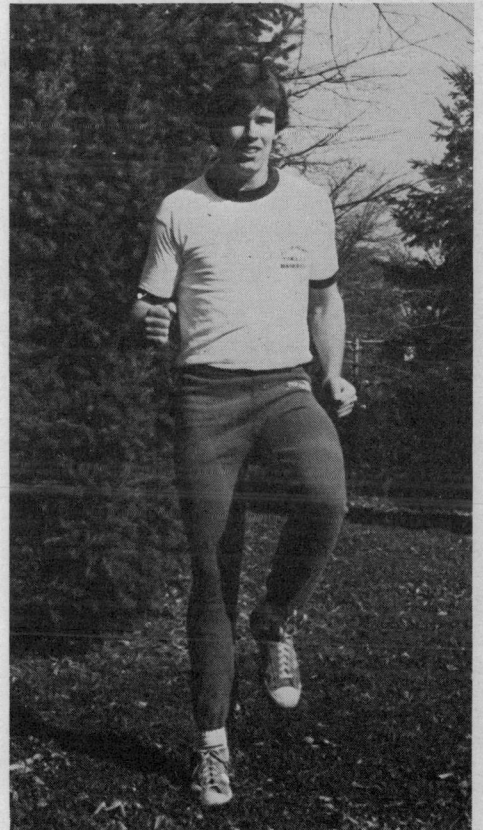

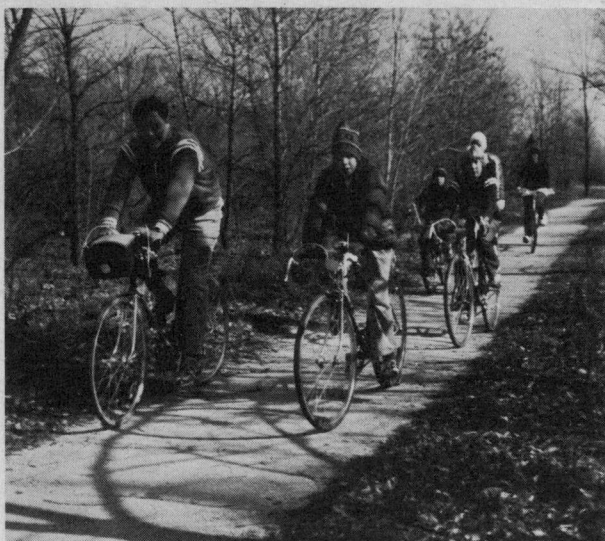

Good bicycle paths or trails are becoming more prevalent all over the United States.

Aerobic Exercises

Aerobic exercise is any rhythmical activity that causes a sustained increase in heart rate, respiration and muscle metabolism. Such exercise will improve the efficiency and the capacity of the cardiovascular and respiratory system—heart, lungs, and blood vessels. Aerobic exercise is essential to any total fitness program because no other exercise method effectively builds the strength and endurance of the cardiovascular pulmonary system. This exercise method includes such activities as jogging, swimming, bicycling, walking, running in place, and jumping rope.

In order to benefit from any aerobic exercise, you must increase your heart beat rate to a training rate (see chart at right) of 110-178 beats per minute depending on your age and cardiovascular fitness evaluation* and sustain that heart beat rate for a minimum of 15 minutes. (For example, if you are 30 years old and rated average on the Step Test your training heart rate according to the Aerobic Fitness Training Heart Rate chart is between 148-159.) The best way to judge if you have reached your training heart rate is to do 5

---

*Your cardiovascular fitness evaluation can be determined by your Step Test rating. Refer to the Personal Physical Fitness Evaluation Chart.

minutes of strenuous aerobic exercise and then immediately take your pulse for 15 seconds. Multiply that number by four. If your heart rate is below that suggested, you should pick up your pace—i.e., if jogging, jog at a faster pace. If your rate is higher than suggested, slow down your exercise pace. You should not over-stress your heart. When you take the count, if your heart rate is around 30 beats over the suggested training rate, you've reached your maximum heart beat rate. Slow down your exercise pace. Take another count after another 5 minutes of aerobic exercise to see if you are within your training heart beat range.

Aerobic Fitness Training Heart Rates

Fitness Level		Training Rate *(in beats/min)*
Excellent		
	Age 20	164-178
	25	162-176
	30	160-174
	35	157-171
	40	154-168
	45	151-164
	50	148-161
	55	145-158
	60	143-155
Average		
	Age 20	153-164
	25	151-162
	30	148-159
	35	145-157
	40	142-154
	45	139-151
	50	136-149
	55	133-146
	60	130-143
Poor		
	Age 20	140-154
	25	137-151
	30	134-148
	35	130-144
	40	126-140
	45	122-136
	50	118-132
	55	114-128
	60	110-124

There are other exercises which will help build cardiovascular pulmonary endurance. Handball, racquetball, basketball and tennis will all produce the desired results if the exercise is steady and continuous over a period of time. The key words here are steady and continuous. If you are playing tennis and after 5 minutes take a breather you are not helping to strengthen your heart and respiratory systems. In that 5 minutes you may have increased your heart beat rate to the proper training level but, when you stop, that rate drops rapidly. It is suggested that these sports activities be used only for maintenance of aerobic fitness, not as a substitute.

Calisthenics

Most of us have done some sort of calisthenic exercise—the jumping jack, pushups, situps, etc. Calisthenics are systematic, rhythmic bodily exercises usually without apparatus. If calisthenic exercises are used to build only strength and endurance then calisthenics is considered to be isotonic exercise. However, calisthenics can be considered an exercise method unto itself and as such can build cardiopulmonary endurance, increase muscle strength and endurance and increase flexibility. In other words, calisthenics, if used properly, can be implemented as a total fitness program although it is not generally recommended. To be used as a total fitness program, the exercise series you choose must be carried out in a steady and continuous fashion with no rest between exercises. If, between exercises, a "rest" period is needed, then only walking or running in place are acceptable.

Calisthenics in combination with other methods of exercise is the most effective way to utilize this exercise method. The reason being, using calisthenics to build muscular strength, for example, would take much longer than a weight training program. The same can be said for calisthenics and cardiovascular pulmonary endurance. The amount and vigor of calisthenic exercises required to increase your heart beat rate to the training level and then sustain that level is much harder work than a 15-30 minute walk, jog, swim or bicycle ride. It is generally recognized that calisthenics are not as effective as aerobic exercises in building cardiovascular pulmonary endurance.

Calisthenics can also be used to correct special problems or to develop selected areas of the body.

Isometrics/Isotonics/Isokinetics

Isometric exercises involve the contraction of muscles *without* movement. In isometric exercises a muscle or group of muscles is exerted against an immovable force such as a wall or another set of muscles. A good example would be putting your hands together in front of you and pushing them together as hard as possible. Isometrics are most effective in building muscle strength and tone. *Isotonic* exercises involve muscle contractions *with* movement. Weight training would be a good example of isotonic exercise. Isotonics are used most effectively in building muscular strength and endurance. *Isokinetic* exercises require movement with a controlled resistance. Usually isokinetic exercises involve the use of exercising machines. The machine controls the amount of resistance—at a slow speed there is little resistance but as you increase in speed, the resistance is also increased. Isokinetics is the best of the three for building muscle strength.

Isometrics, isotonics and isokinetics will build muscular strength, endurance and all over body tone. However, none of these should be considered a total fitness program because they do not stimulate the cardiovascular system and therefore do not build cardiovascular pulmonary endurance. They also do not provide any flexibility improvement. These three exercise methods, however, can be effective as an integral part of a total fitness program.

Hopefully, you're now eager to start a total fitness program—but don't be impatient. Before we give you any actual programs, we want to give you a basic knowledge of the four aspects of physical fitness—flexibility, muscular strength, muscle endurance and cardiovascular pulmonary endurance—why you need to develop each aspect and what exercises you can do to attain fitness in each aspect.

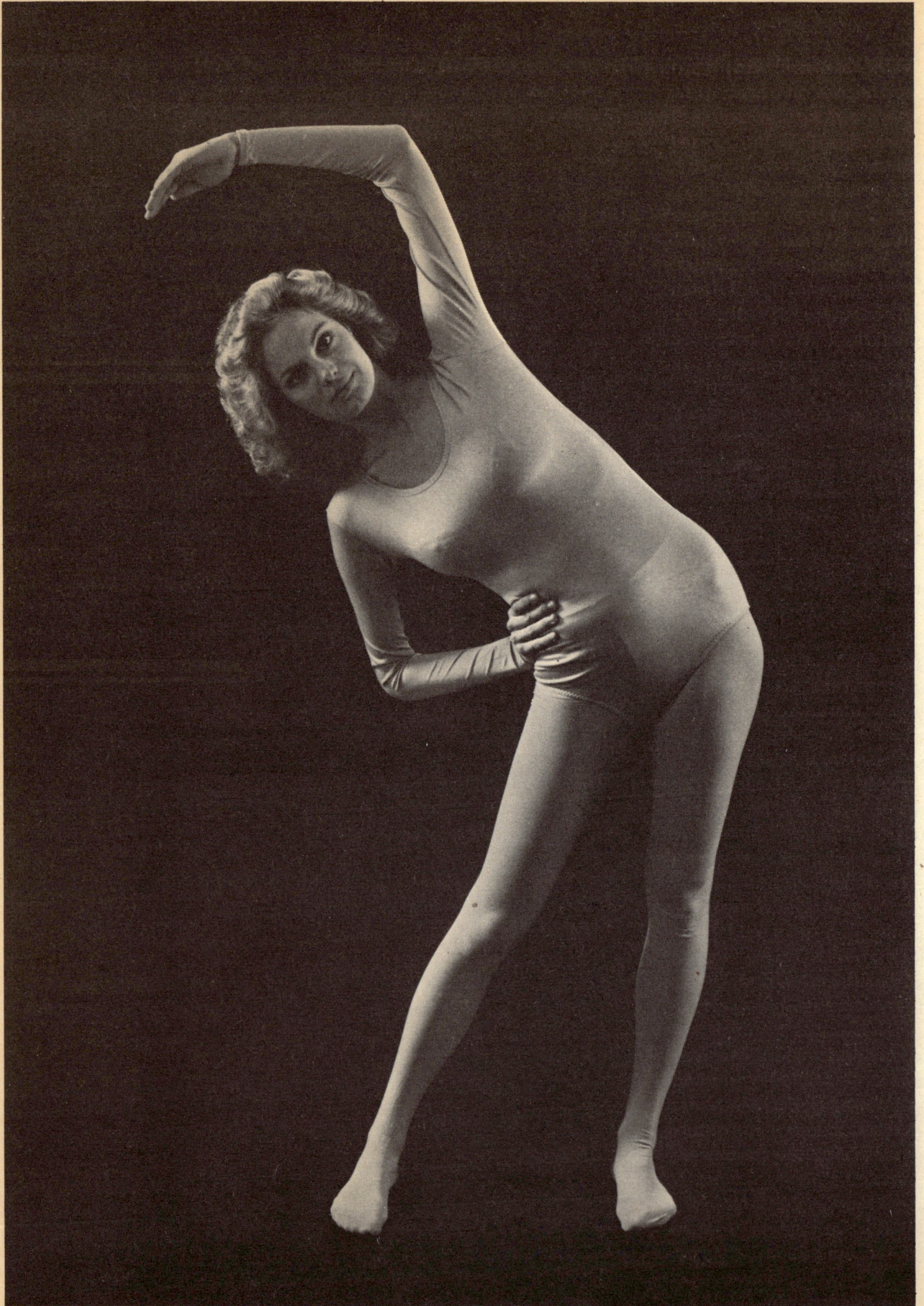

chapter 2

Flexibility

AS STATED IN CHAPTER 1, flexibility pertains to the range of motion you have in a particular joint or series of joints. That range of motion is controlled by the degree the muscles, connective tissue, tendons, ligaments and skin associated to that particular joint can be stretched. In doing flexibility exercises the purpose is to increase the elasticity of the muscles and connective tissue surrounding a particular joint so you get the maximum range of motion.

IMPORTANCE OF FLEXIBILITY

All-Over Fitness

Good flexibility fitness contributes to your overall fitness—your movements become more graceful and your chances of injuring yourself in everyday life are lessened. However, for many of us our inactive life-style has lead to inflexibility in major joints in the body. The areas of the body which lose flexibility first are the hamstrings, lower back, neck and pectoral areas. These are the joints most susceptible to injury by being forced beyond their normal range of motion. Your "normal" range depends on your flexibility fitness. Millions of Americans are beset by lower back problems which in most cases are caused by the lack of physical activity, poor posture, inadequate flexibility and weak abdominal and/or lower back muscles. We've all encountered situations when we've had to make a sudden movement which overstressed a muscle—perhaps lifting something that was really too heavy for

Flexibility is but one of the four basic elements of the total physical fitness spectrum – but it is an essential element for development of strength and endurance. Inadequate flexibility when performing strength and endurance exercises can prove harmful and in some cases such exercises performed without proper warm-up can actually reduce the range of motion you have in your joints. It's not necessary that you possess above-normal flexibility – in fact, extreme flexibility coupled with inadequate muscular strength can be detrimental. But a reasonable or average range of motion in each body joint is important for everyday living and essential for participation in a total fitness program.

us—which resulted in either muscle soreness or something more serious such as a torn ligament or a sprained or torn muscle. Good flexibility fitness will neither prevent muscle soreness nor prevent a more serious muscle or tendon injury. But it will reduce your chances of such an injury by increasing the degree to which your muscles and tendons can be stretched before injury is incurred.

Graceful body movement and better posture can also be benefits of flexibility fitness. As we grow older, our muscles, ligaments and tendons begin to lose some of their elasticity and connective tissues become stiff and actually shorten. The result is a loss in the range of motion in the joints. Without adequate joint flexibility, body movements, whether walking, sitting or a sports activity, become jerky and lack smoothness of action. In addition to poor body movement our posture can suffer from a combination of muscle strength loss and inadequate flexibility. Chest and shoulder muscles which become weak rely on connective tissue to keep the shoulders from pulling forward. However, connective tissue becomes stiff and shortens, only aggravating the problem—and a round shouldered posture results.

The good news is that if you do suffer from poor posture and lack a gracefulness in movement, it is reversible. If you already possess good posture and move smoothly, that *also* is reversible. Flexibility exercises are essential to improve and maintain our physical appearance.

Flexibility Exercises for Warm-Up

In any fitness program there are four periods of exercise which make up the total program—warm-up, conditioning activities, circulatory activities and cooling-off. All are vital—none should be ignored. The *warm-up period,* which should last from 5-10 minutes, stretches and limbers up the muscles and speeds up the action of the heart (hopefully to training rate) and lungs. It prepares the body for greater exertion and reduces the possibility of unnecessary strain. The *conditioning period* builds and increases flexibility, muscle strength and endurance and tones up abdominal, back, leg, arm, and other major muscles. The *circulatory activity period* produces contractions of large muscle groups for relatively longer periods than the conditioning activities—to stimulate and strengthen the circulatory and respiratory system. The *cooling-off period* is essential in helping the body—in particular, the muscles, heart and lungs—return to its normal activity level.

The most effective way of using flexibility

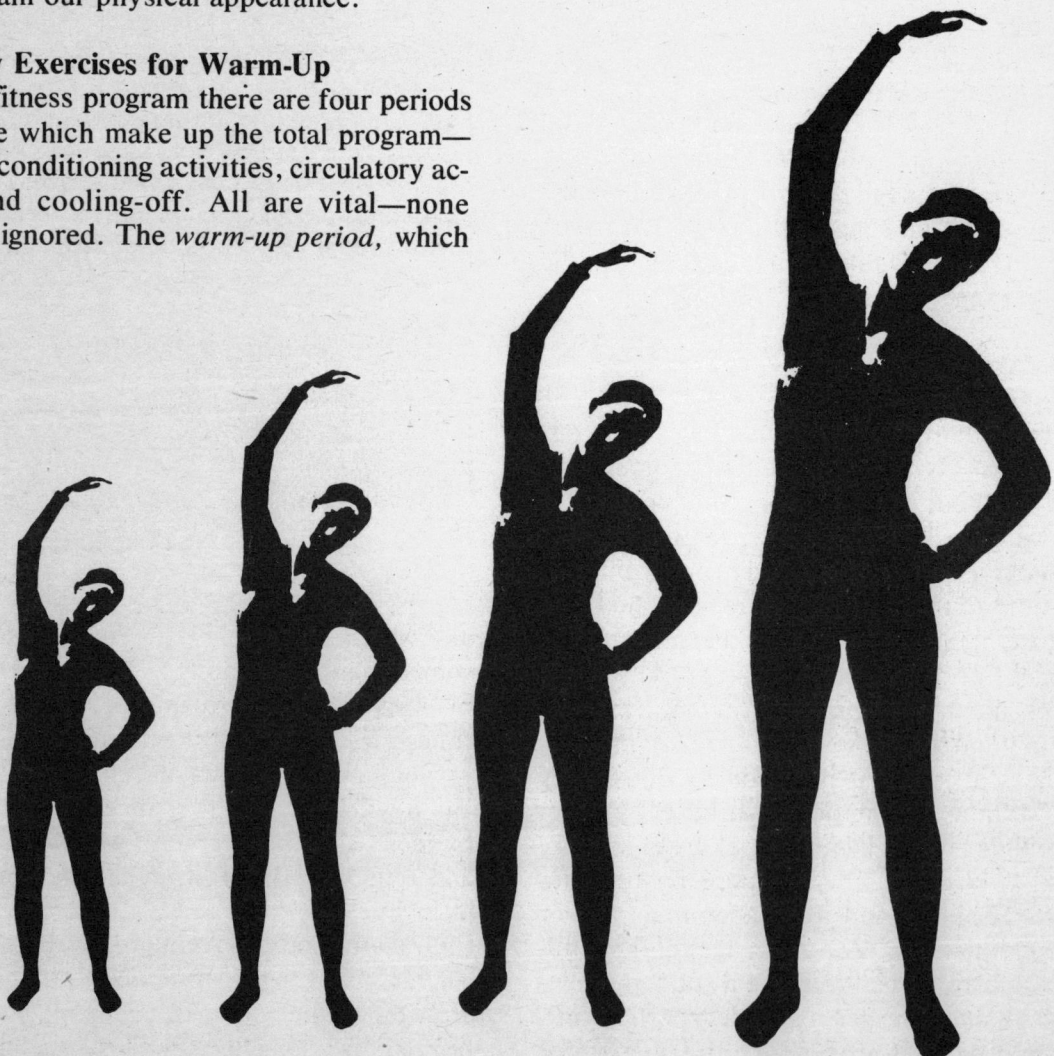

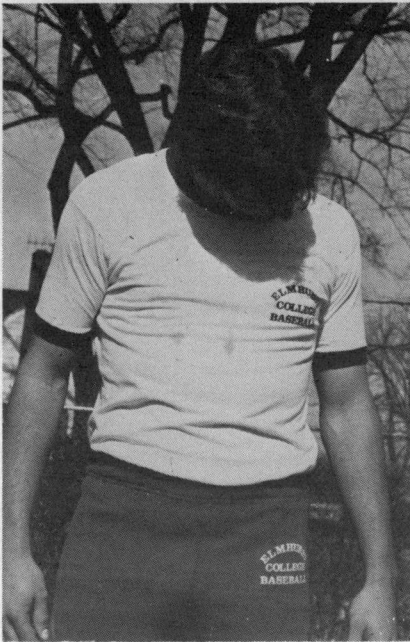

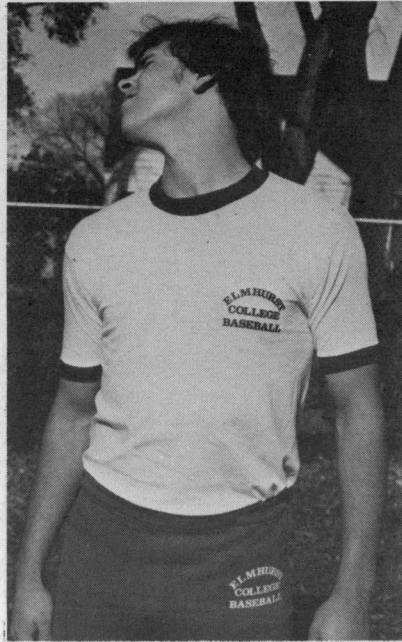

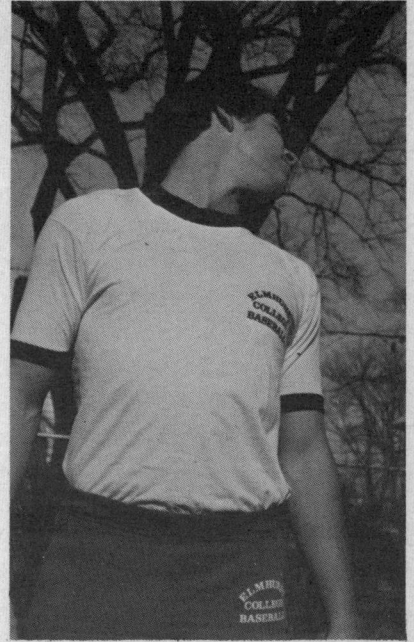

When using flexibility exercises for warm-up, you should work from the neck down. Neck Circles help stretch and limber up your neck muscles. Begin by bending your neck forward until your chin touches your chest. Turn your head slowly to the right as far as possible and then repeat to the left. Then bend your neck back and stretch. Gently roll your head in a full circle.

exercises is to include them in the warm-up and cooling-off periods. Flexibility exercises used in warm-up activities prepare you for the vigorous conditioning period by stimulating blood circulation, increasing your heart rate and raising your body temperature. But most importantly, flexibility exercises stretch and limber up your muscles and joints so they can adapt to the increase in activity. The warming up of your muscles and joints increases your range of motion. If you ignore the warm-up and go head-long into vigorous exercise—e.g., jogging or weight lifting—you'll be much sorer the next day than you would have been had you done warm-up exercises—and that's if you are in decent physical condition. If you are in poor physical condition and you ignore a warm-up period before those same vigorous exercises, you could come away with something more serious than muscle soreness. Sudden vigorous stretching of a muscle causes the muscle to protect itself by a reflexive contraction or tightening up. Restretching that same muscle in a burst of activity can overstretch the muscle and result in a muscle tear or worse. Most of us have experienced to a much lesser degree the unpleasant effects of this reflexive contraction when, after a long period of inactivity, we decide to go out for a long run. The next day finds us virtual cripples. How much wiser to have spent a few days doing flexibility exercises and then preceded the run with a warm-up exercise period.

When selecting flexibility exercises for your warm-up period, keep in mind that flexibility is specific to each joint. Each joint should be exercised with particular attention to those joints you know will receive the most strain when you begin your conditioning period of exercise.

Flexibility Exercises for Cooling-Off

Flexibility exercises used in the cooling-off period following vigorous exercise do the reverse of the warm-up exercises. Instead of preparing your body for vigorous activity, they help your body return gradually to its normal working level. Failing to do cooling-off exercises can result in lightheadedness, dizziness and sometimes even nausea. The reason for this is simple. While engaged in vigorous activity your heart beats rapidly, supplying the extra oxygen the muscles need for the stepped-up activity. When you suddenly stop exercising with no cooling-off period, your heart rate drops rapidly but is still beating far above its normal level. The additional blood is still being pumped to the now inactive muscles. This leaves less blood to supply the brain with oxygen—therefore the lightheaded or dizzy feeling. A cooling-off period following vigorous exercise allows your heart to slow down gradually and your circulatory system to adapt to the lesser demands of normal activity.

If you want the greatest possible benefit from flexibility exercises, the cooling-off period is ideal. Your muscles, tendons and ligaments are warmed up and stimulated by the conditioning and circulatory periods. In this condition your muscles are more pliable and can most easily be stretched. By doing flexibility exercises in the cooling-off period you can work on stretching your muscles so that a reflexive muscle contraction is prevented. This post-conditioning stretching not only speeds you to flexibility fitness but will help reduce muscle soreness and cramps.

FLEXIBILITY EXERCISES

In doing the following flexibility exercises, it is important you remember to move slowly. You want to stretch your muscles, not pull or tear them. For example, when doing the Seated Toe Touches, lean *slowly* forward, trying to touch your fingers to your toes and then gently pull forward further to stretch the muscles. A jerking or vigorous bobbing will only tighten the muscles through the muscle's protective reflex contraction. If, when you begin, you're not sure if you are doing the exercises too vigorously—wait 24 hours. You'll get your answer.

The two exercise methods which best help build flexibility fitness are **calisthenics** and **Yoga**. Yoga was not covered in Chapter 1 as an exercise method, as you've probably noted. We are covering Yoga and the Yoga exercises separately because Yoga is more than a method of exercise; it is a philosophy.

After the name of each exercise is the muscle or groups of muscles that the exercise helps. Between the calisthenic exercises and Yoga exercises there will be considerable overlapping with exercises in each method that help the flexibility fitness of the same muscle or groups of muscles. This allows you a choice of exercises—after all, we all have our personal preferences.

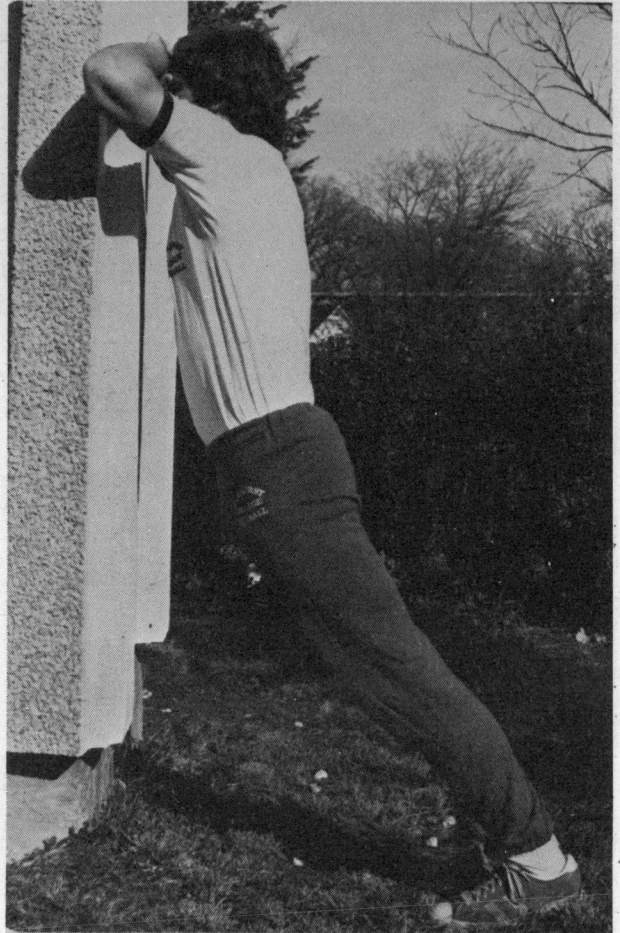

The Wall Stretch promotes flexibility of your calf and hamstring muscles. Remember when doing flexibility exercises to do them smoothly and not jerkily. When a muscle is suddenly stretched too far it fights back and actually shortens causing muscle soreness.

This Yoga exercise, Hand-To-Foot, will help stretch your leg and lower back muscles.

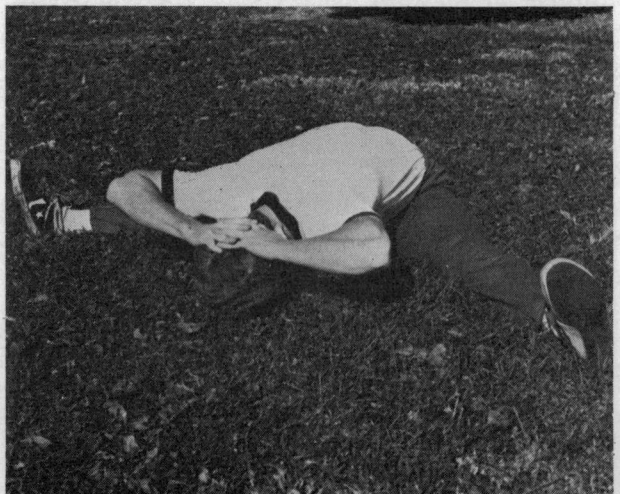

Calisthenic Exercises

Hamstring Stretch (lower back and hamstring muscles, hip joints)

1. Stand erect. Cross your right leg over the straight left leg and plant your right foot firmly on the floor.
2. Put your right palm firmly on your left shoulder with the right elbow projecting downward toward your navel. Your left arm should be hanging at your side.
3. Keep your left leg straight, bend slowly forward, bringing your right elbow as close to your crossed legs as you can get it. The straight left arm arcs backward as you do this. Tighten your abdominal muscles as you bend forward.
4. Return to starting position.
5. Repeat the exercise to the opposite side, with left palm on right shoulder and left leg crossed over the right.

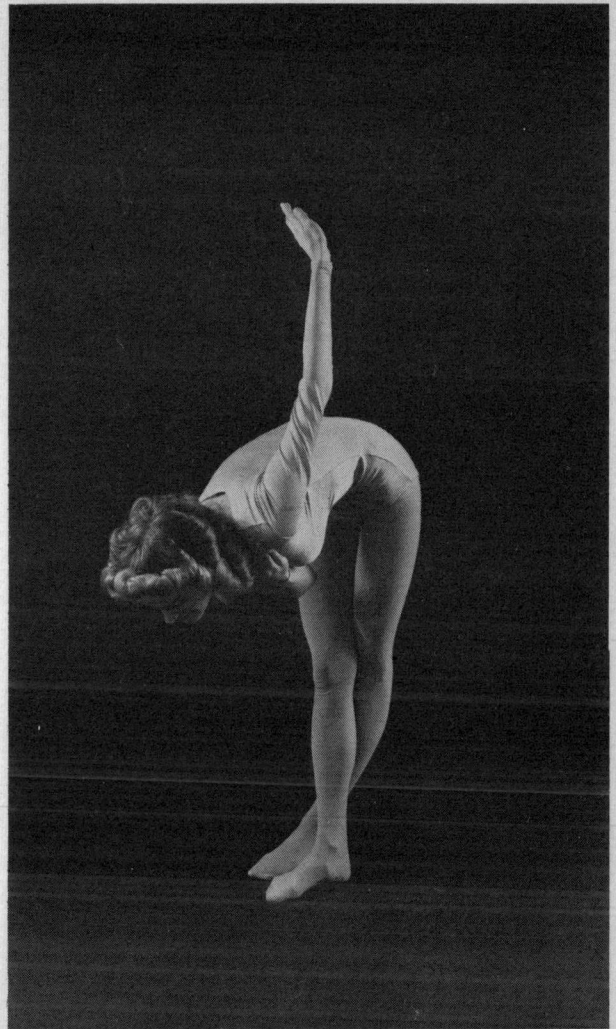

3

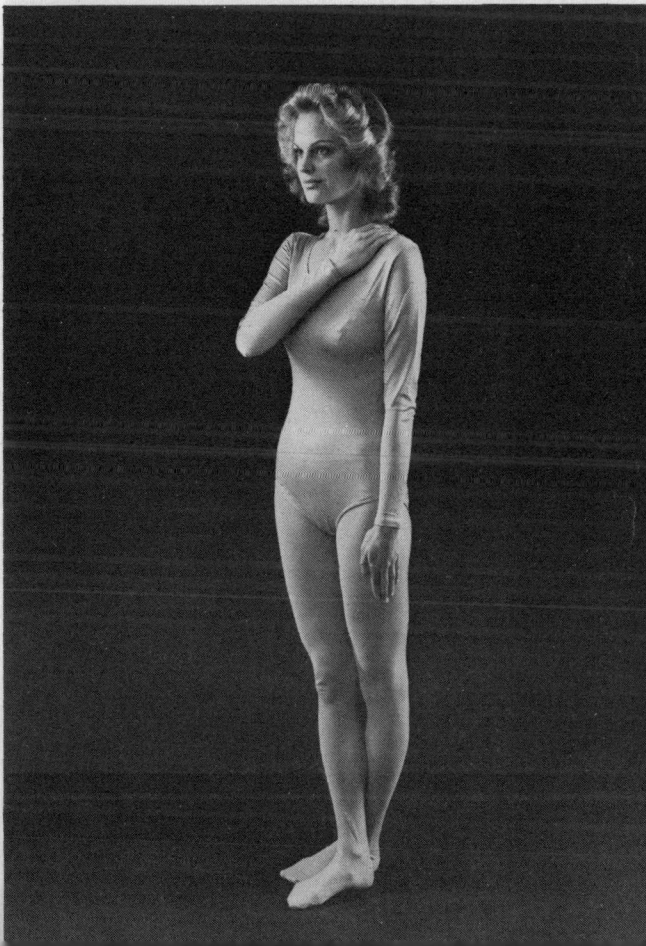

1

Flexed Leg Back Stretch (thigh, hamstring and lower back muscles)

1. Stand with knees slightly flexed, feet shoulder width apart, hands at sides.
2. Slowly bend over, touching the floor with the palms of your hands.
3. Now slowly try to straighten your legs without lifting your palms off the floor.
4. Return to starting position.

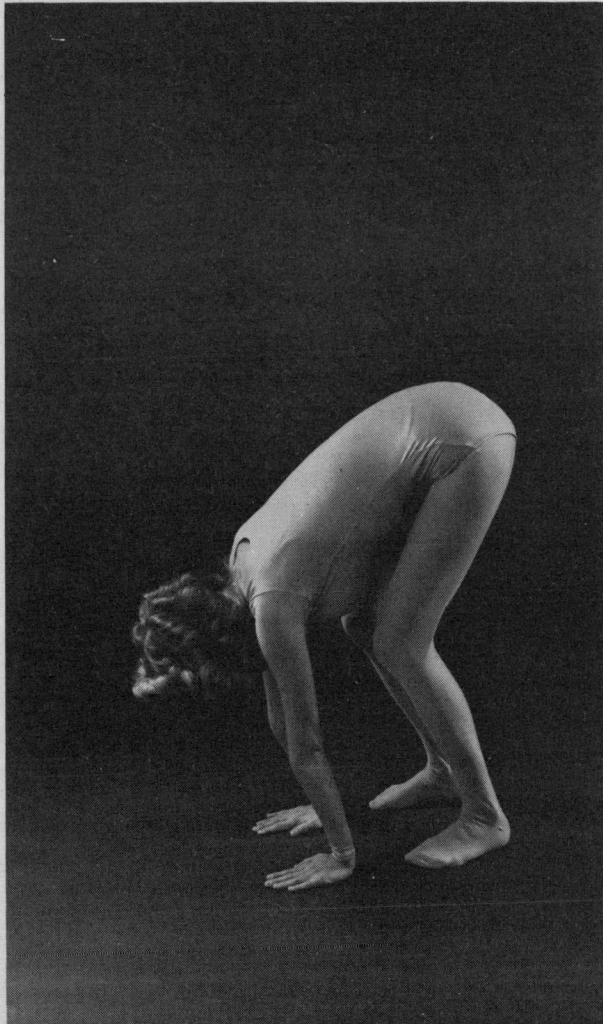

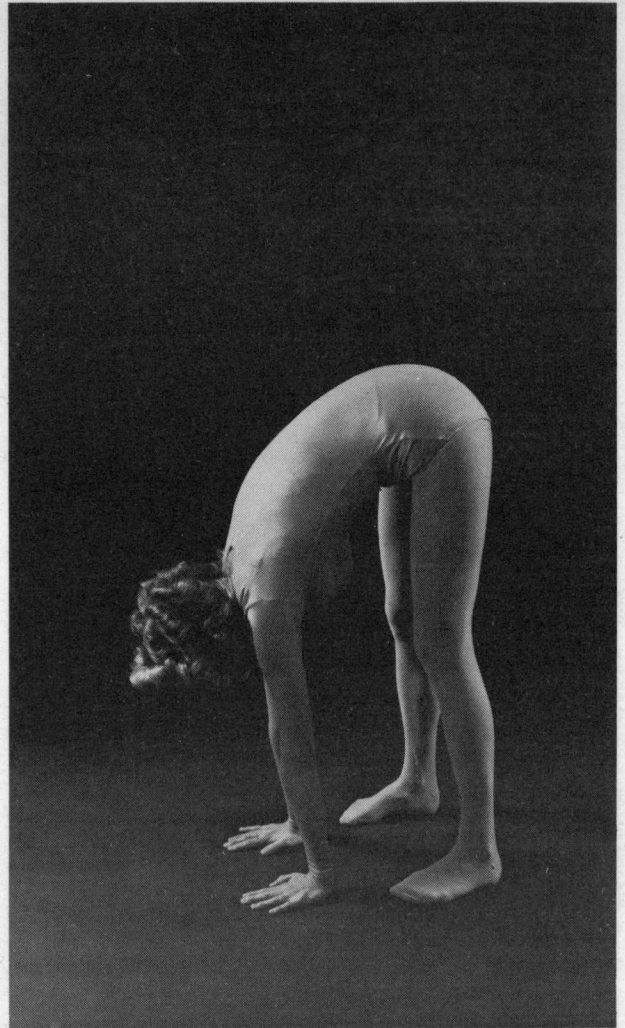

3

2

Lower Leg Stretch (ankles, calf and thigh muscles)

1. Stand on a thick book, stair step, or block of wood (approximately 6 inches high) with your weight on the balls of your feet and your heels raised.
2. Lower heels trying to touch the floor.
3. Return to starting position.

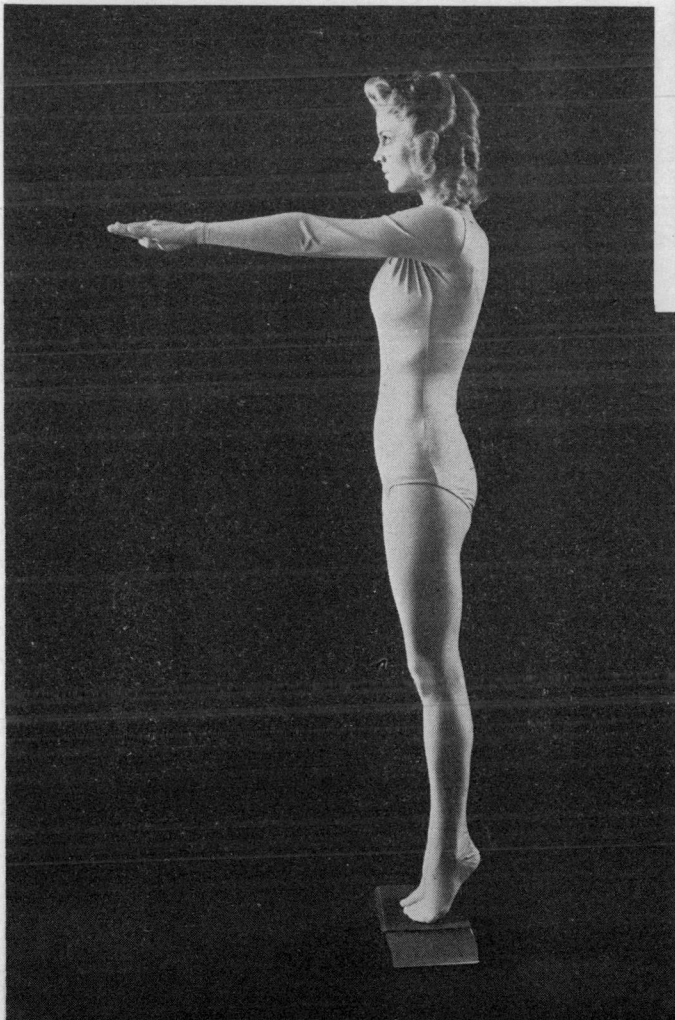

1

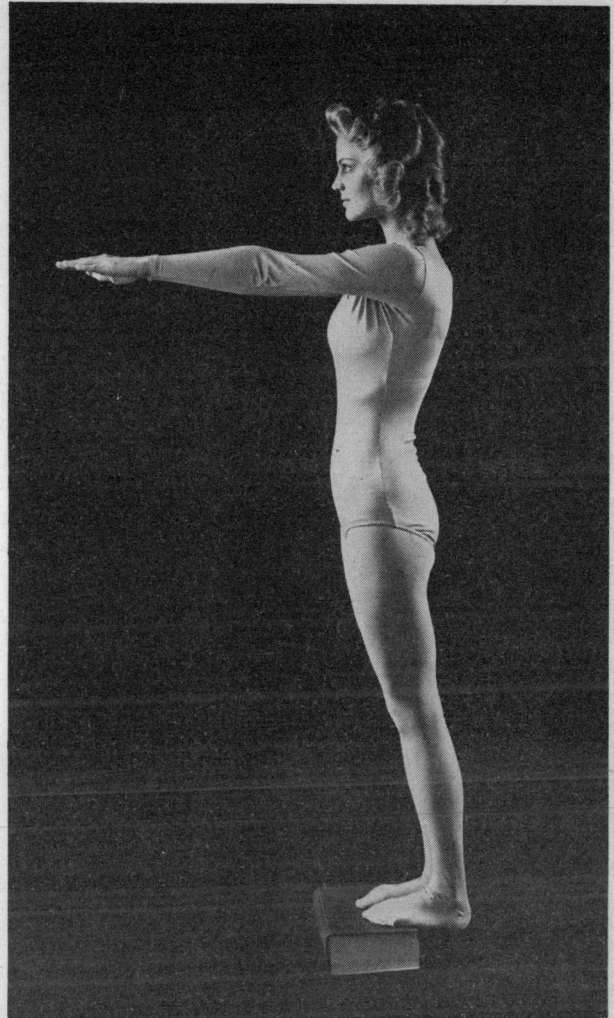

2

Step and Stretch (achilles tendon, calf and hamstring muscles)

1. Stand erect with right foot directly in front of left foot with a minimum of 12 inches between them. Hold hands at your side.
2. Bend right knee forward. Keep left foot flat on the floor.
3. Return to starting position.
4. Repeat exercise, putting your left foot forward and right foot back.

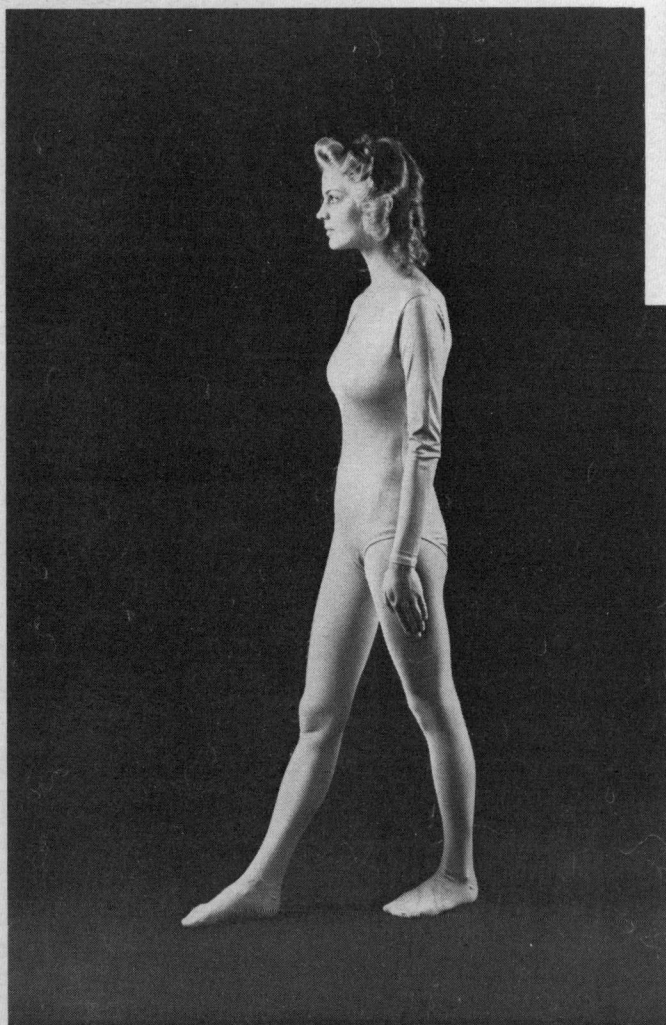

2

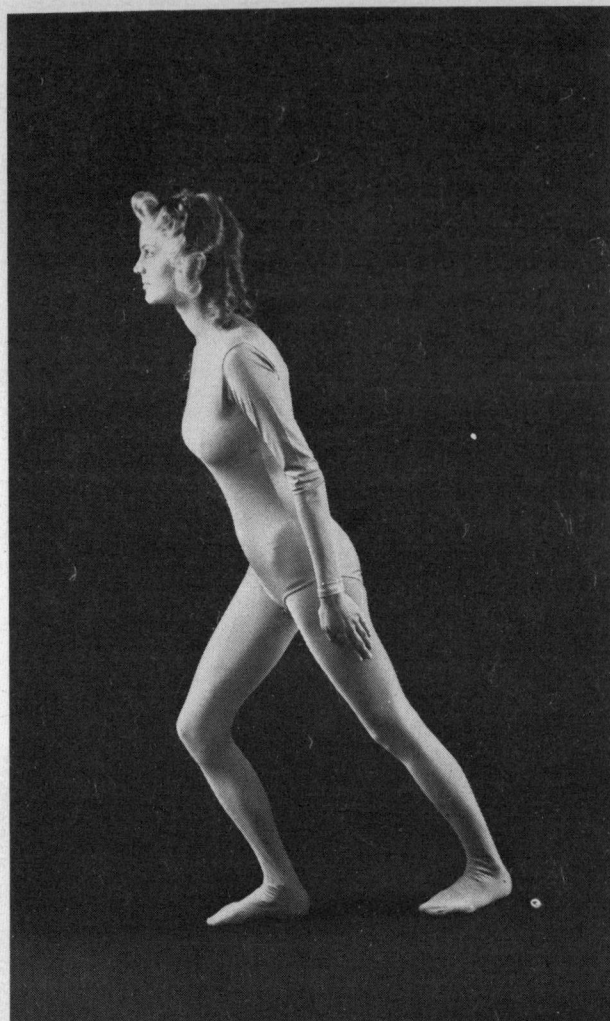

1

Half Knee Bend (leg, thigh and buttock muscles)

1. Stand erect, shoulders squared, feet slightly apart with hands on hips.
2. Bend knees until you reach a half-squat position while extending arms forward, palms down.
3. Return to starting position.

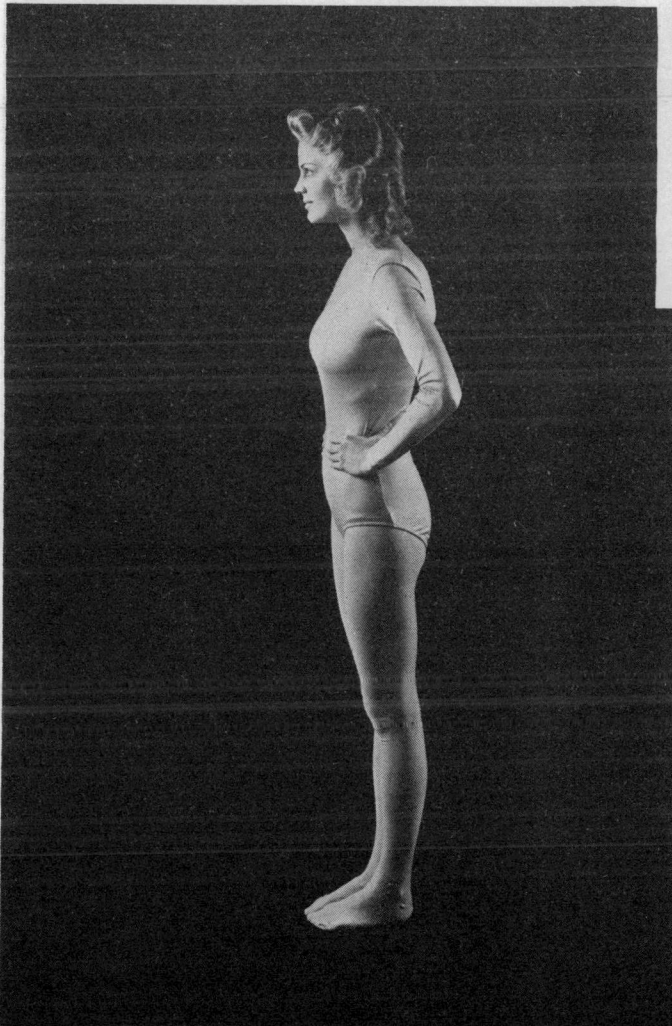

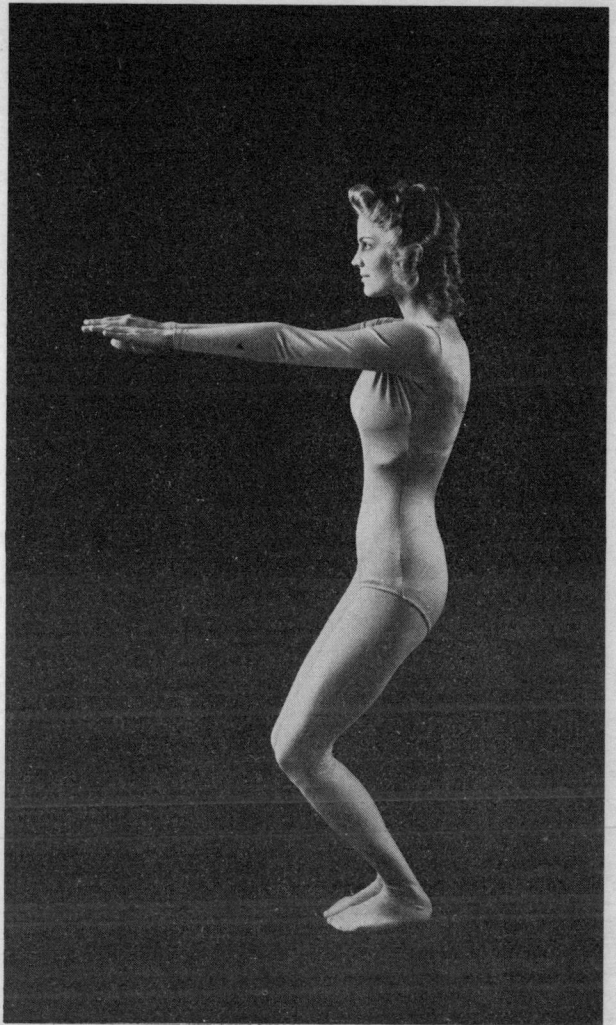

2

1

Windmill (lower back, hamstring, thigh and abdominal muscles)

1. Stand erect, knees slightly flexed, with feet spread shoulder width apart. Arms are extended out to the sides of the body.
2. Bend and twist trunk, bringing right hand to left toe keeping arms straight and knees flexed.
3. Return to starting position.
4. Twist and bend trunk bringing left hand to right toe.
5. Return to starting position.

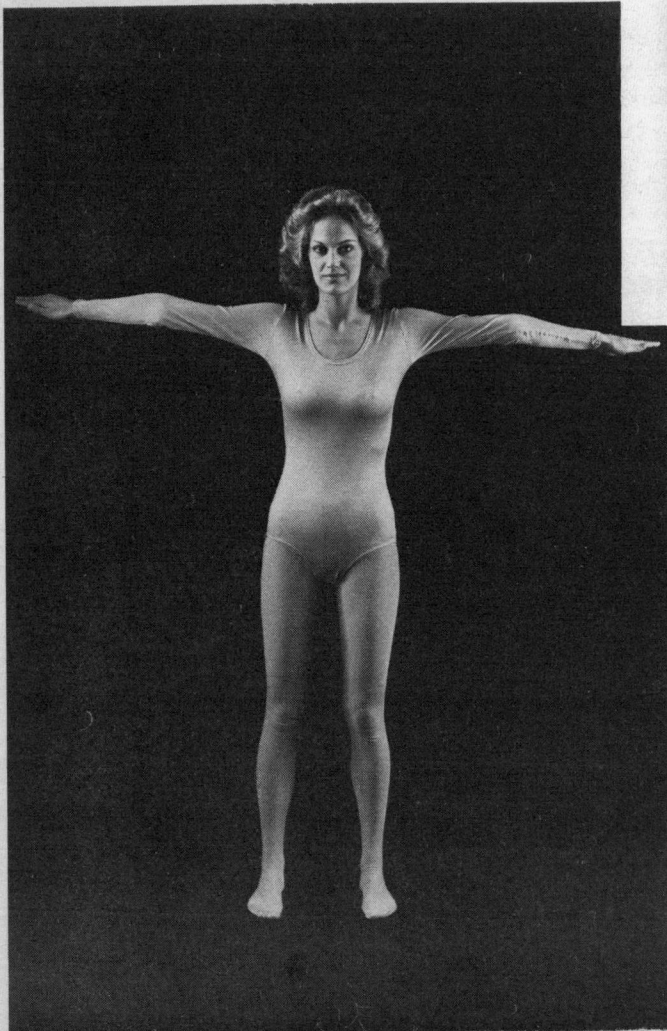

2

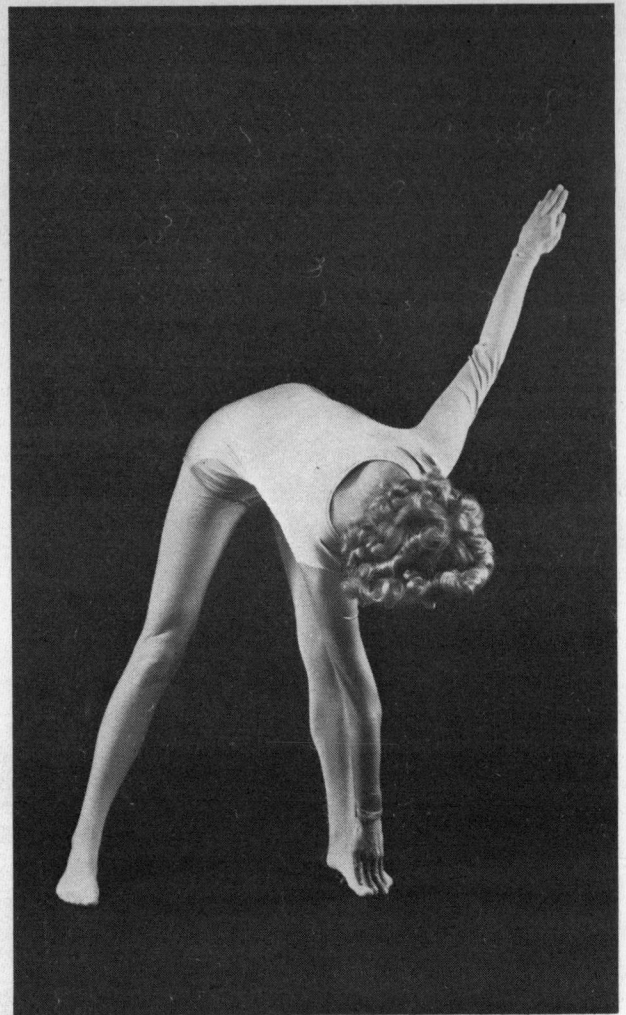

1

Stride Stretch (wrist, hip, groin, leg and lower back muscles)

1. Squat on floor with buttocks touching heels, body bent forward, hands on floor on either side of knees.
2. Move right leg straight back, keeping back rigid.
3. Try to press left knee toward the floor.
4. Return to starting position.
5. Move left leg straight back, trying to press right knee to floor.
6. Return to starting position.

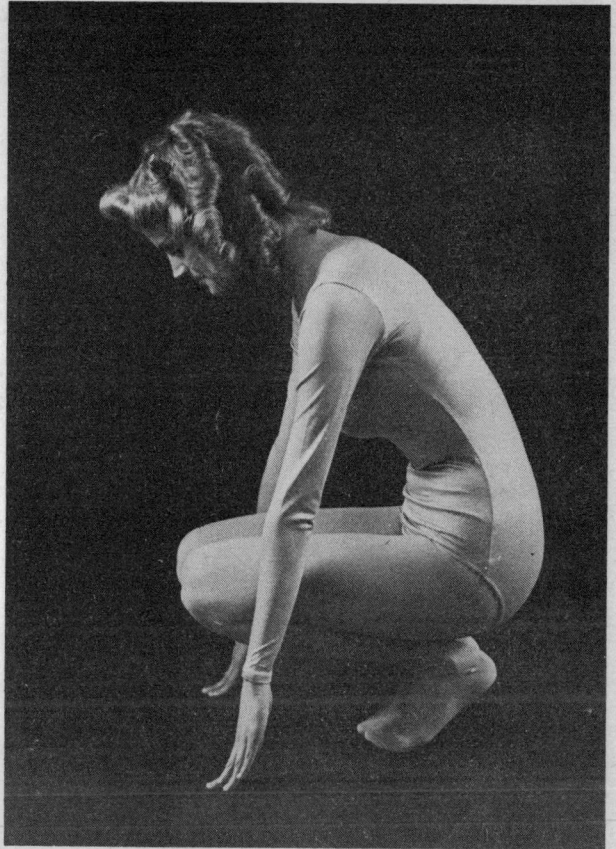

1

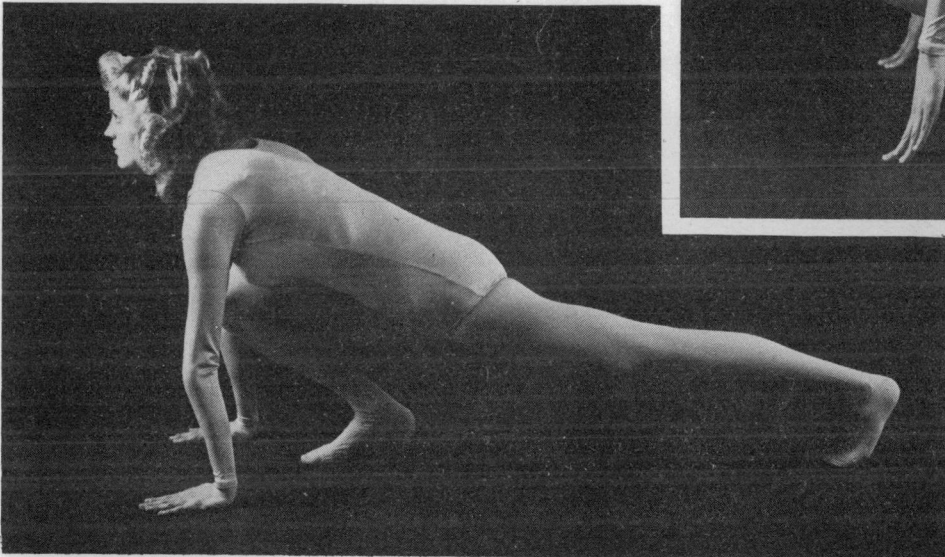

2

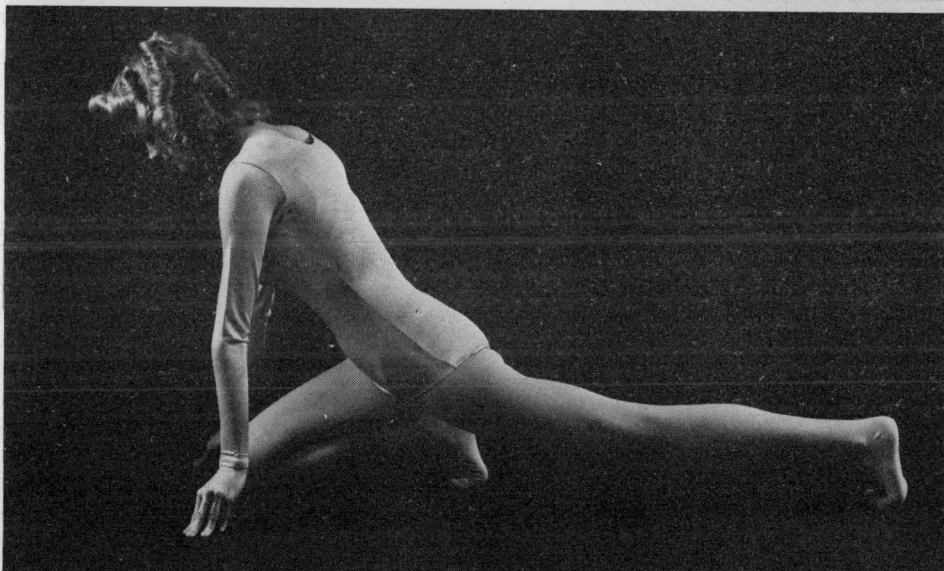

3

Side Twister (trunk, shoulder and back muscles)

1. Stand erect, feet about 12 inches apart, arms extended out to the sides with palms down.
2. Twist torso as far as possible to the left keeping arms extended.
3. Repeat, turning torso as far as possible to the right, keeping arms extended.
4. Return to starting position.

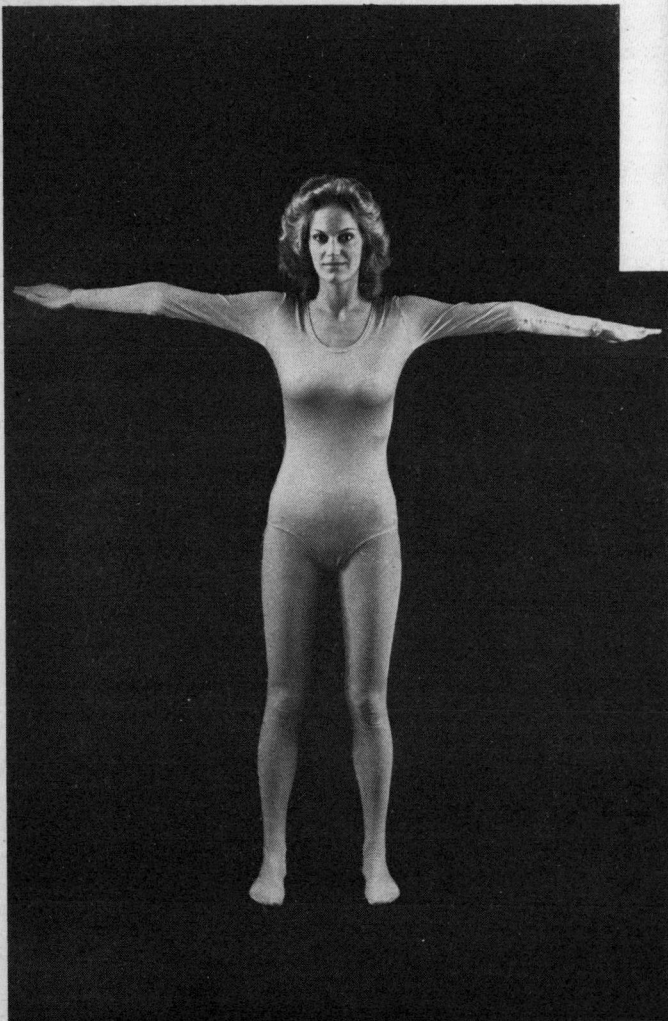

2

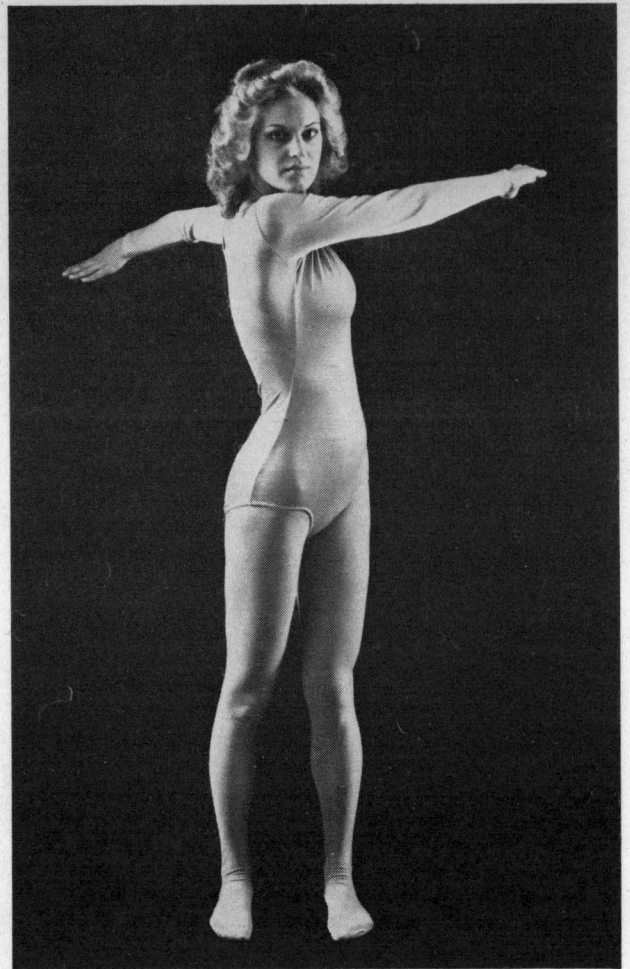

1

Side Bender (trunk, arm and neck muscles)

1. Stand erect with hands on hips and feet about shoulder width apart.
2. Extend left arm overhead, keeping right hand on hip.
3. Bend to the right side as far as possible and gently pull.
4. Return to starting position.
5. Extend right arm overhead, keeping left hand on hip.
6. Bend to the left side as far as possible and gently pull.
7. Return to starting position.

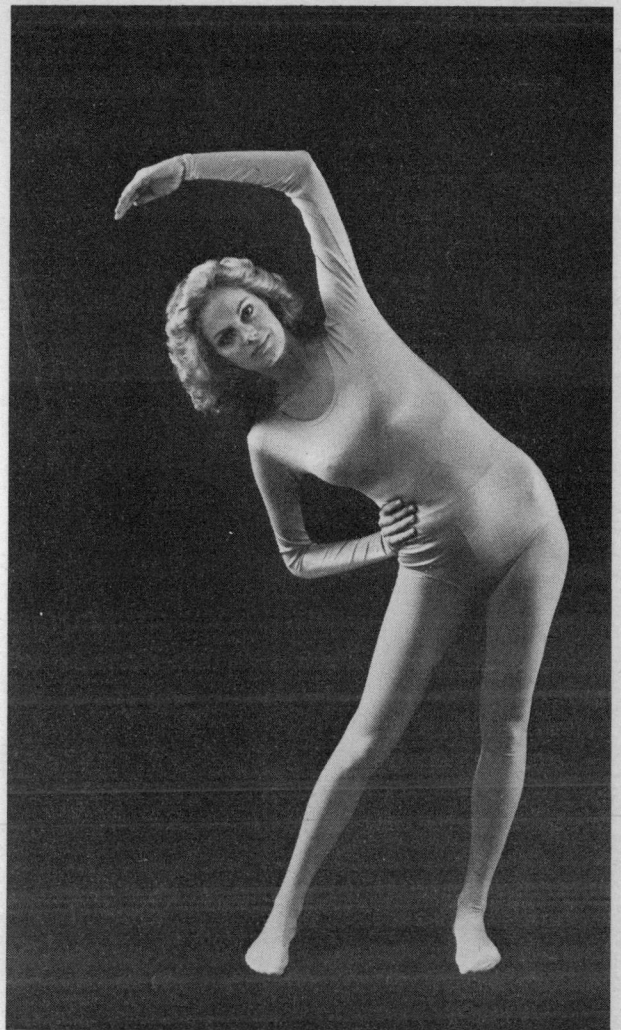

3

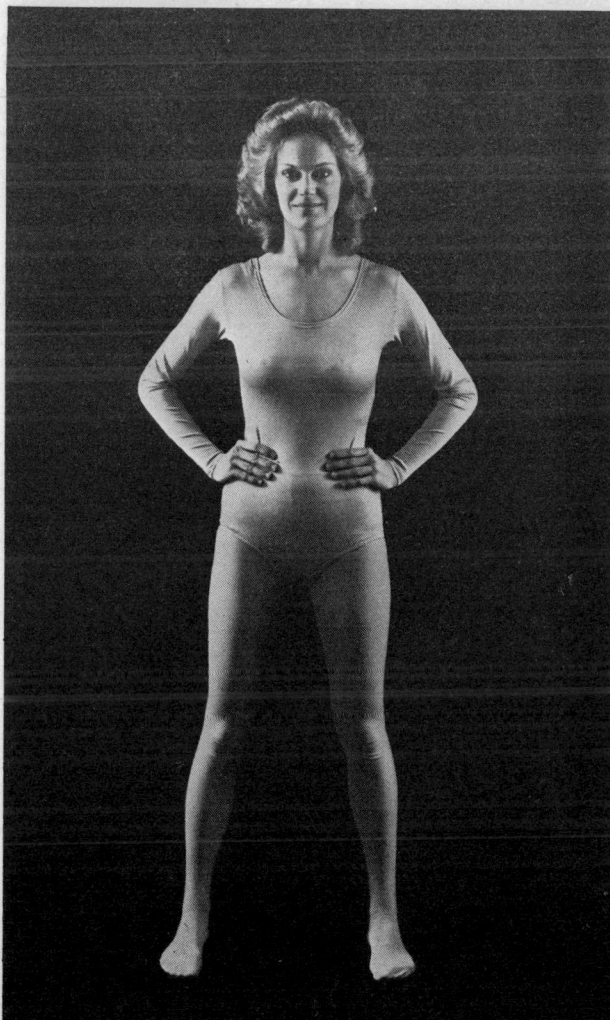

1

Wing Stretcher (pectoral, shoulder and upper back muscles)

1. Stand erect, feet about 12 inches apart, arms bent, elbows out to each side at shoulder height.
2. Slowly push elbows backwards as far as possible.
3. Return to starting position.

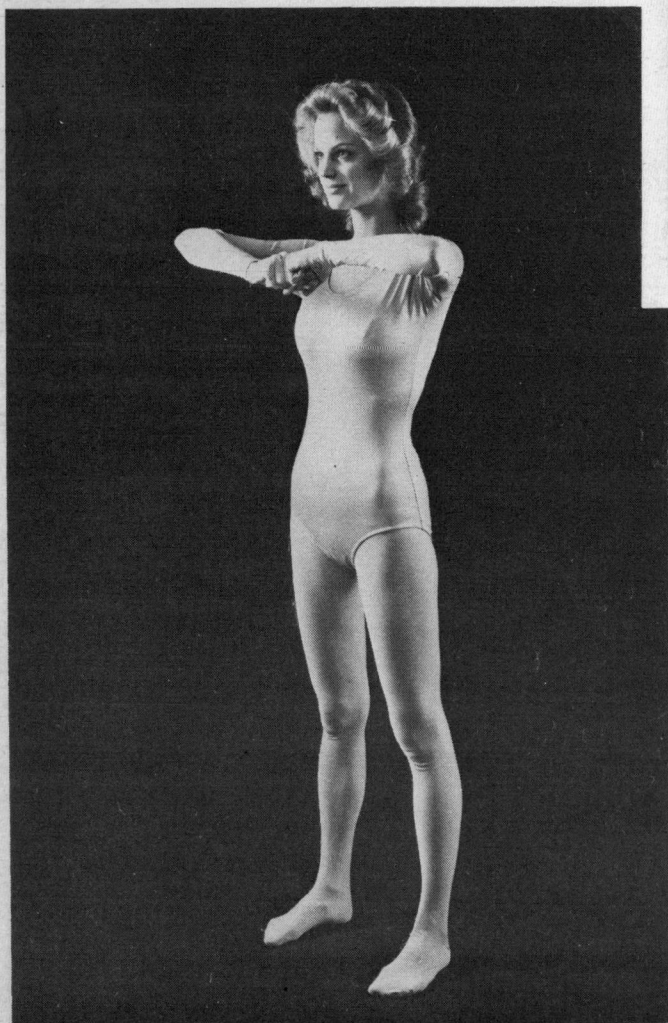

2

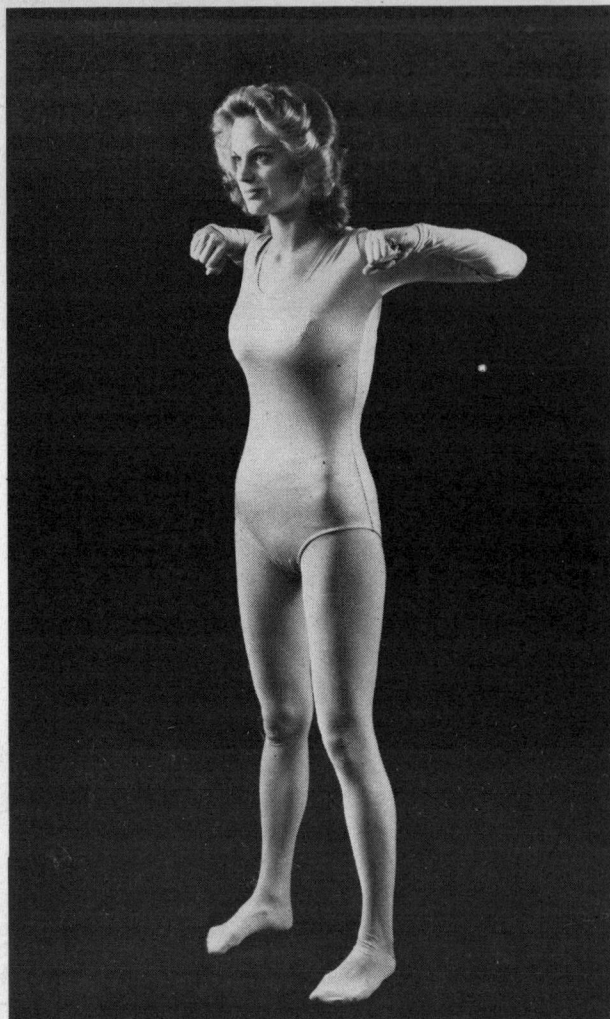

1

Neck Circles (neck muscles)

1. Stand erect with arms hanging loosely at sides.
2. Bend neck forward until chin touches chest.
3. Turn head to the right as far as possible.
4. Bend neck backward as far as possible.
5. Turn head to the left as far as possible.
6. Gently roll head in full circle, first to the right and then again to the left.

2

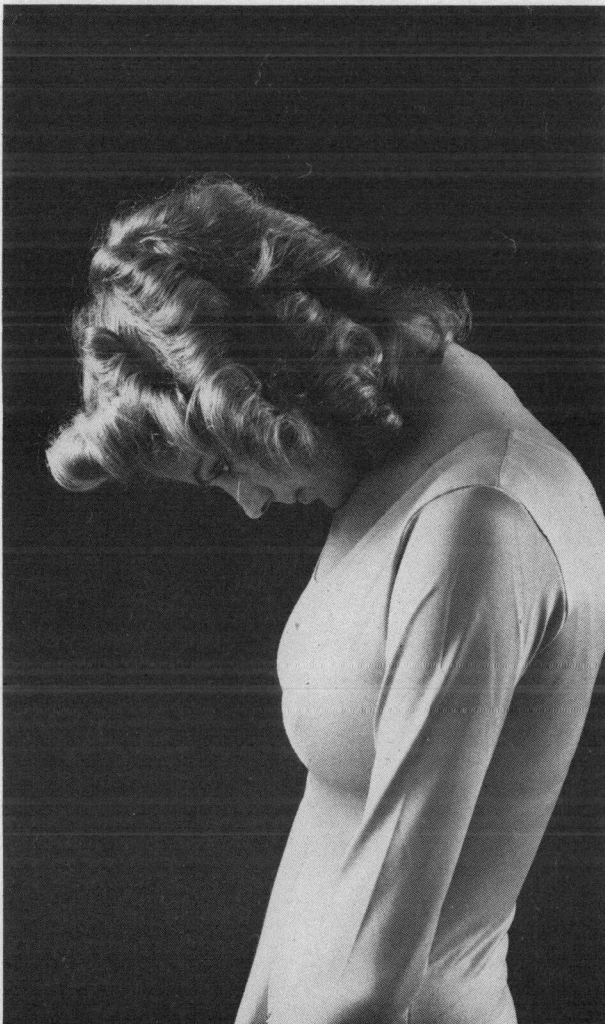

4

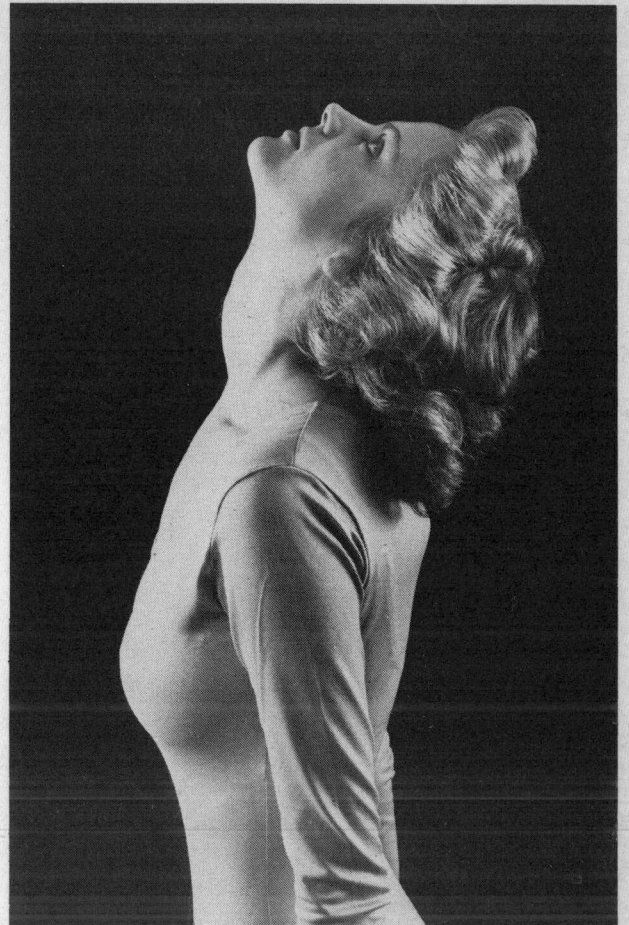

5

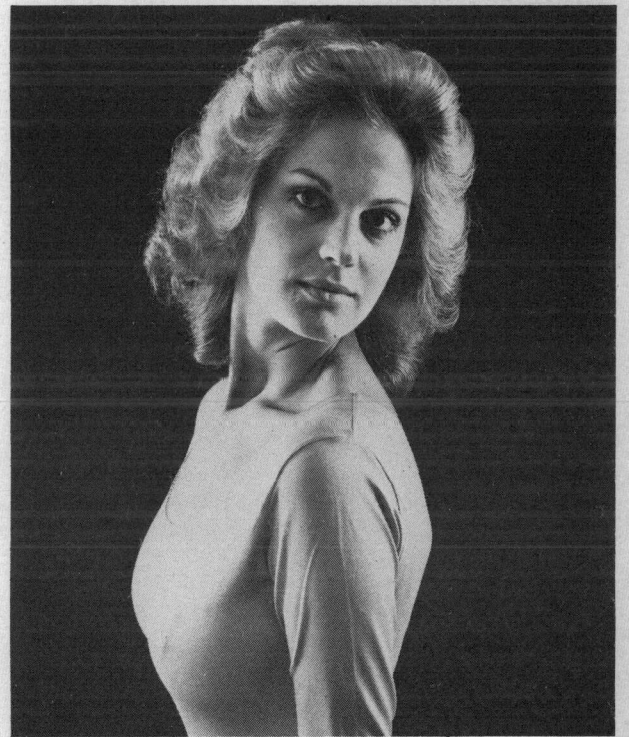

Hurdle Stretch (lower leg, thigh, abdominal and back muscles)

1. Sit on floor with left leg extended out front and right leg bent at knee and out to the side. Hands should be at your sides.
2. Reach out with right hand and touch extended left toe.
3. Return to starting position.
4. Reverse position of legs with right leg extended and left leg bent at the knee and out to the side.
5. Reach out with left hand and touch extended right toe.
6. Return to starting position.

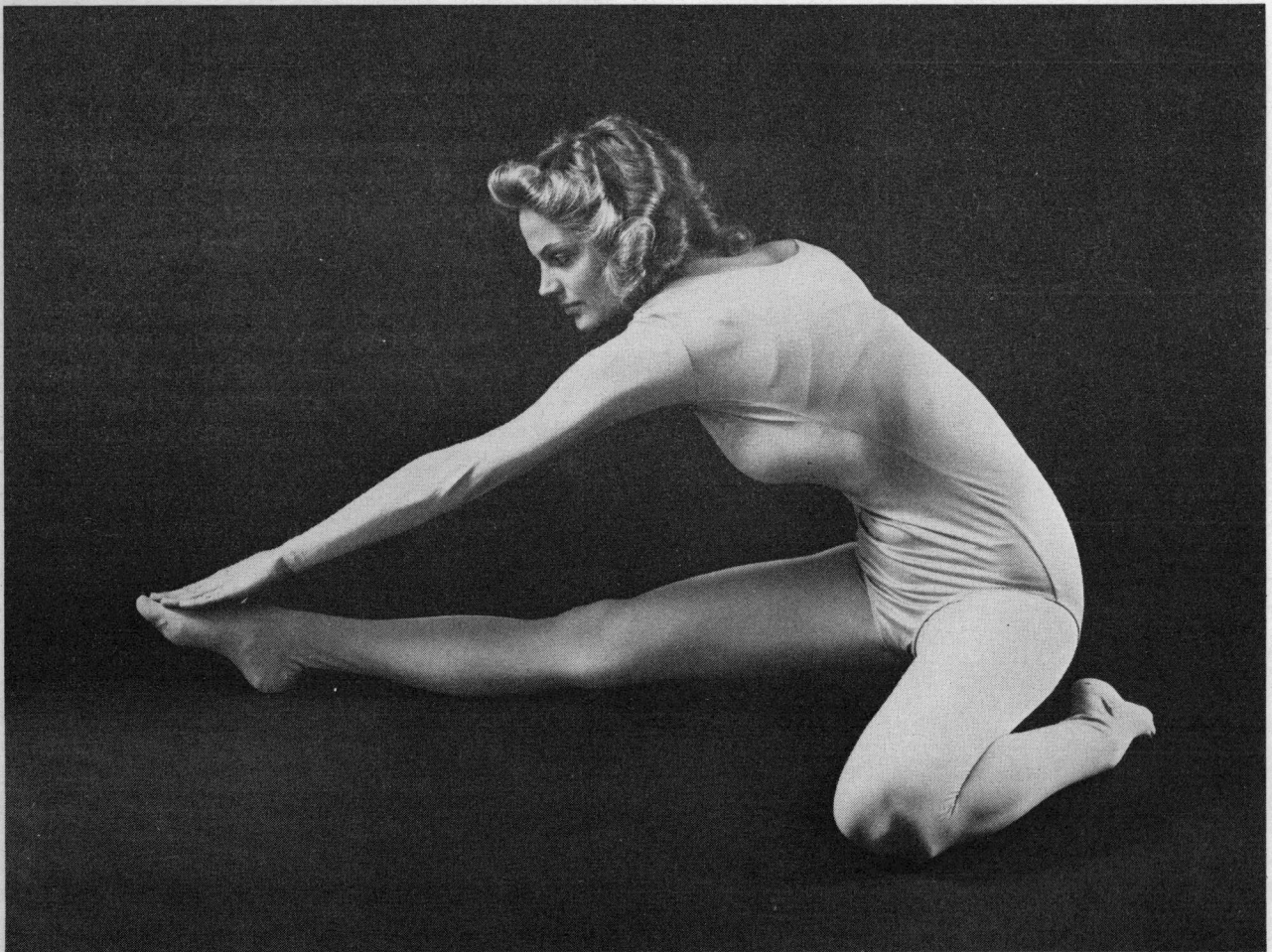

Sit and Stretch (lower back, inner thigh and hamstring muscles)

1. Sit on floor, legs apart with knees straight. Clasp hands behind neck.
2. Bend forward at waist as far as possible.
3. Gently stretch, trying to touch elbows to floor.
4. Return to starting position.

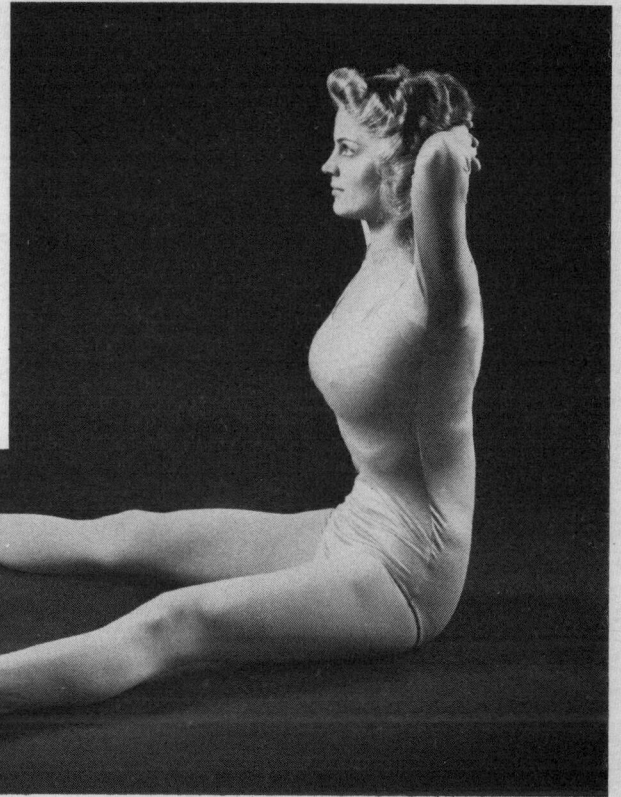

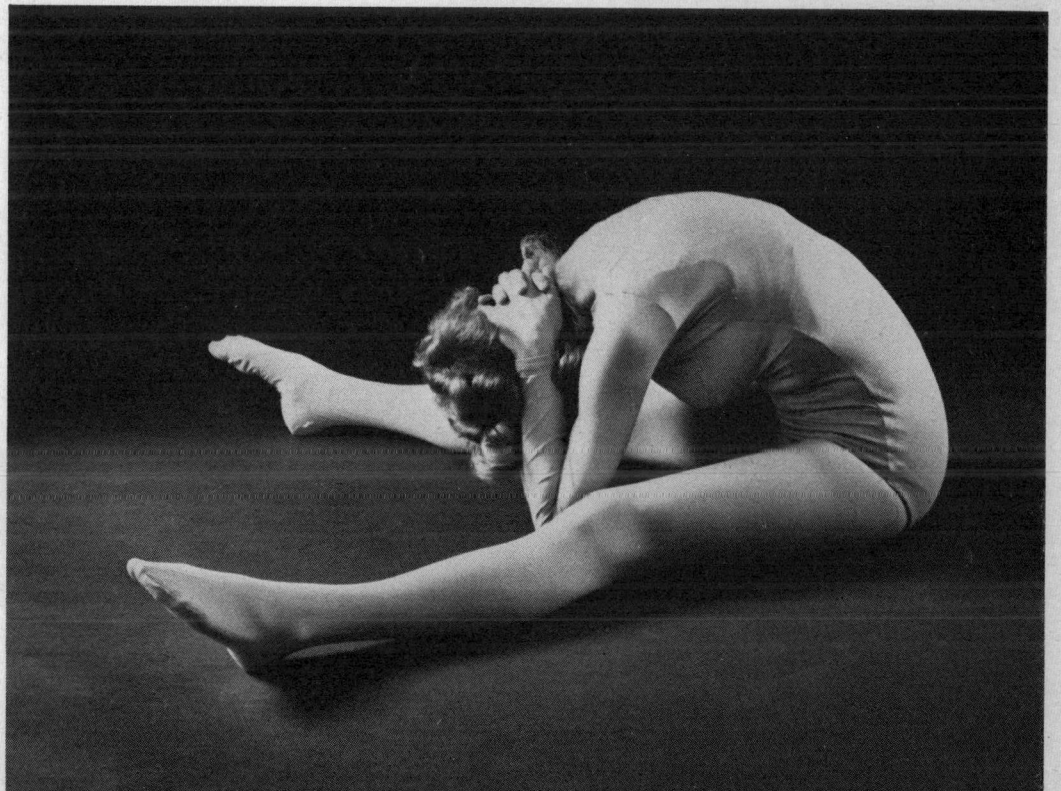

1

3

Side Lunge (inside and outside thigh muscles)

1. In a squat position, move your right leg out to the side.
2. Keeping your right leg straight, gently push right leg out as far as possible.
3. Return to squat position.
4. Extend left leg out to the side.

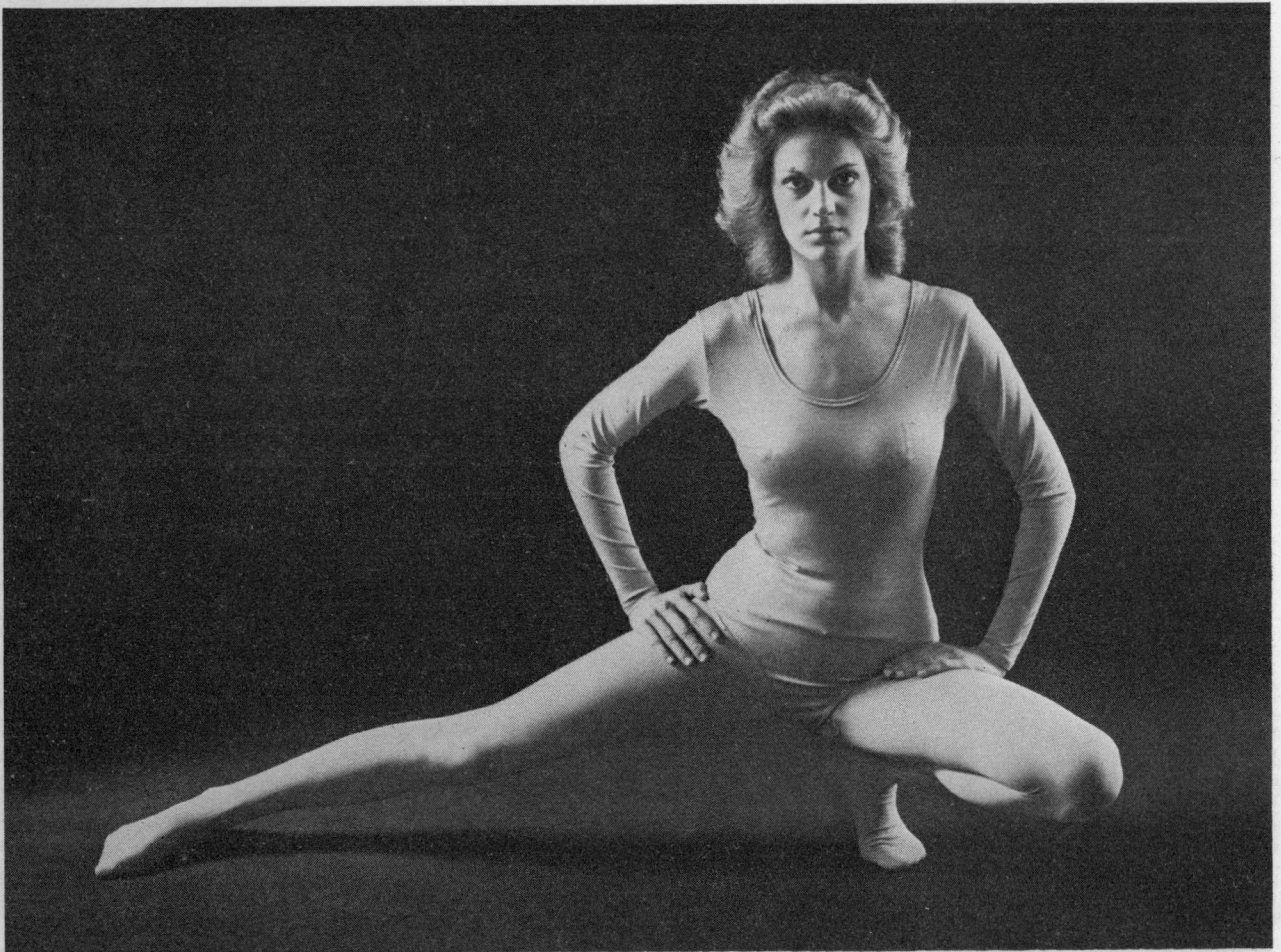

Knee Pull (thigh and trunk muscles)

1. Sit on floor, back straight, both legs extended straight ahead.
2. Keeping back straight, pull right leg as close to chest as possible.
3. Return to starting position.
4. Pull left leg as close to chest as possible.
5. Return to starting position.

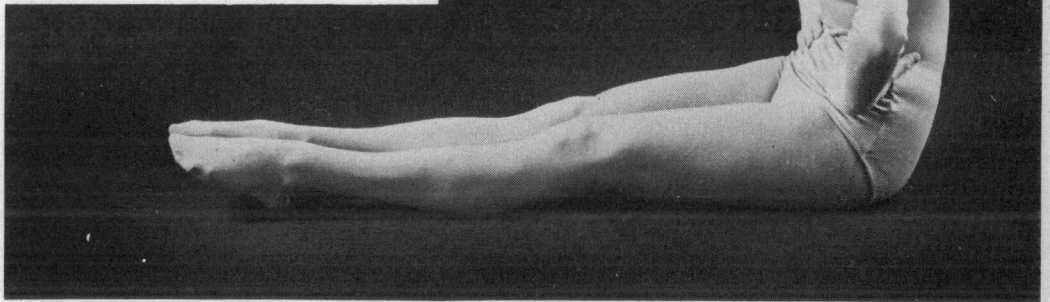

1

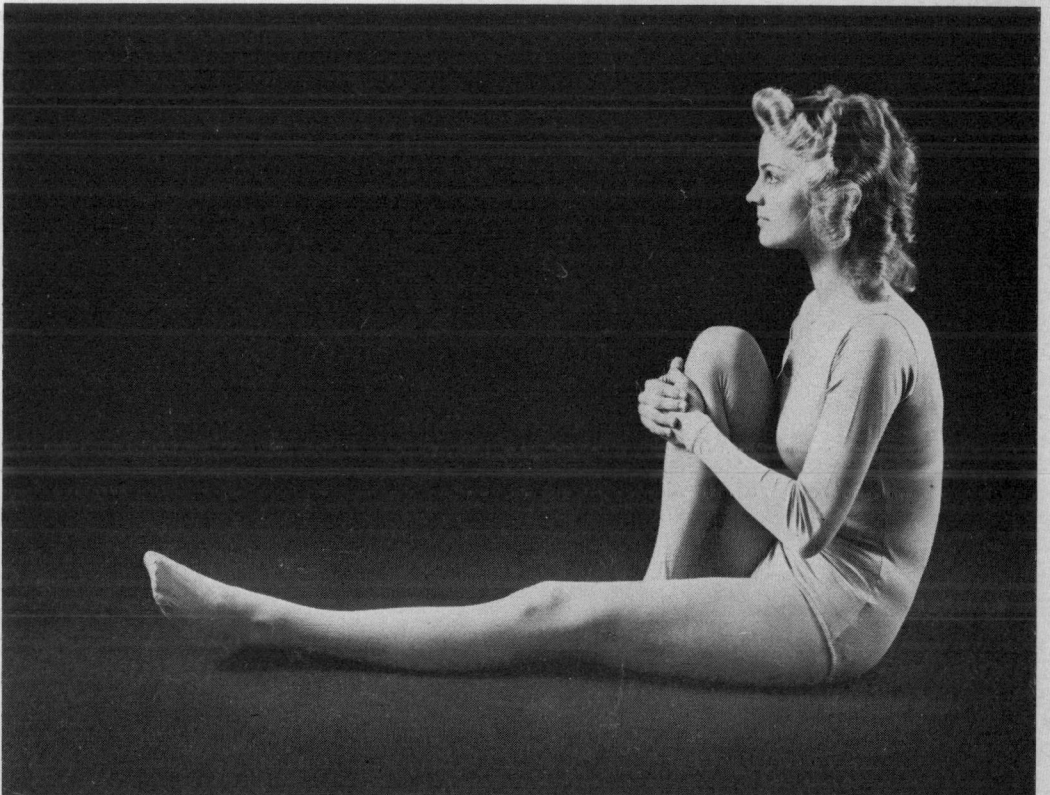

2

Toe Pull (groin and thigh muscles)

1. Sit on floor, knees bent and out to each side with the bottoms of your feet together and drawn as close up to your body as possible.
2. Grasp feet with both hands and pull on toes while pressing knees toward the floor with your elbows.

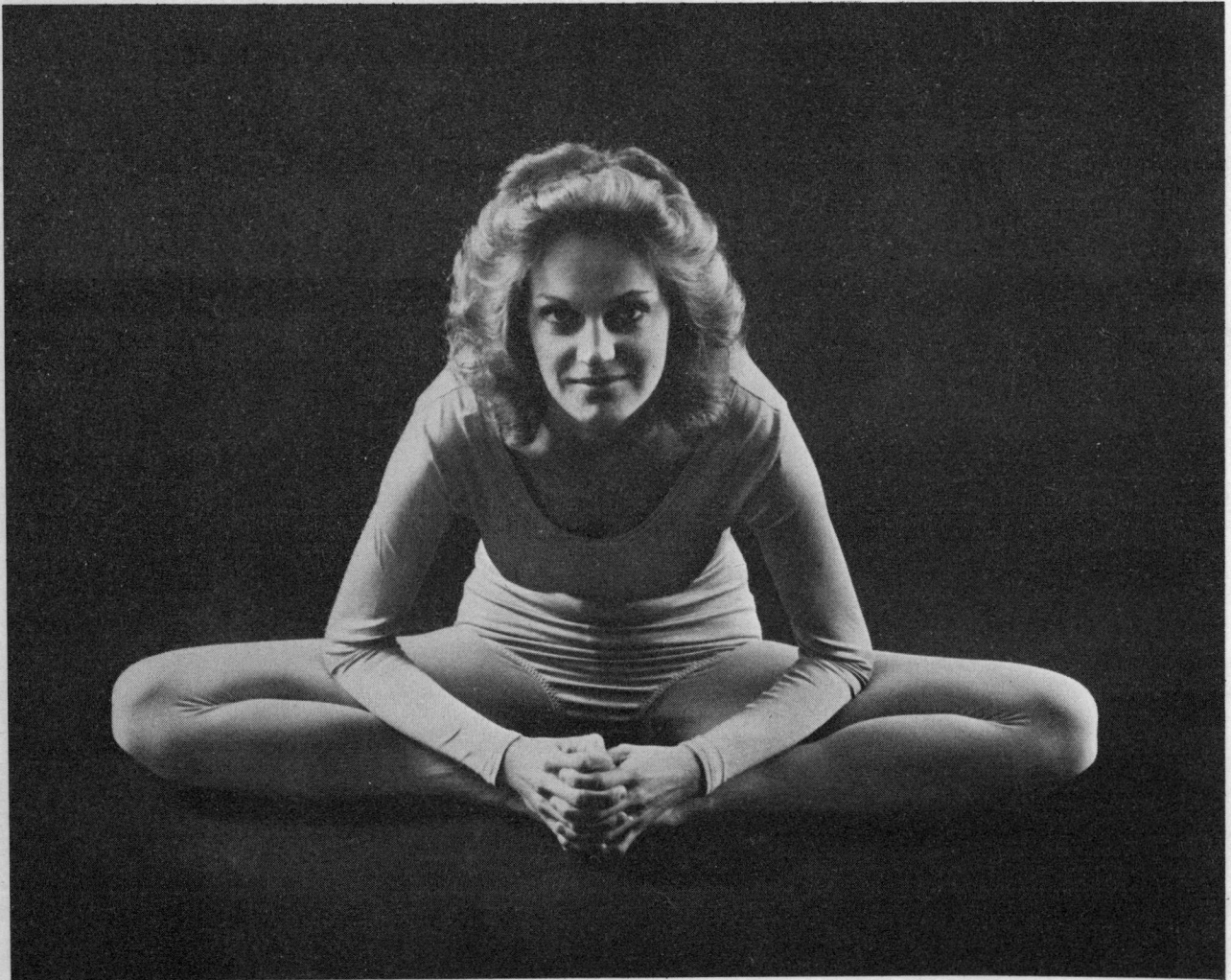

Wall Stretch (calf and hamstring muscles)

1. Stand erect, 3 feet from a wall with feet slightly apart.
2. Put both hands on wall.
3. Keeping heels on the floor, lean forward, slowly trying to touch head to wall.
4. Return to starting position.

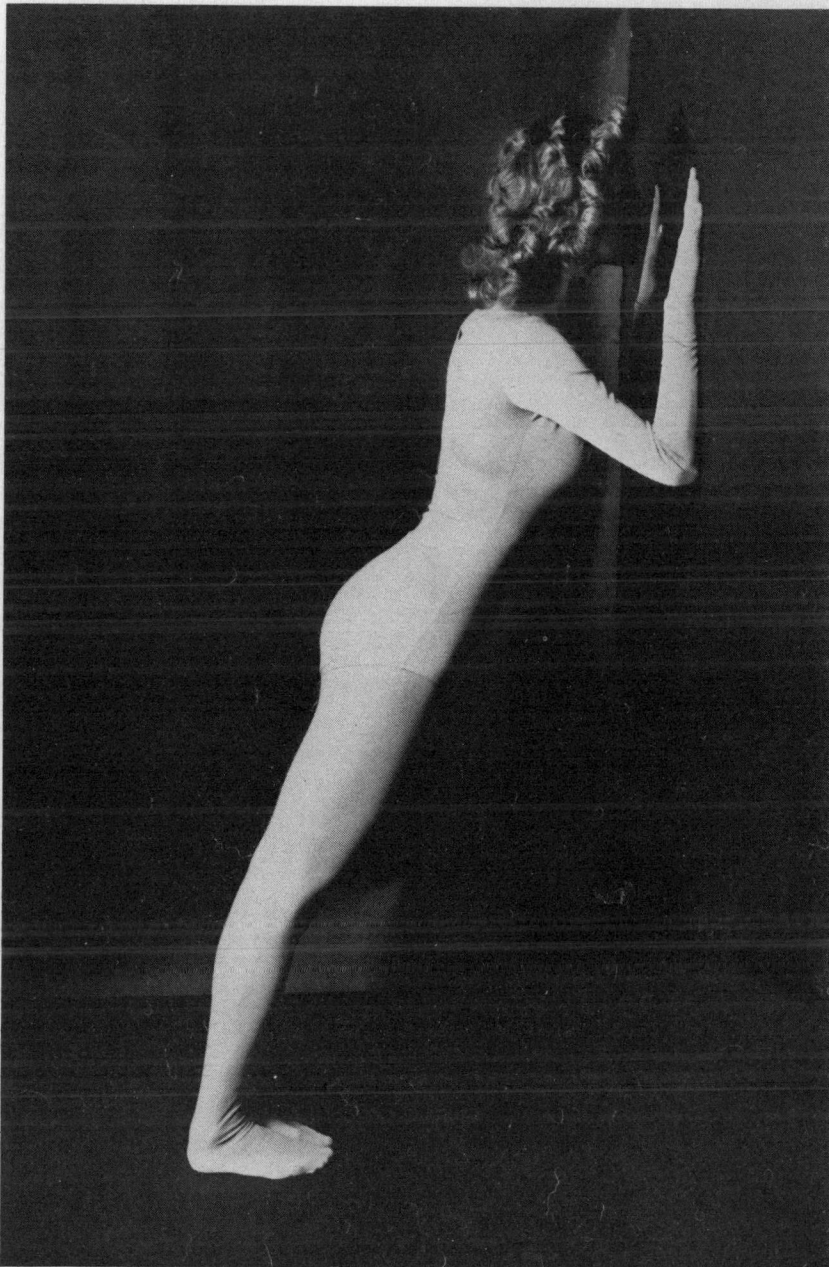

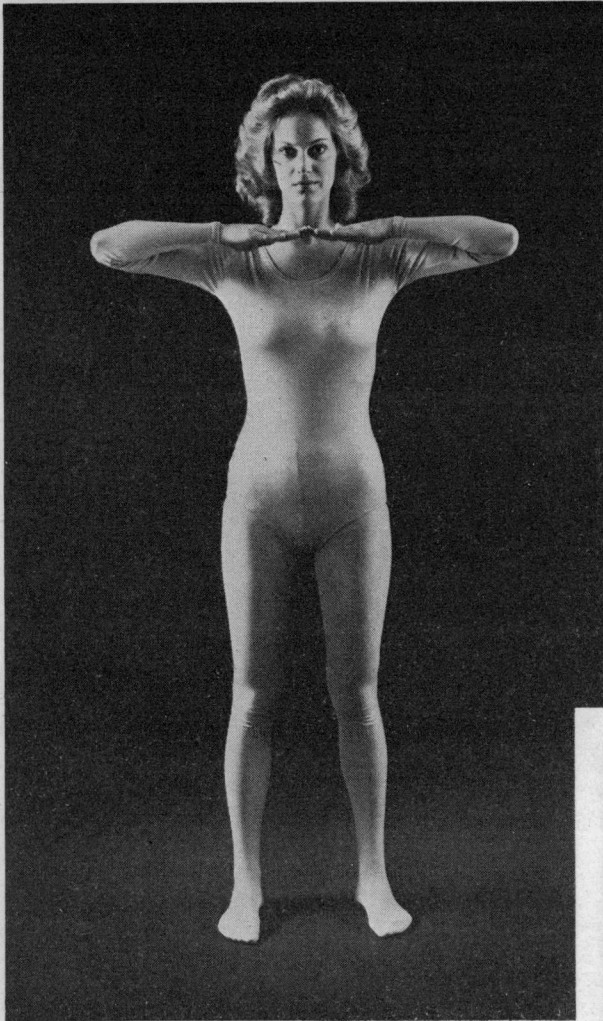

1

Bicep Stretch (biceps and upper back muscles)

1. Stand erect with feet about 12 inches apart, arms bent, elbows out to each side held at shoulder height.
2. Slowly extend arms straight out to sides and push them back behind the body as far as possible.
3. Return to starting position.

2

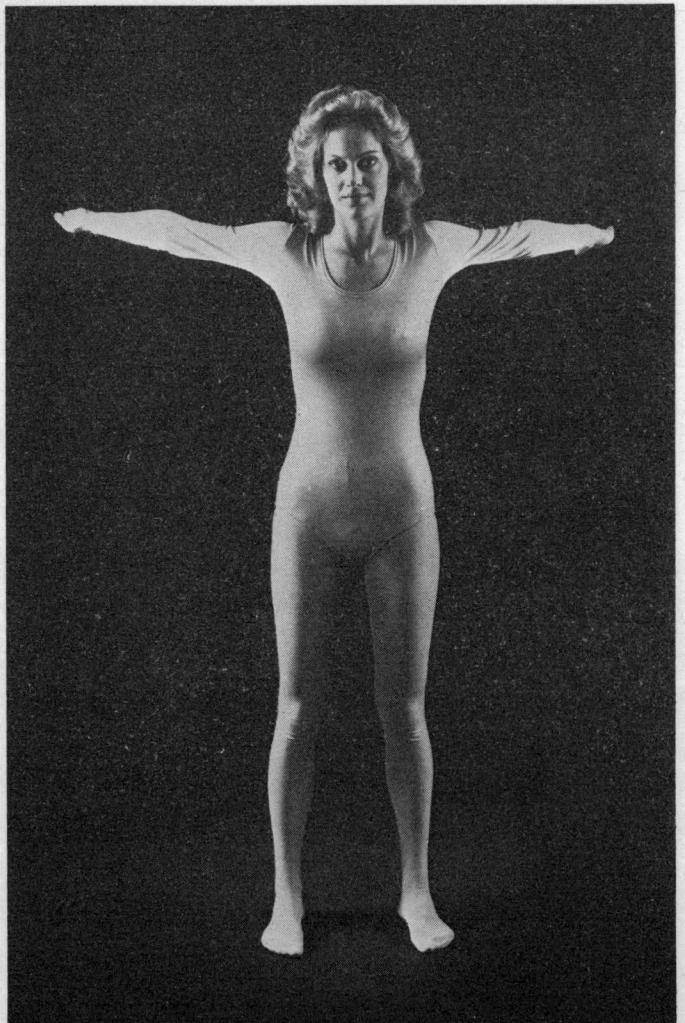

Cross-Legged Twist (trunk, shoulder and back muscles)

1. Sit cross-legged on the floor, hands clasped behind neck.
2. Twist your body slowly to the right as far as possible.
3. Return to starting position.
4. Twist your body slowly to the left as far as possible.
5. Return to starting position.

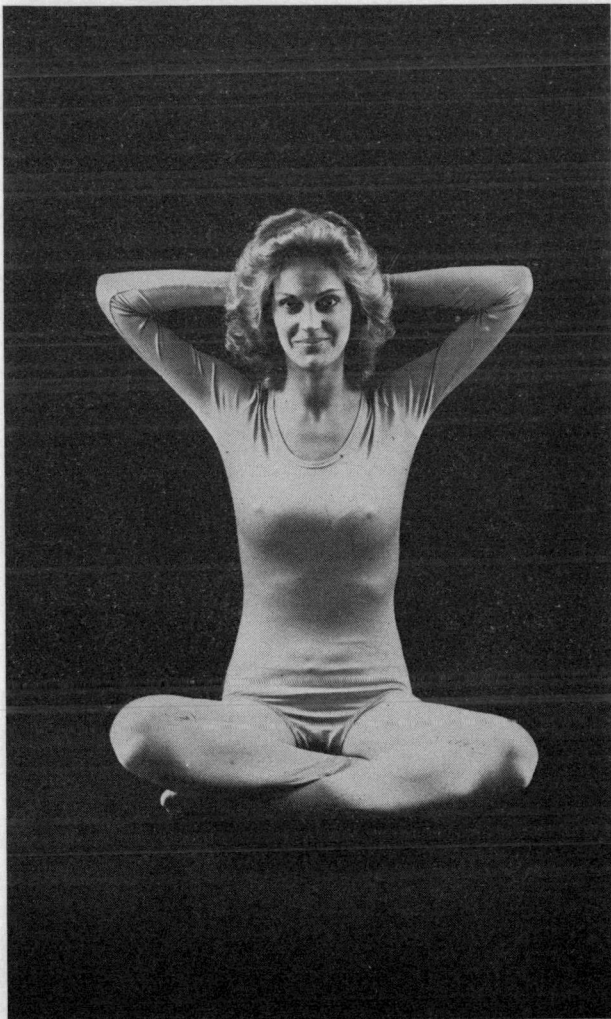

2

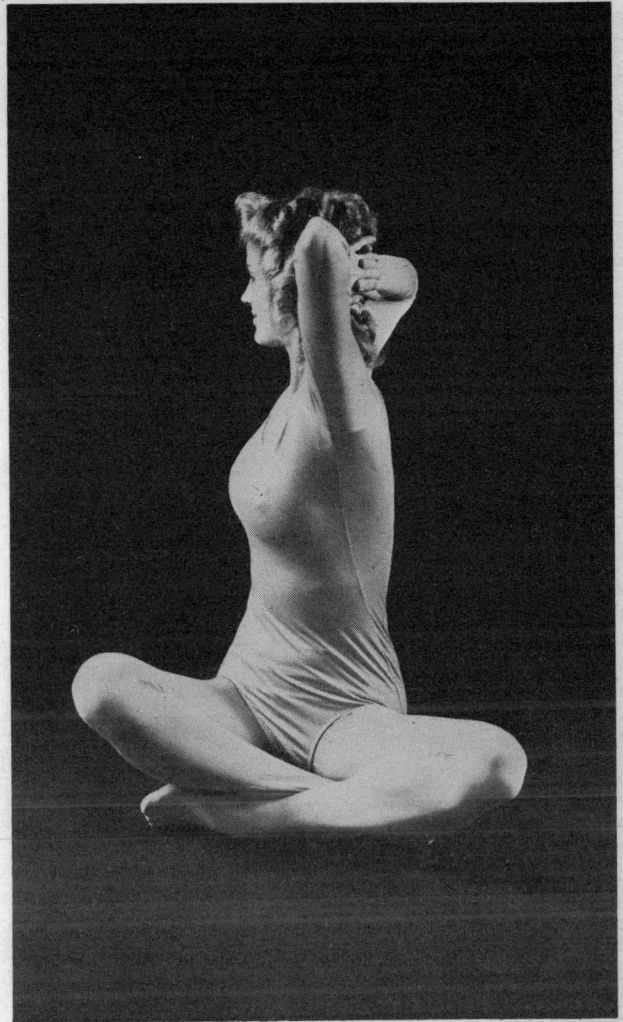

1

Seated Toe Touches (lower back and hamstring muscles)

1. Sit on floor, legs extended straight out in front, feet together, arms outstretched in front of body.
2. With toes pointed, bend at waist, trying to touch hands to your toes.
3. To increase stretch, grasp ankles and pull head as close to legs as possible.
4. Return to starting position.

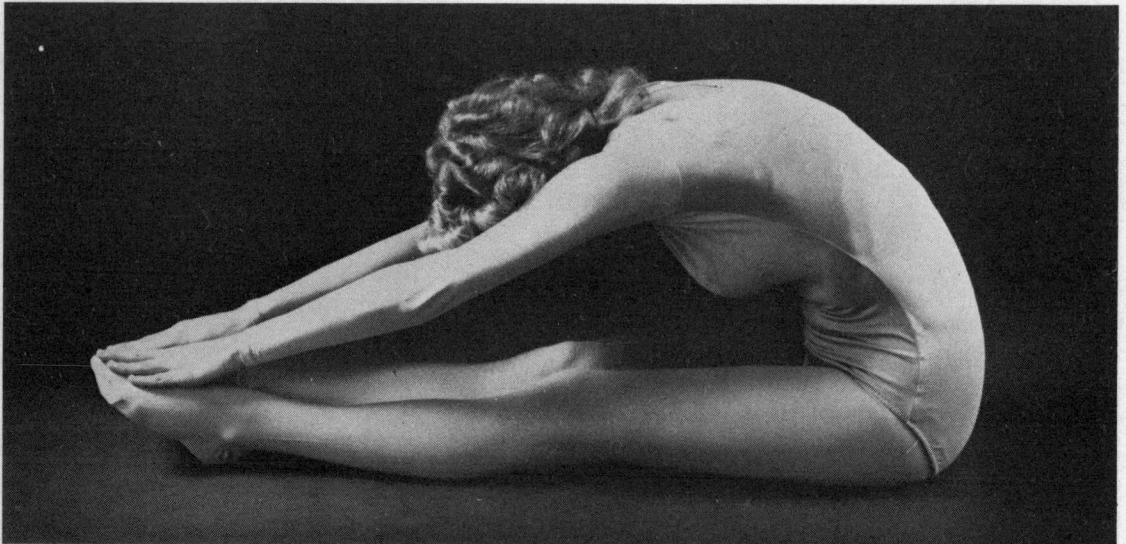

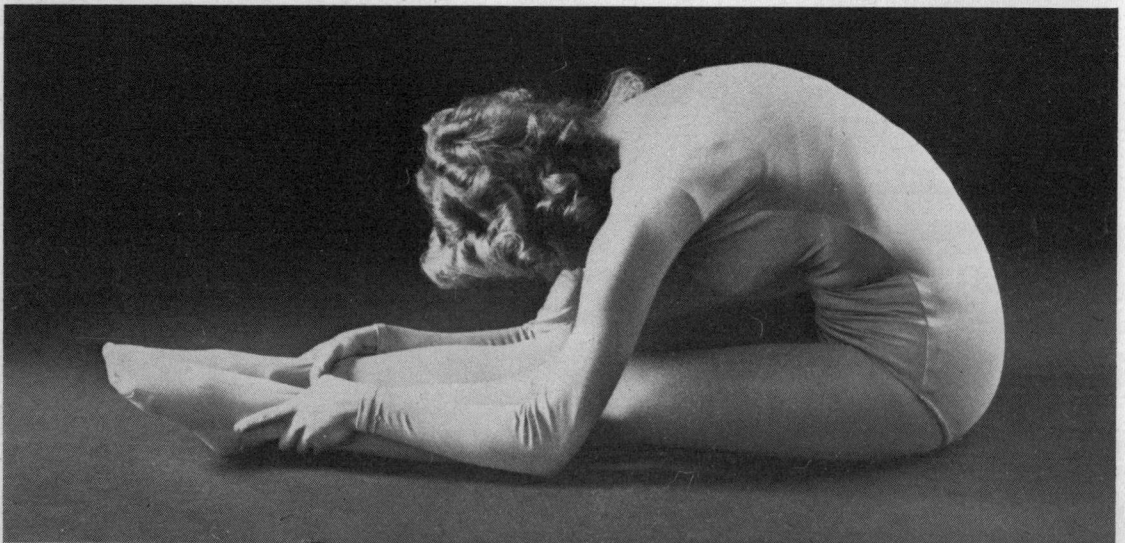

YOGA PHILOSOPHY

There is certainly nothing new about Yoga, which is described by its advocates as exercise for the whole person—mental and spiritual as well as physical. Millions of Easterners have followed it for at least 6,000 years. By comparison, the growing popularity of Yoga in the Western World within the past 50 years is recent. Ancient gurus felt that the body, mind and spirit of a person were seldom united into a harmonious whole, with each phase receiving adequate attention. That concern prompted the development of Yoga to its present state. There are several major types of Yoga, each of which employs different techniques to achieve the same unifying goal. We are primarily concerned in this book with Hatha Yoga, the kind of Yoga that is concerned with the physical. The other basic type of Yoga with which you may be familiar is Raja Yoga, concerned primarily with meditation.

Since one does not have to embrace Yoga in totality to enjoy its benefits, the discussion in this book will deal with the most logical and practical phases of it.

The various Yoga postures or poses (*asanas*) are intended to be done smoothly and rhythmically in "slow motion" movements. Let me say at the outset that the beginning Yoga practitioner should *not* stretch to the point of pain and won't if each exercise is done slowly and rhythmically as intended. You should stretch only as far as is comfortable. Some doctors report an increasing number of patients who are practicing Yoga and have stretched too hard, too soon, developing bursitis and tendonitis.

In Yoga, the exerciser concentrates on the exercise, thinking of nothing else at the time. It is this concentration that makes the exerciser feel to the utmost what is happening to him as the exercise progresses—awareness, stimulation and relaxation.

YOGA AND BREATHING

Yoga puts great stress on proper breathing. (Some Yoga exercisers tell me that they had tried time after time, without success, to give up cigarettes. With the practice of Yoga breathing, they have been able to do it. One reason is that smoke fills a nervous need for the chronic chain smoker and that proper breathing and relaxation

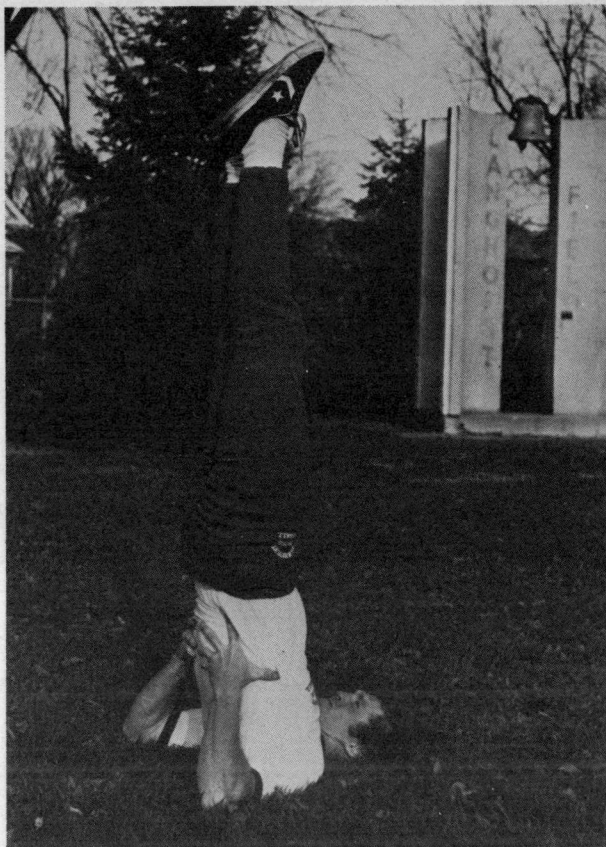

Above is the Shoulder Stand and below is the Half Plough. Both of these exercises help stretch your back muscles.

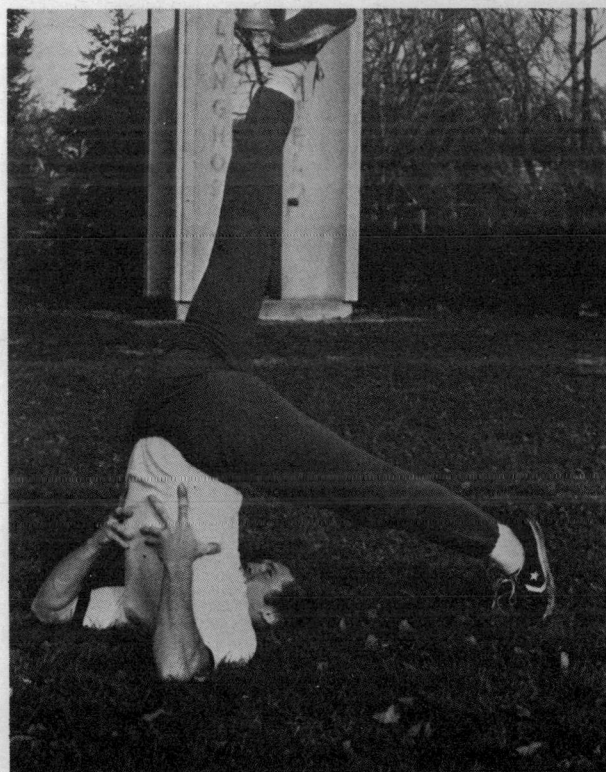

eliminate that nervousness.) One of the first things we have to learn about the Yoga method of breathing is quite contrary to habit. We've gotten into the habit of pulling in the stomach and only expanding the chest while inhaling deeply, which, according to Yoga practitioners, is all wrong. Pulling in the stomach shrinks the diaphragm and thus results in a shallow breath, our lungs taking in much less air and oxygen. The correct procedure is to *expand* the abdomen while inhaling and pull it in while exhaling. This method utilizes the lungs in their entirety. This technique may require some practice, and while the breathing exercises are usually done from the Perfect Posture, the Lotus Posture and the Easy Posture, all of which take a bit of getting used to, you may want to practice your breathing first while lying down.

If the Lotus posture is difficult for you and not necessary, when you're ready, try the Easy Posture, in which you sit with both legs stretched out straight in front of your body. Then you bend your right knee so that your foot touches your left thigh. Following that, you bend your left knee and put it under the right one. With a little perseverance, the soles of both feet should touch the inside of the thighs.

And if that's difficult, try the Tailor Posture. You simply sit cross-legged like a tailor. Every time you do it, try to bring your knees a little bit closer to the floor.

Once you've picked a position and are sitting at ease with your hands on your knees, it's time for your first real exercise, full Yoga breathing.

First, inhale into the abdomen through the nostrils by expanding the abdomen as far as you can. Following that, expand the thoracic cage so that the ribs expand outward and the chest measurement increases. Lift your collar bones as far as possible without hunching up.

You do these three things in order, on one inhalation of air, filling each section of the lungs. Then you exhale slowly.

The exhalation should take twice as long as the inhalation. A pause may be taken between the inhalation and the exhalation, but holding your breath long enough to cause discomfort is not only unnecessary but also forces you to exhale with too much speed. One Yoga expert, Karen Ross, author of the excellent book, *New Manual of Yoga,* published by the Arco Publishing Company, New York, recommends following this up by doing Yoga breathing through one nostril at a time, alternating nostrils.

A further Yoga breathing exercise she encourages is one she calls Bellows Breath. It's a rapid chain of quick inhalations and exhalations, keeping the one-to-two ratio on inhalation and exhalation but doing both in 1 second. I found it impossible to complete a breath in 1 second. One thing that speeds up the process is to take your pause after the exhalation instead of between inhalation

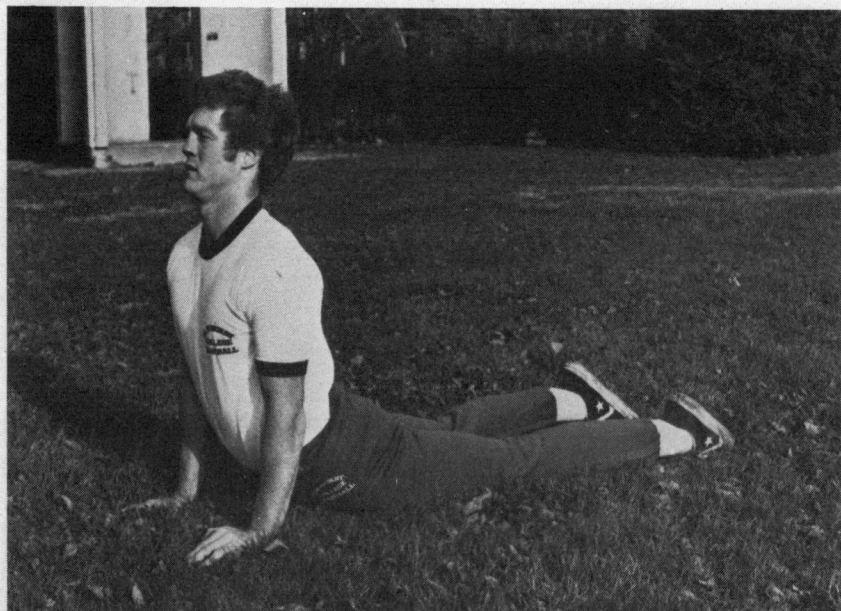

This is the Cobra. If your spine starts to hurt on the first trials, don't go any further, but aim for eventually holding the position for a count of 10 breaths.

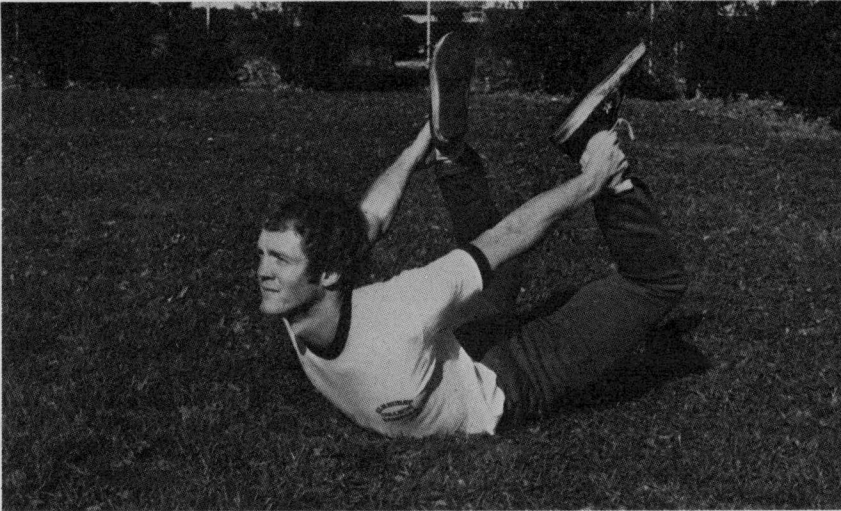

Inorder to successfully do the Bow, you must have flexibility in your abdominal, upper and lower back and leg muscles.

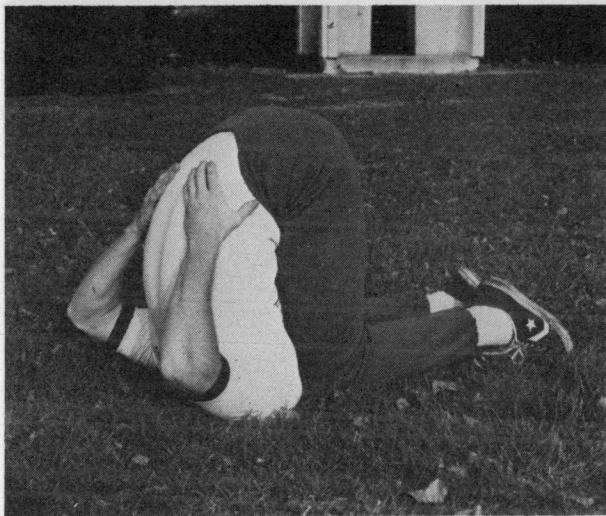

The final position of the Plough called Knee-To-Ear is not recommended for beginners.

and exhalation. Ten of these bellows breaths, done at your best speed, is about right for the beginner.

There's no reason why you can't do Yoga breathing while you're standing or walking. You'll find that you can walk at a stiffer pace and a longer distance without tiring.

People working in offices can do Yoga breathing for about 2 minutes when mid-afternoon letdown hits them. They will find that the breathing will not only get rid of the tired feeling but will make them more alert.

The sooner you learn to make a practice of Yoga breathing, the more beneficial it will become.

YOGA AND RELAXATION

Yoga exercises call for complete relaxation before and after each Yoga session, and relaxing isn't easy for most people in our hectic world. It's something we have to learn, and most of us don't learn the art of relaxation because in trying to relax we force tensions to work on the body. An important exercise in Yoga is one in which the human body is taught to relax.

You lie flat on the floor on your back in much the same position as that from which you start doing straight leg situps, except that the feet are slightly apart and the hands are at the sides, palms up with fingers bent slightly in what should be their most natural position. If any part of the body is uncomfortable, it's advisable to do the exercise on a spread-out bath or beach towel. If the neck feels uncomfortable, you can start by putting a folded towel under it at a position that makes it comfortable.

The exercise is one of *progressive* relaxation, starting with the toes, one at a time. After you've concentrated on relaxing the toes, you relax the ankles one at a time, then the knees, one at a time, and then the hips.

Once that's accomplished, you concentrate on relaxing the abdomen and its muscles, all the way around from the belly button to the back.

Then you relax the neck, which is usually one of the tensest parts of the body, since the head it supports usually weighs close to 40 pounds. You start by relaxing the neck, the lower jaw and then the face. You think of relaxing every muscle in the face, feeling the frown lines fade away.

Then you relax the eyes by closing the eyelids

softly, without pressure. You even concentrate then on relaxing the scalp.

Then you relax the fingers one at a time in turn, including the thumbs. You move from there progressively to the hands, the wrists and the arms up to the shoulders. Then you relax the shoulders all the way around from front to back, relaxing the face again as you do it.

Don't expect to reach complete relaxation on your first trial. You may find that after relaxing your legs, when you move up to the abdomen, your legs become tense again. Because you're concentrating, properly so, your facial muscles will tighten up.

For that reason, it's advisable to go through the complete relaxation routine twice at every session when you're starting to practice Yoga exercise. Before long, you'll be able to relax as you never could before.

While you're doing the relaxation exercise from the supine position, your breathing should be helping. Since you're relaxed and physically inactive, you don't require much oxygen so your breathing will be gentle. Slow the speed of your breathing while maintaining the ratio of one-to-two between inhalation and exhalation.

You'll find that if you also practice the relaxation exercise after going to bed, it will help you to go to sleep, even if you've been troubled with insomnia.

Yoga experts can control their internal organs, even regulating the pulse beat. It's impractical for us to attempt advancement that pronounced, but we should get well acquainted with our bodies.

Start by thinking about your skin. As in the relaxation routine, start with the feet, feeling the hard skin on the soles and the closeness of the skin between the toes. Think about your skin progressively, in the same order as was followed in the relaxation routine.

Then think progressively about the muscles beneath the skin, starting again with the toes. Feel every muscle in action, all the way up to and including the head. Feel your facial muscles move. Smile broadly; then frown. At the outset, do the body recognition exercise routine every day for a few minutes.

What you've been doing so far is really preparation for the Hatha Yoga exercise routine. As a routine, Yoga can improve flexibility, muscle

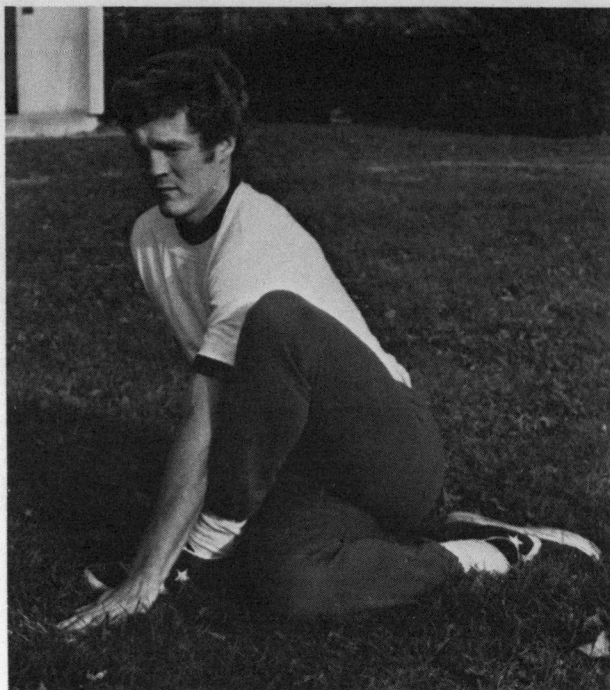

The Half Spinal Twist is a great exercise for trunk, lower and upper back and arm muscles. At first your waist and legs may feel tight but with practice you will have no trouble at all.

strength and body tone. If you choose to use a Yoga routine apart from a total fitness program, there's the matter of when to do it. It should never be until 3 hours after a meal or 2 hours after a snack. You should always wait until emptying the bladder after drinking. Women who are plagued with severe menstrual pains should skip practice during the first few days of a period.

Immediately after getting up in the morning is probably the best time to do a routine, having breakfast afterward and then going to work. Just prior to going to bed at night would be the second best time. Many housewives prefer late afternoon.

Yoga exercises should not be done while wearing clothing that restricts movement. Men usually prefer wearing nothing but a pair of shorts without a restrictive belt. Most women prefer leotards.

Prior to performing a routine of Yoga exercises, it's advisable to start with a few warm-up exercises which will make the muscles more limber. Then choose a series of Yoga exercises for each joint in the body.

Neck Roll: Let the head fall forward and down,

Complete Relaxation

1. Lie on a flat surface on your back in the pose of relaxation. Let your eyes be closed and maintain awareness.

2. Tense and relax the limbs in the following order: right leg, left leg, right arm, left arm.

3. Tense the buttocks and anal muscle. Then relax.

4. Take a deep breath into the abdomen only, hold the breath, tense the abdominal muscles, then let the air out through an open mouth.

5. Do the same with the chest only.

6. Raise just the shoulders off the floor, tense them, and relax.

7. Gently roll the head from side to side, then center it.

8. Tense up your facial muscles, then relax.

9. Without moving any part of your body, bring your awareness over all the parts once again, checking to make sure that all the tension has left in the following order: the feet; the legs; the back and spine; the abdomen; chest; fingers, hands, arms and shoulders; face and head.

10. Be aware only of your breath, and without trying to control the breathing, watch the breath as it flows freely and easily in and out of the body.

11. Bring your awareness to your mind, and watch the thoughts as they enter and leave your mind. Without trying to control or stop any of them, be aware of the thoughts.

12. The thoughts are like ripples in a pond. As they fade out, the mind becomes still. Be aware of the stillness, the silence and peace which is present. Feel at one with this peace.

13. When you are ready, bring the awareness back to your body, and first be aware of the top of your head. Feel energy pouring into the body through the top of your head, filling the head and face. Feel your face aglow with energy.

14. Feel the energy come into your neck and shoulders; arms, hands, and fingers; chest; back and abdomen; legs, feet and toes. Feel the entire body filled with energy and refreshed.

15. To awaken completely, gently move your head and limbs. Then stretch like a cat waking up, sit up, and breathe deeply.

HINTS: Practice the Complete Relaxation after doing the Yoga postures or *asanas.* Or practice it anytime to attain a state of relaxation deeper than in sleep. Practice it before going to sleep, for better sleep. You will soon require less sleep and have more energy in the day.

Robert C. Fellows

the chin almost touching the upper chest. Inhale and, as you do so, lift the head while turning it as far to the right as you can get it. Hold the position for a count of five, exhale, turn the head forward again and repeat the exercise, turning the head to the left as far as it will go this time. After bringing it back to the front, again force the head to drop back as far as possible. From that position, again lower the chin to the upper chest. Next after inhaling, roll your neck around in a circle, first clockwise and then counterclockwise, exhaling each time the chin comes to rest on the upper chest. Repeat this exercise four or five times in a session, or until neck tension is stopped.

Back/Buttocks Roll: Lying on your back, you raise your knees as far up and back as possible, grasping the toes in your hands. Then you rock back and forth, developing a steady rhythm.

Swinger: Sitting on the floor, legs straight out in front and held together, hands at sides, lift both feet 7 or 8 inches up from the floor and swing them together to the right side while inhaling. Then swing the legs as high as you can, holding them for a count of five while you exhale. Return to the starting position and do the exercise to the opposite side. Repeat the exercise three times to each side.

YOGA AND WEIGHT REGULATION

Yoga has some interesting approaches to the weight problem. We can't vouch for their efficiency because we haven't tried them, but we have noticed that most people who have gotten into Hatha Yoga exercise and have stayed with it have trim bodies.

The first thing Yoga says about weight regulation is that different human bodies have different metabolism responses. So you start out by determining the weight at which you perform best and feel best—not the weight recommended for your age and height in a chart. A heavily-boned, stocky person shouldn't try to emulate a fashion model. The Yoga answer is to proportion your weight over your body so that it's right for you.

Yoga disapproves of high protein diets and appetite depressants. It frowns on heavy use of cigarettes and coffee to dull the appetite, along with the synthetic liquids that are substituted for food. It teaches that weight reduction through the various fads and "trick" diets doesn't last. It believes that if you think seriously about what you eat, your native instinct will tell you what you should have and what you shouldn't.

Here are a few of its guidelines:

1. Never stuff yourself. Make your meals light but nourishing.

2. Try to get as much "natural" food as possible into your diet. Try to eat fruits raw or lightly baked, with the same thing applying to vegetables. For protein, cottage cheese and legumes are better than poultry, meat and fish.

3. Coffee, intoxicants and refined sugar should be regarded as stimulants to be avoided.

4. Confine a meal to as few different types of food as possible.

5. Once a week, on a day when you can get plenty of rest, confine your intake to nothing but water.

As you consider your whole being while progressing in Yoga, you'll find that some meals make you dull and listless, while others seem to give you energy flow. Overeating is responsible for a great many problems and is certainly a major cause of obesity.

While Yoga is not specifically designed to take off weight, it aims at a well-proportioned body, and some of the exercises not only limber and tone up specific parts of the body but slenderize them in the process.

Before you begin the Yoga practice of fasting one day a week, with no intake except water, you should certainly consult a physician. It may be that you have some medical problem which would be aggravated by the fast.

YOGA AND ARTHRITIS

Arthritis, an excruciatingly painful inflammation of the joints, has become a national problem that continues to grow. Where it once affected only the elderly, it's now crippling middle-aged and even young people. The sole effects of most drugs prescribed for arthritis sufferers is simply to temporarily lessen the pain without doing a thing to stop the cause. Heat treatments and massage have only a temporary effect.

Elimination of foods that cause deposits in the joints can certainly be helpful, but the most effective thing seems to be self-exercise. A serious problem here is getting the sufferer to exercise, because he or she finds exercise painful.

Yoga's slow, graceful, rhythmic movements, done only to the point of mild temporary discomfort but never to the point of actual pain, may be the answer. The variety of stretches and pulls are intended to reach deep into the joints and break loose the deposits.

The arthritis victim should start with only a few mild exercises, holding the positions for as little as 4 or 5 seconds. With the same overloading principle that's been successful in other exercise programs, the sufferer should try to first move another inch without undue pain and hold the position for another second or two. Regular daily Yoga exercise may well be able to prevent the occurrence of arthritis in those who don't yet have it and arrest its progress in those who do suffer from it.

Anyone with severe arthritis should, of course, get a physician to okay.

YOGA AND GLANDULAR PROBLEMS

Certain Yoga exercises have highly salutary effects on the various glands in the human body, glands which may be malfunctioning. Before trying any of the Yoga corrective measures, you should see a physician and have him determine whether the gland is simply sluggish from lack of exercise or is seriously malfunctioning in a way that could cause serious trouble. Yoga practitioners say that once a malfunctioning gland is corrected with drugs, Yoga exercises for the gland will keep it stimulated and healthy.

YOGA AND FLEXIBILITY FITNESS

Used individually, Yoga exercises are excellent for building flexibility fitness. Where calisthenics require considerable movement with one part of the body actively moving to stretch a muscle, Yoga uses static stretching in which you move into position slowly and hold or sustain that position to stretch a muscle. Both methods bring about substantial gains in flexibility; however, there are three advantages to the Yoga method.

1. *There is less probability of overextending the tissues and muscles involved.* Yoga exercises are meant to be executed with slow and controlled movements. Moving slowly is important because you are aware of your body and you can feel when you've stretched a muscle far enough—at which point you stop. In exercises requiring motion for stretching, on the other hand, you know when you've stretched too far only when it's too late and you've pulled a muscle or ligament. Thus there is a greater chance of incurring a muscle injury when doing motion stretch exercises than when doing Yoga stretch exercises.

2. *Energy requirements are less.* Since Yoga exercises are performed with slow, controlled movements, the energy expended to execute the exercises is much less than for calisthenics.

3. *Static stretching relieves muscle soreness where motion stretching sometimes causes it.* Static stretching of muscles prevents sudden reflexive contraction of muscles and therefore reduces muscle soreness.

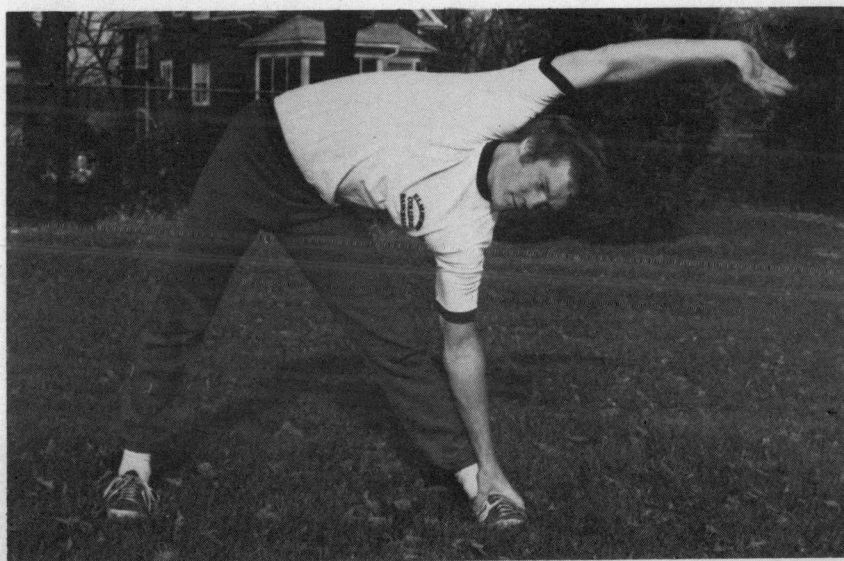

Graceful, smooth movements are the key to Yoga exercises. Remember to stretch only as far as is comfortable. This final position of the Triangle may require quite a few practice sessions before it can be mastered.

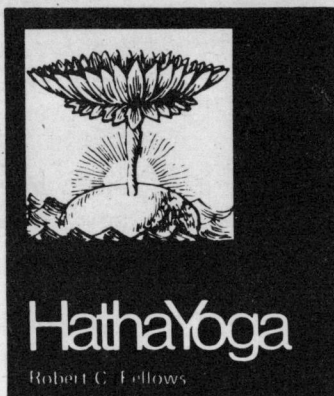

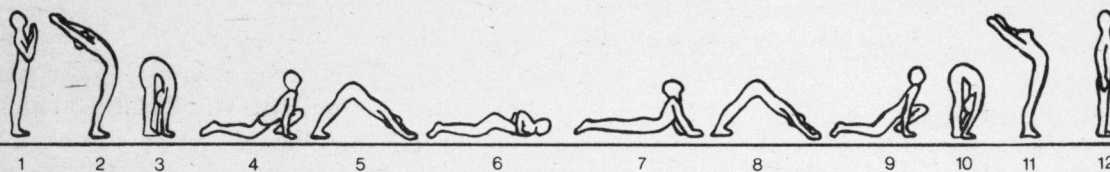

HathaYoga

Robert C. Fellows

Sun Salutation

1 2 3 4 5 6 7 8 9 10 11 12

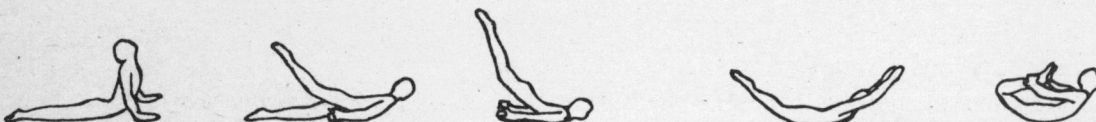

Cobra   Half-Locust   Locust   Boat   Bow

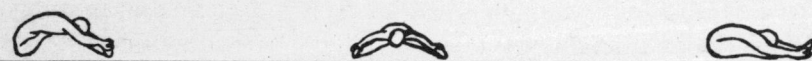

Head-to-Knee   Hand-to-Foot   Back Stretch

Shoulder Stand   Half Plough   Plough   Knee-to-Ear

Fish   Half Spinal Twist   Triangle   Lotus

Robert C. Fellows

PHYSICAL HEALTH AND YOGA

Robert C. Fellows

Yoga is a spiritual technique and system of philosophy, but it is also the oldest and most thoroughly tested form of physical and mental exercise known to humanity. There is clear evidence that Hindus practiced Yoga over 4,000 years ago.

Hatha Yoga is the form of Yoga which has developed a system of physical exercise that integrates the mind and emotions with the body. The goal is to develop these three aspects of the personality simultaneously and harmoniously through the discipline of Yoga.

This self-development is accomplished by means of physical postures (asanas), breathing exercises (pranayamas), diet, and techniques of relaxation, concentration, and meditation. Hatha Yoga is a gentle technique which emphasizes that there must be no strain in the physical practice, but this emphasis is foreign to many American students. Therefore, it is necessary to systematically discuss the physical health benefits of Hatha Yoga to show how it works.

Primarily, the benefits of a regular practice of physical postures (asanas) and breathing exercises (pranayamas) are an improvement in general health, an increased ability to control tension, and increased awareness.

The Muscular System. By practicing a varied series of postures, the student tones many muscles which would not otherwise be used in work or sports. By stretching the muscles and articulations without straining them, they become more flexible. The stretching of many muscles reduces the basal tension of the muscles. The postures bring a physical harmony to the body by reducing useless antagonistic muscle contractions. One learns to sit, stand, and lie down in more relaxed positions.

It is important that many of the poses strengthen the abdominal muscles and diaphragm, increasing the vital capacity as well as the strength and coordination of the entire body. Students who dance, sing, practice body building or the martial arts understand the importance of a strong, controlled abdomen. By concentrating on the muscles that are being stretched and contracted in each posture, one increases awareness of the muscle system and learns to control isolated muscles and muscles which often fall into disuse. After long practice, this awareness can expand to increased awareness of internal organs, with a corresponding increase in control over bodily functions.

The Spine. In the postures, the spine is put through tractions, stretchings, and torsions of varying degrees. This makes the spine more flexible and prevents or corrects wrong attitudes of the spine in normal standing, sitting, and lying down positions. The stretching of the ligaments of the spine in all directions also gives greater freedom to the nerves and small blood vessels which pass from the body into the spine. One of the most common ailments among Americans is lower back pain; the Yoga poses keep the back and spine in a supple condition.

The Respiratory System. The strengthening of the diaphragm by means of breathing exercises increases the vital capacity. The chest is expanded and the lungs are strengthened. There is greater control in breathing so that with less effort the practitioner obtains more air with each breath. The techniques of deep breathing which are taught in Yoga are the basis for breathing techniques which are taught in natural childbirth methods and to patients with respiratory diseases.

The Circulatory System. Through practicing the poses, the student increases the circulation to all parts of the body and can learn to control the heart rate and the flow of blood to specific parts of the body. By placing the body in an inverted position, such as in the head stand or shoulder stand, the blood is allowed to flow more freely to the upper parts of the body, benefiting the throat and head. The inverted poses must, however, be practiced with caution or not at all by persons with very high or very low blood pressure. Expert advice is necessary in such cases.

By sitting in a cross-legged position, the flow of blood is inhibited to the legs which causes an increased flow of blood to the visceral organs, stimulating them. By strengthening and learning to use the diaphragm, the venous circulation is improved.

The Endocrine System. The endocrine glands are developed primarily by practicing poses which cause accelerated circulation to the glands, stimulating their functions. The thyroid gland is stimulated and developed by practicing the shoulder stand pose in which the heart is placed directly above the gland. Since this gland controls the metabolism of the entire body, the shoulder stand is beneficial to all parts of the body. The parathyroids, pineal, pituitary and adrenals are also benefited by an increase in blood supply brought by various poses.

The Nervous System. The nerves are calmed by the regular practice of postures and breathing exercises. The nerves and sensory organs also become more acute. The brain cells are developed by an increase in blood supply brought by the inverted poses. The balancing poses improve the balance and equilibrium.

Yoga Exercises

Neck Roll (neck muscles)

1. Sit erect in cross-legged posture on the floor with eyes closed and hands on knees.
2. Bend head slowly forward and rest chin on chest. Hold for count of 10.
3. Very slowly roll head to extreme right. Hold for count of 10.
4. Very slowly roll head to extreme backward position. Hold for count of 10.
5. Very slowly roll head to extreme left. Hold for count of 10.
6. Return to starting positon.

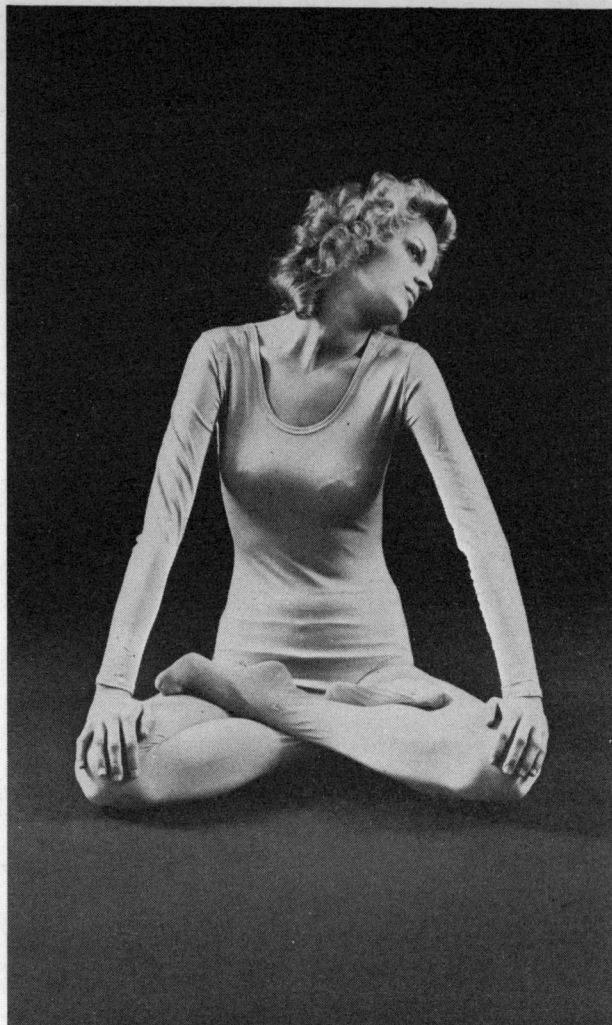

5

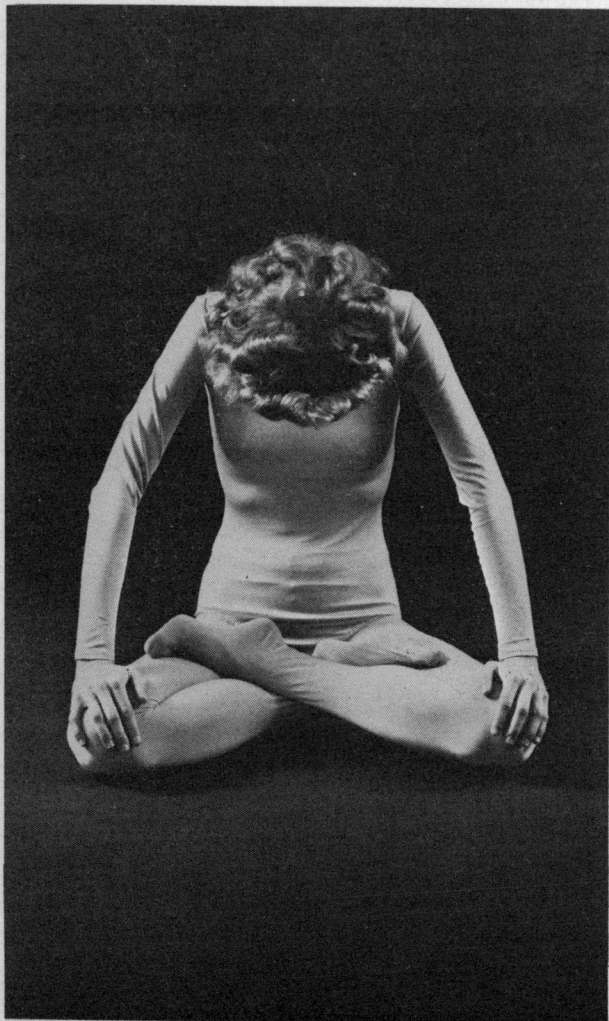

2

Shoulder Stand (upper and lower back and leg muscles)

1. Lie face up on the floor with legs together and palms of hands on floor.
2. Tense abdominal and leg muscles.
3. Slowly raise legs to 45-degree angle to floor keeping knees straight and feet together.
4. Gently swing legs back with enough momentum for hips to leave the floor. Hold hips up by putting elbows on floor and bracing hands against hips.
5. Straighten legs, press chin against chest and hold for as long as possible.
6. To return to starting position, bend knees and lower them toward head. Place hands on floor.
7. Slowly lower body with knees bent.
8. When hips touch floor, straighten legs to 90-degree angle to floor.
9. Slowly lower legs to floor.

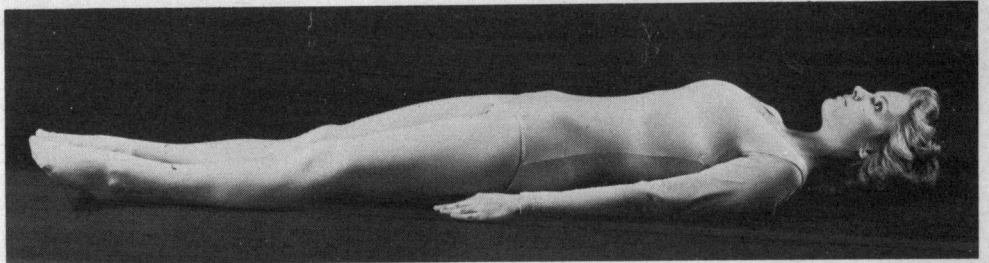

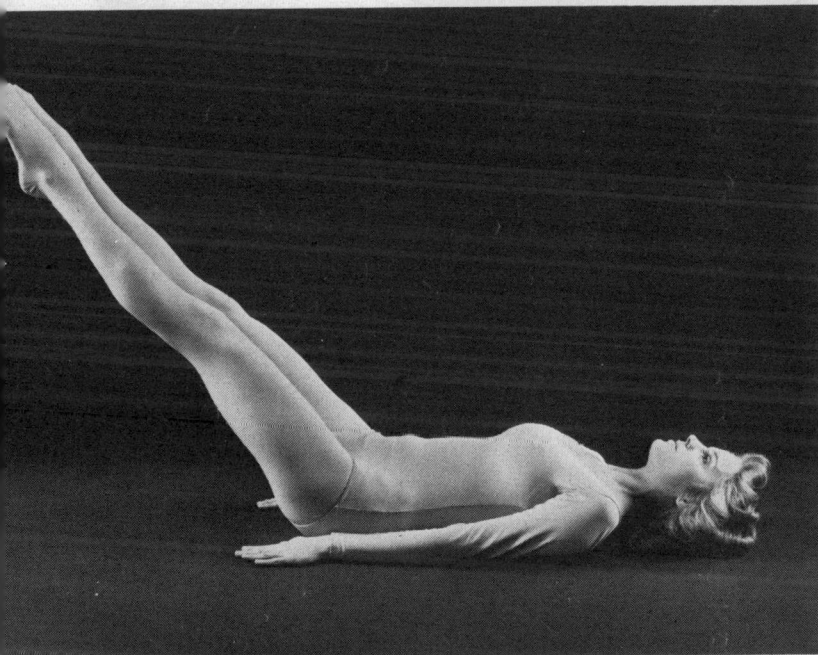

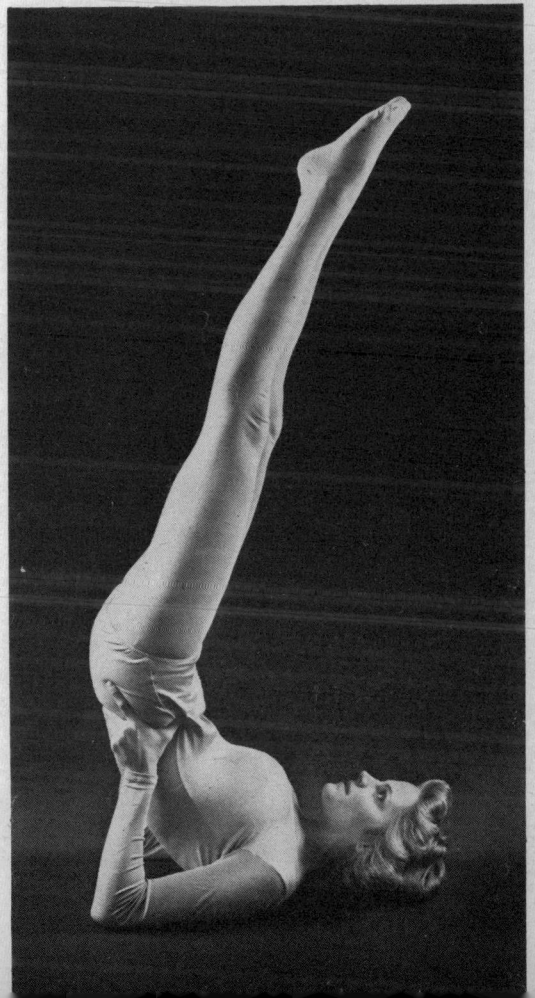

The Plough (upper and lower back and leg muscles)

1. Lie face up on the floor with legs together and palms of hands on floor.
2. Tense abdominal and leg muscles.
3. Slowly raise legs to 45-degree angle to floor keeping knees straight and feet together.
4. Gently swing legs back with enough momentum for hips to leave the floor, bringing legs over your head until they are parallel to floor.
5. For completed first position of the Plough,

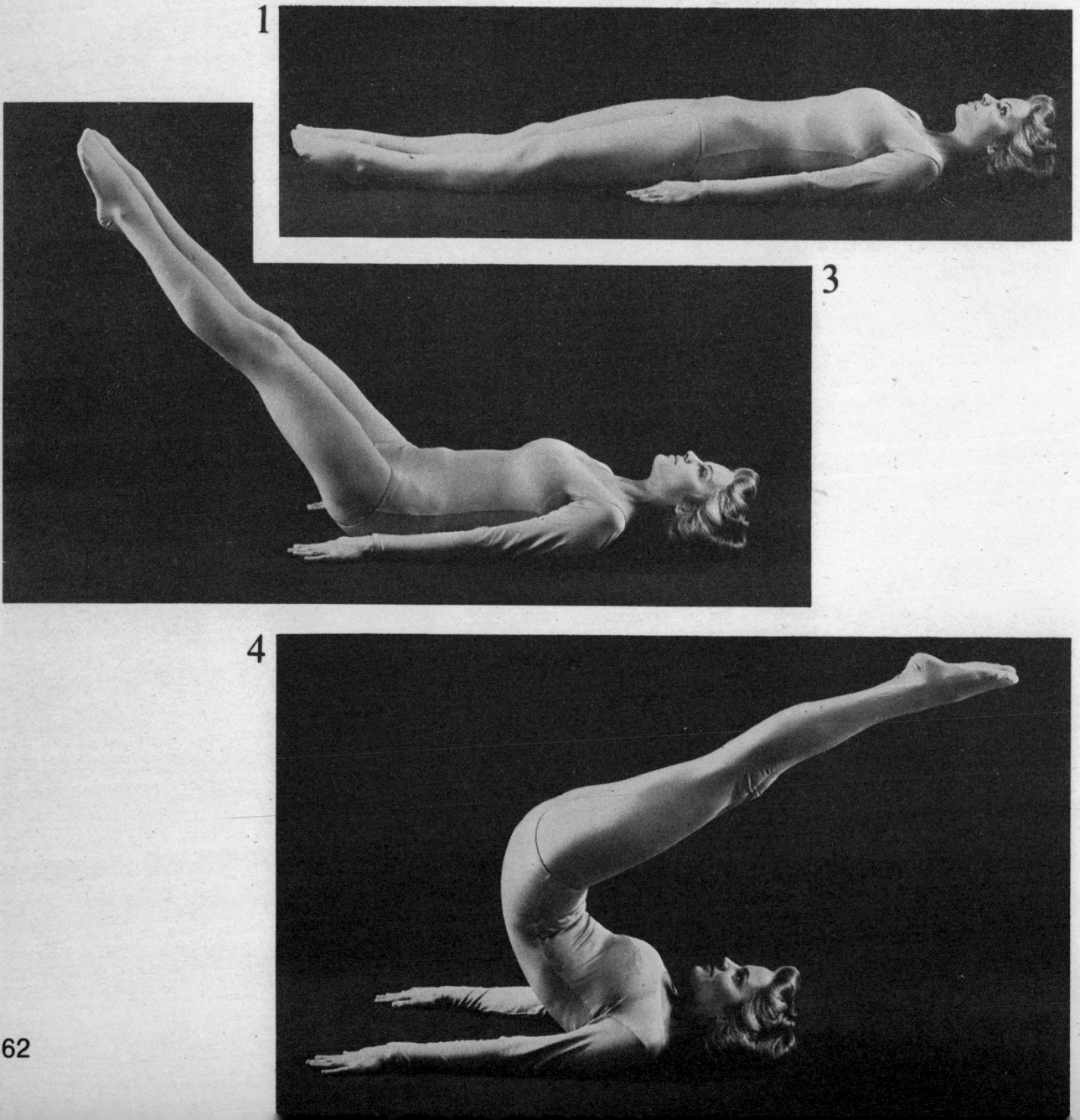

you slowly lower your legs, stretching them as far behind you as possible with toes touching the floor. Hold for count of 10. (The final position, which we don't recommend for the novice, is the Knee-To-Ear position. See chart on page 58.)

6. To return to starting position, raise legs to parallel position with floor and then bend knees in toward the chest.

7. When hips touch floor, legs should be in 90-degree angle to floor. Slowly lower legs to floor.

5

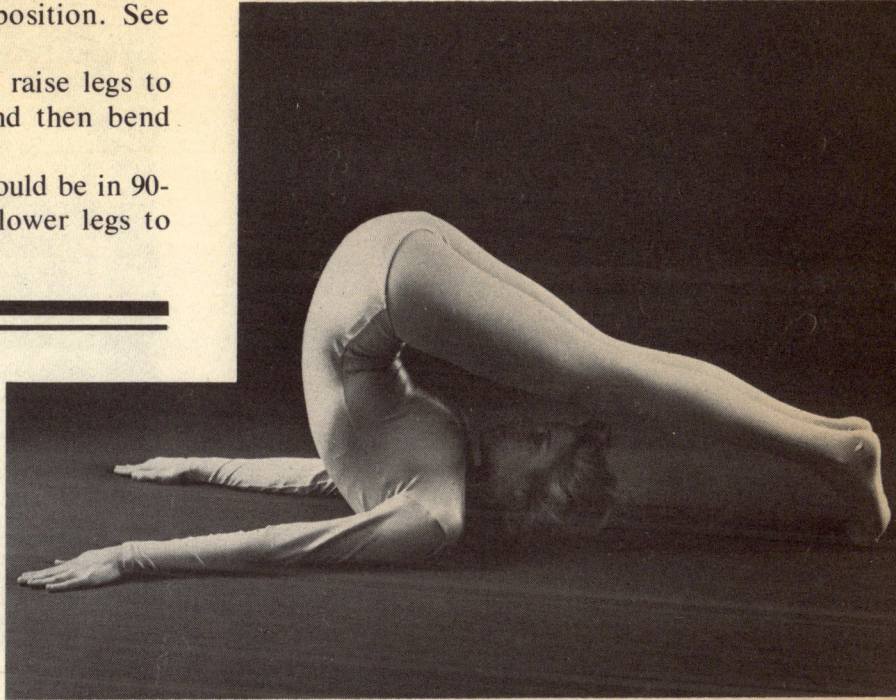

6

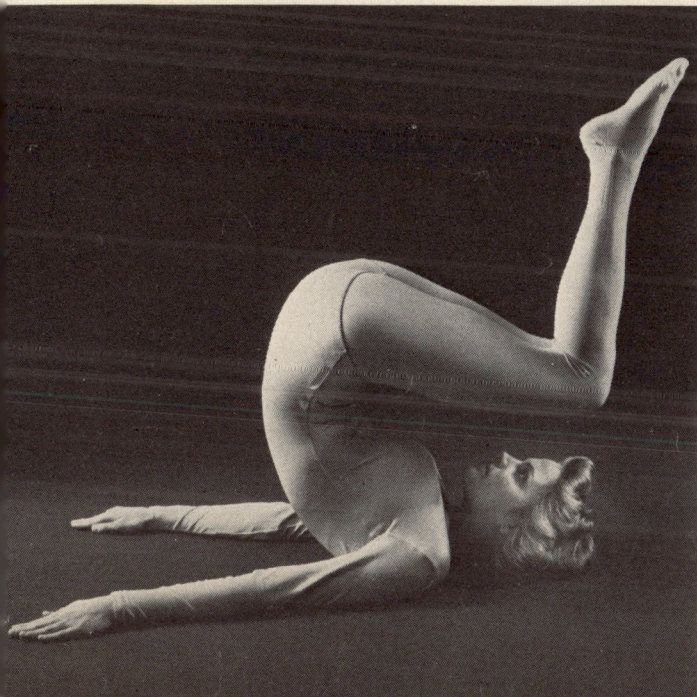

7

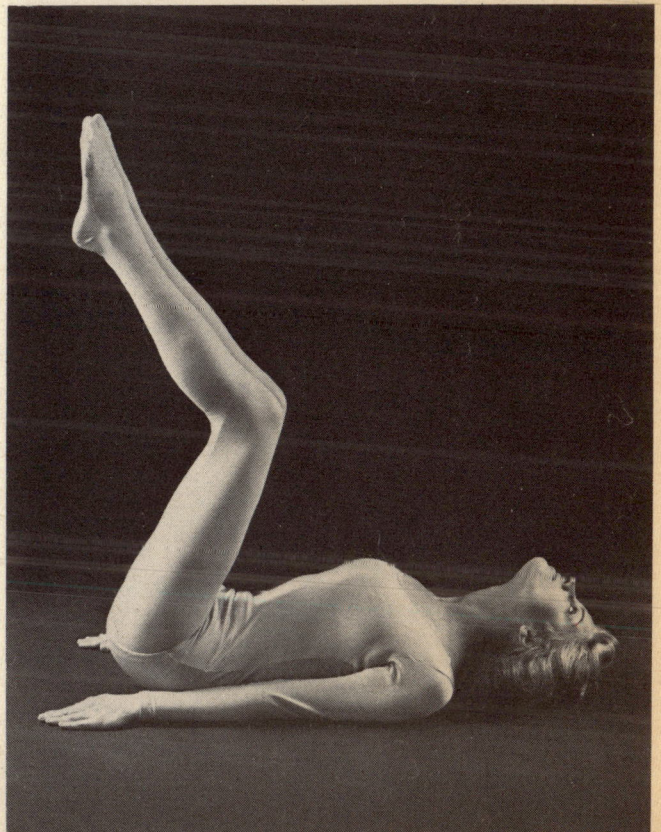

Triangle (trunk, arm and neck muscles)

1. Stand erect with feet 2 feet apart, arms held outstretched at shoulder level, palms downward.
2. Bend slowly to the right, keeping arms outstretched.
3. With right hand, firmly grasp right knee and bring left arm overhead as far as possible, keeping elbow straight. Hold for count of 10.
4. Slowly return to starting position.
5. Repeat to the left side and hold for count of 10.

Note: As you increase your flexibility fitness, grasp lower and lower on the leg until you can comfortably grasp your ankle and hold for a count of 10. See picture below.

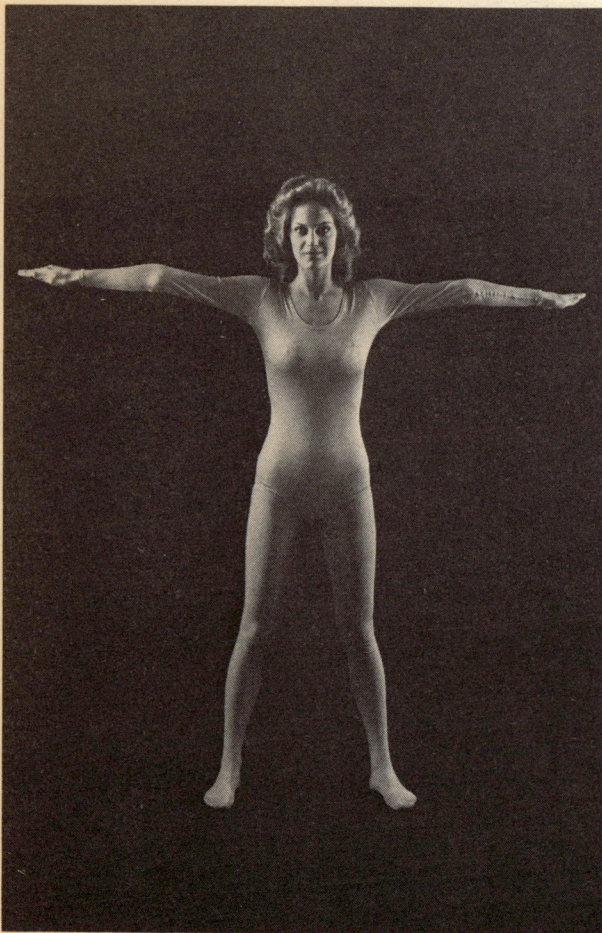

1

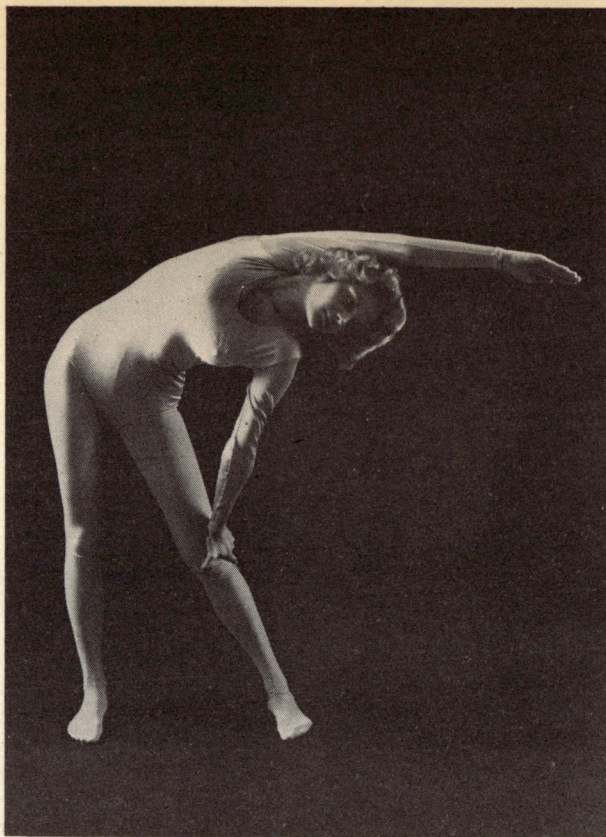

3

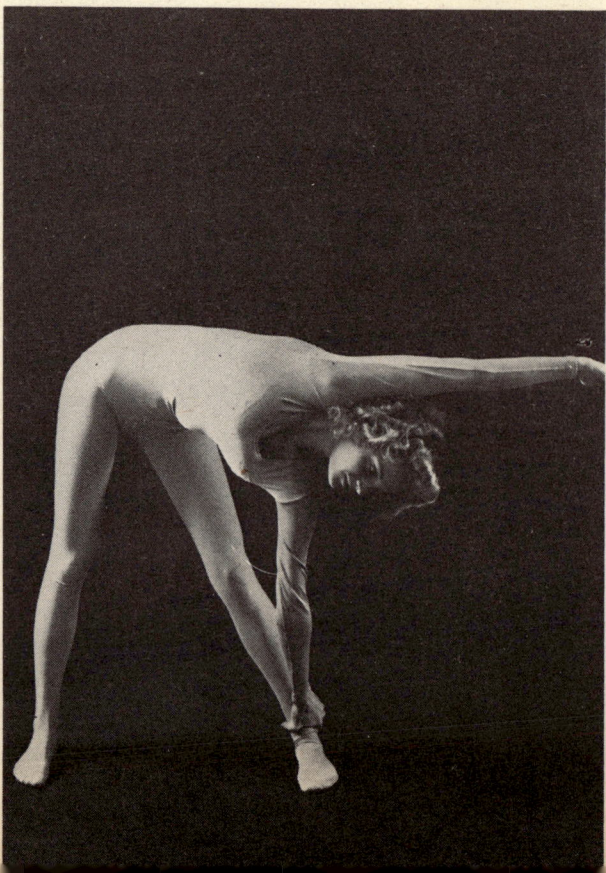

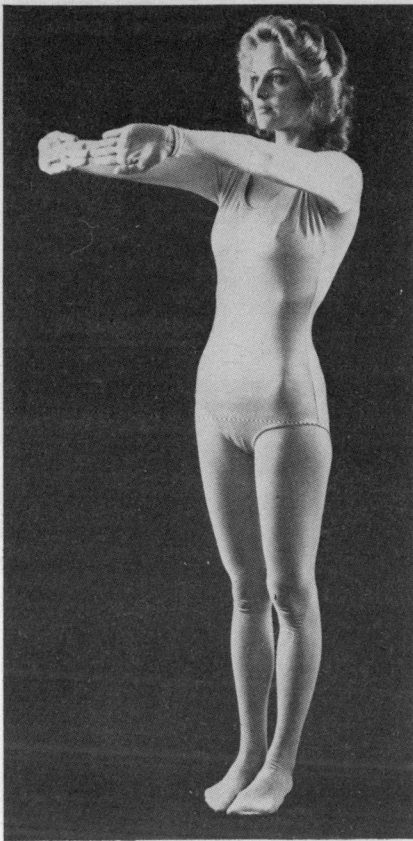

Chest Stretch (arm, pectoral, upper and lower back muscles)

1. Stand erect, feel together, arms at sides.
2. Slowly bend elbows and bring hands up in front of chest, palms facing outward.
3. Straighten arms slowly, keeping them at chest level.
4. Move arms slowly behind you, keeping them at shoulder level.
5. Lower arms slightly so that the fingers can be interlaced.
6. Bend backward slowly, letting head drop back and keeping arms high. Hold for count of 10.
7. Bend forward slowly, head forward, arms kept up high. Hold for count of 20.
8. Return to upright position and unclasp hands.

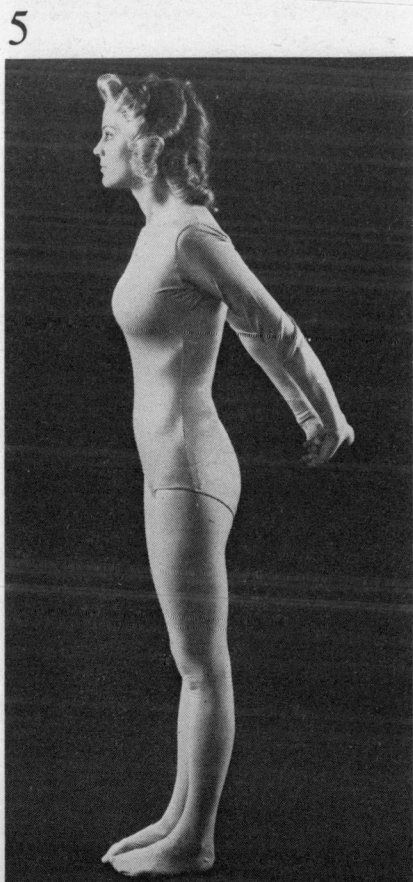

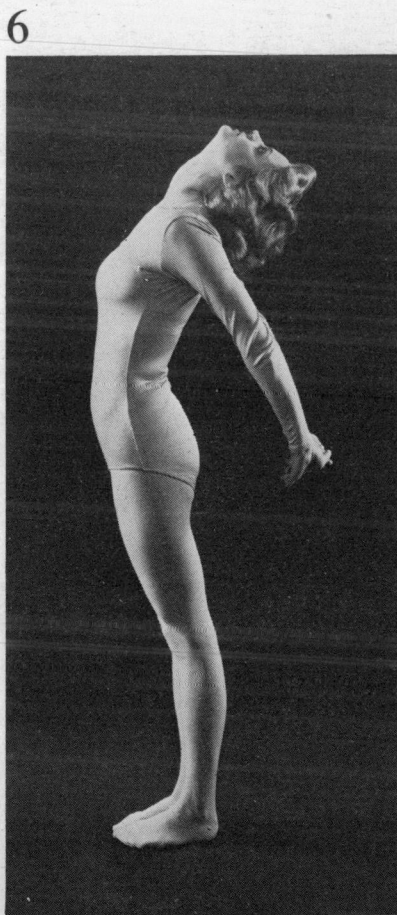

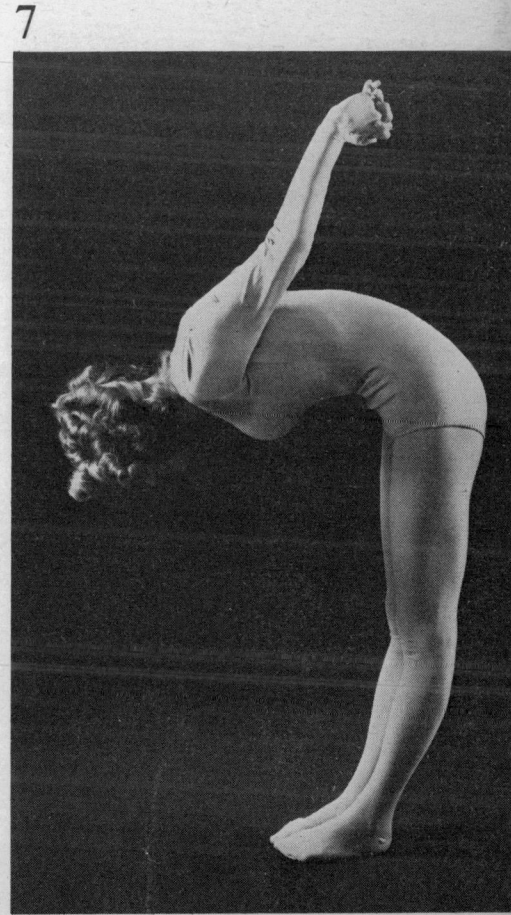

Arched Back Bend (upper back, pectoral, neck muscles)

1. Sit on floor, legs together and straight in front of you.
2. Slowly lean back and to the right to place right elbow on the floor.
3. Slowly lean to the left to place left elbow on floor.
4. Push chest forward slowly, forming a hollow at small of back and let head fall back to touch the floor. Hold for count of 15.
5. Now remove elbows from floor and place hands on thighs. Hold for count of 10.
6. To return to starting position, place elbows on floor, straighten head and slowly pull yourself back into sitting position.

3
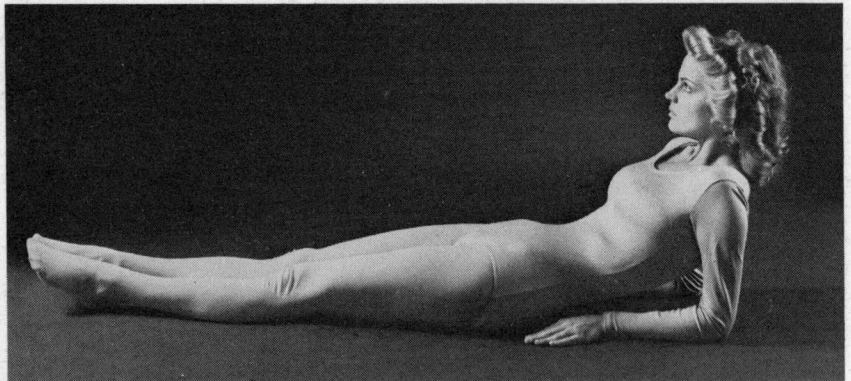

4
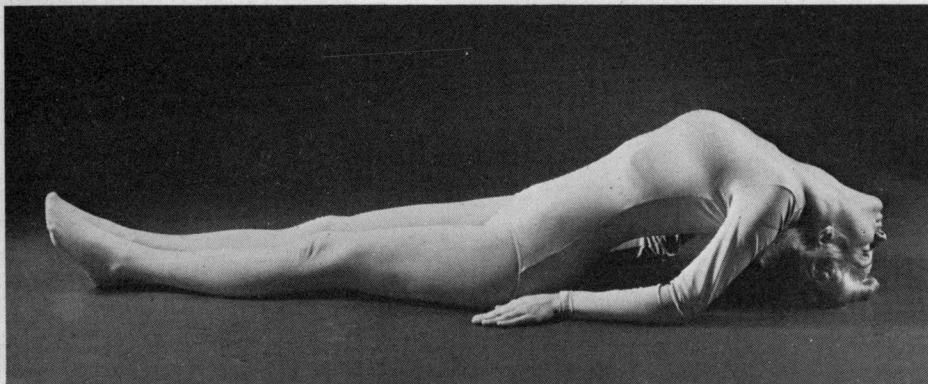

5
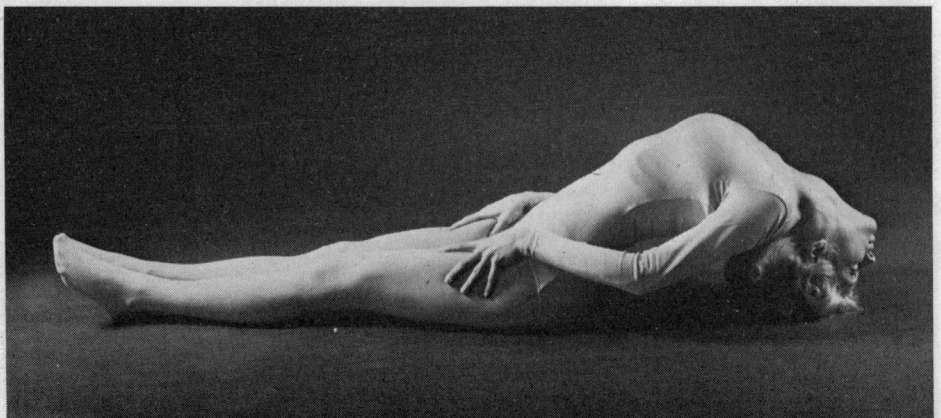

Forward Back Bend (lower back and hamstring muscles)

1. Lie face up on the floor with feet together, toes pointed, and arms extended back behind head.
2. Slowly raise arms to 90-degree angle to floor. Then move arms down and forward while lifting your head.
3. Slowly continue forward movement, raising first shoulders, then back, off the floor until in sitting position.
4. Lowering hands to knees, slide hands forward as far as possible while keeping knees straight. Lower head as far as possible and hold for count of 10. (The final position of this exercise is to slide hands down legs, finally grasping feet with head touching knees.)
5. To return to starting position, reverse procedure, bringing hands to shoulder level, slowly lowering back to floor, and then bringing hands to extended position behind head.

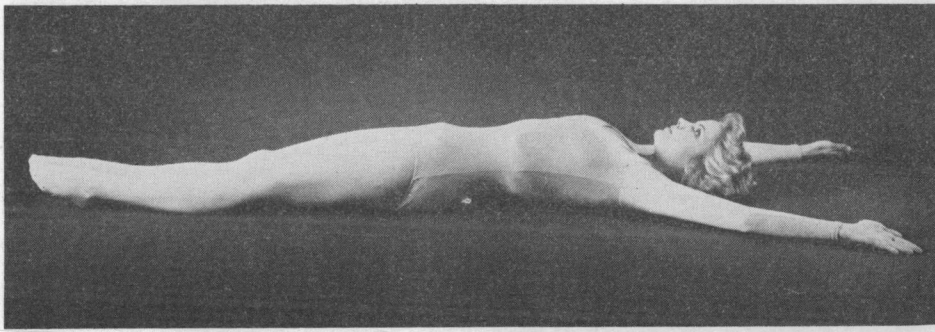

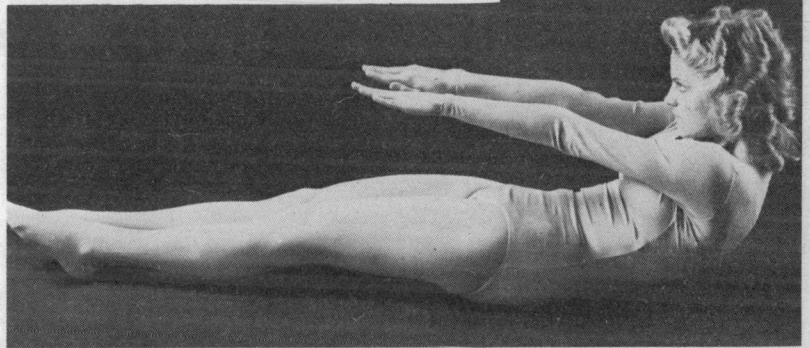

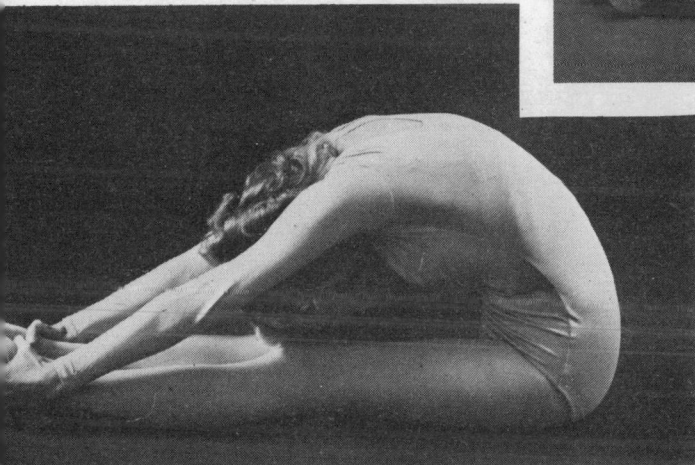

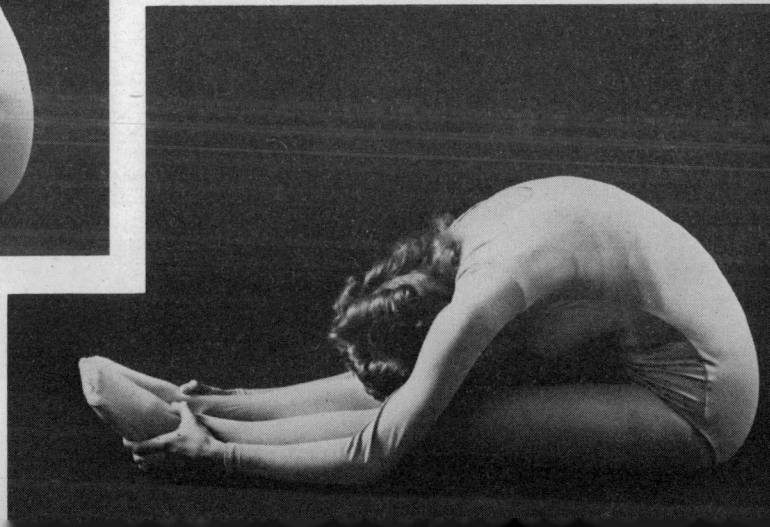

Hand-To-Foot (leg and lower back muscles)

1. Sit on floor, legs extended out to sides as far as possible, feet pointed upward. Hands on thighs.
2. Slowly slide hands along legs, bending forward.
3. Slide hands as far as possible, keeping knees straight.
4. Bend head forward, trying to touch floor with head and hold for count of 10. (The final position of this exercise is with hands grasping ankles and head touching floor.)

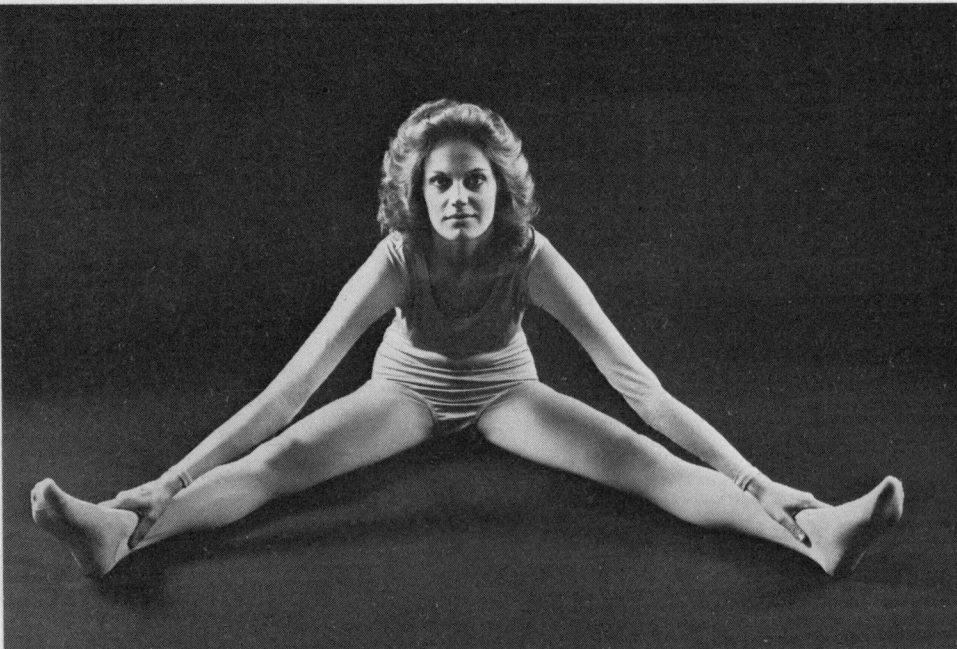

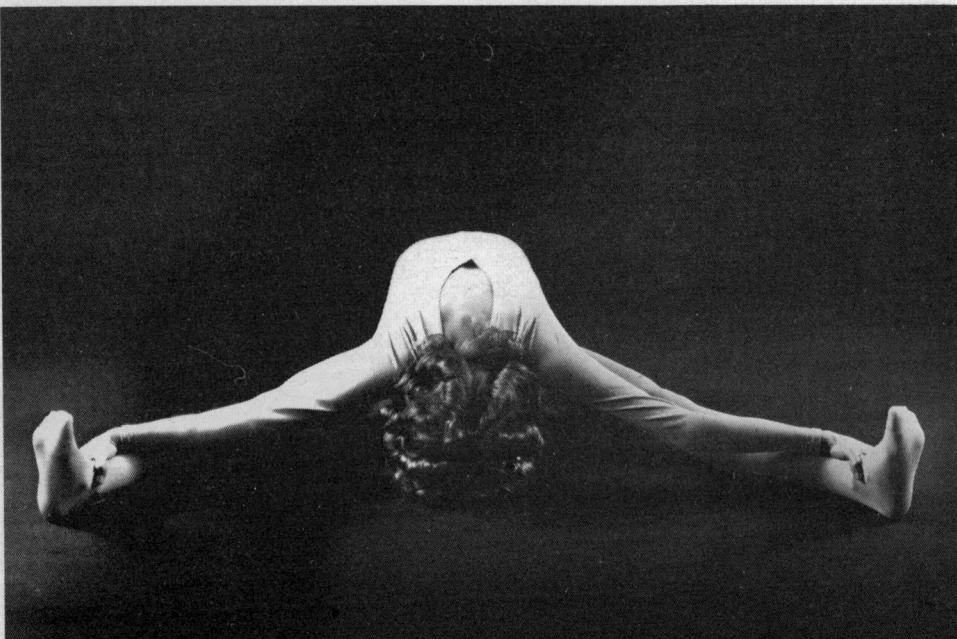

The Bow (abdominal, trunk, pectoral, leg and arm muscles)

1. Lie face down on floor, with head resting on chin, legs together, hands at sides.
2. Bend knees bringing feet toward the body.
3. When feet are as close to the body as possible, reach back with your hands, keeping elbows straight and try to grasp feet.
4. Raise your head and gently push the feet back toward the floor, pulling your shoulders back.
5. Pull head backward and up. Hold for a count of 5.
6. To return to starting position, bring feet toward body, letting your body sink slowly until chin is resting on floor.
7. Slowly release grasp on feet and lower legs to floor slowly.

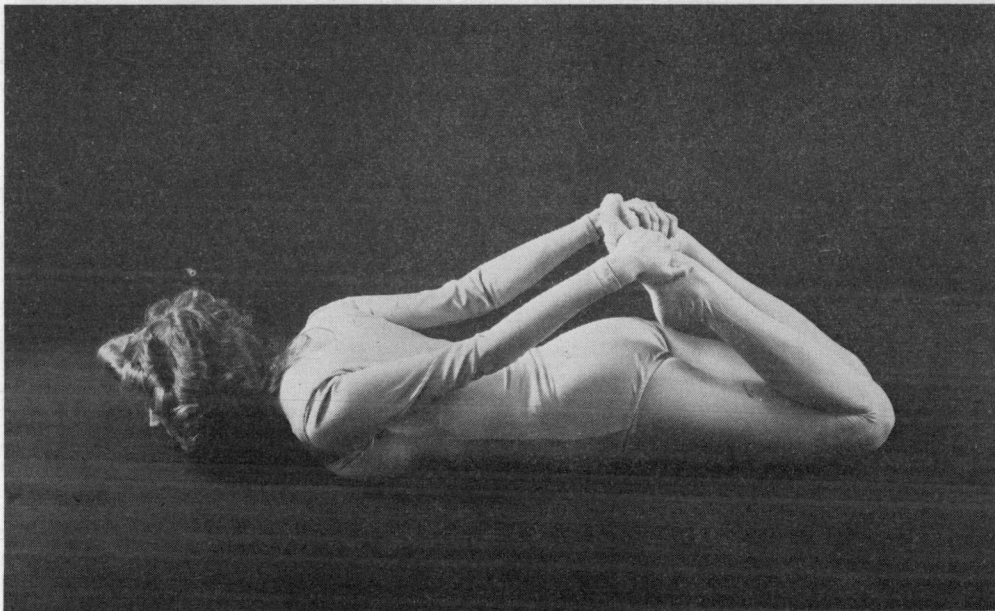

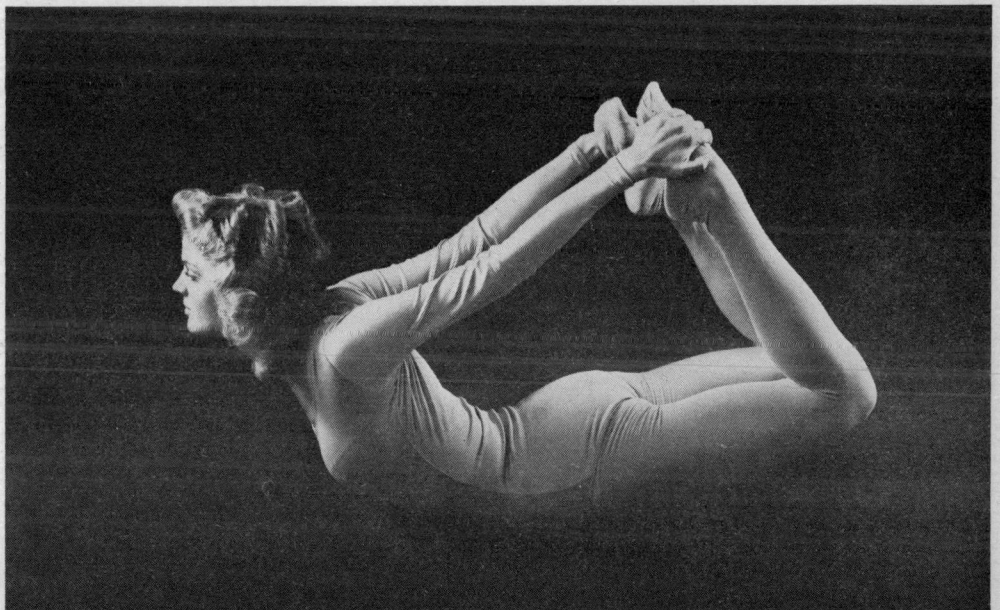

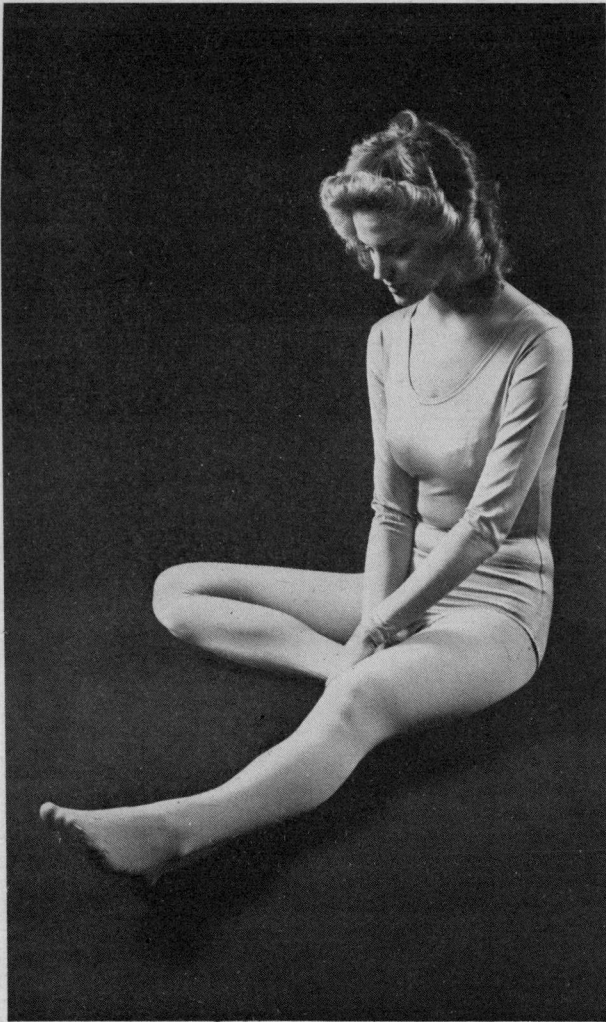

2

Half Spinal Twist (trunk, lower and upper back and arm muscles)

1. Sit on floor, legs extended straight outward.
2. Place sole of right foot against inside of left thigh.
3. Firmly grasp left ankle and slowly raise left

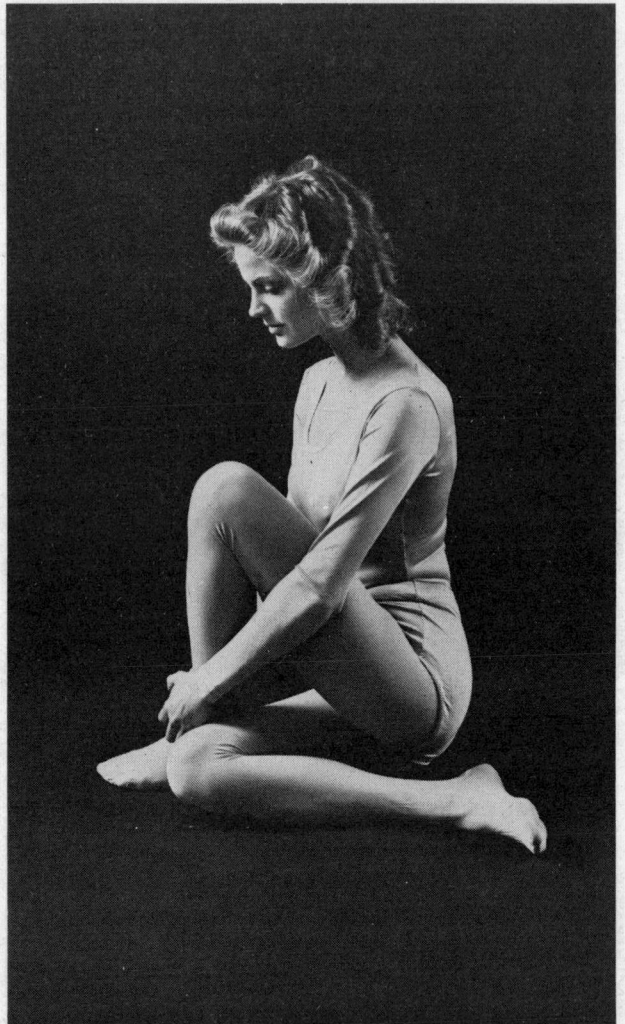

3

foot over right knee and place sole of left foot on floor.

4. Bring right arm over left leg and grasp right knee.

5. Slowly twist trunk and head as far as possible to left with left hand extended back behind you to right as far as possible. Hold for count of 10.

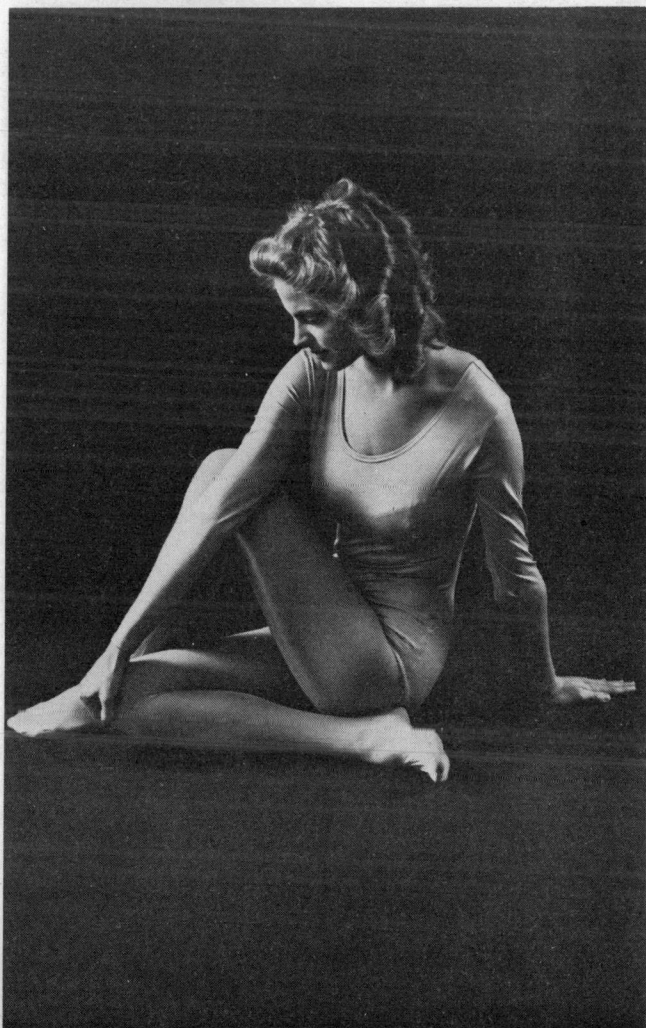

4

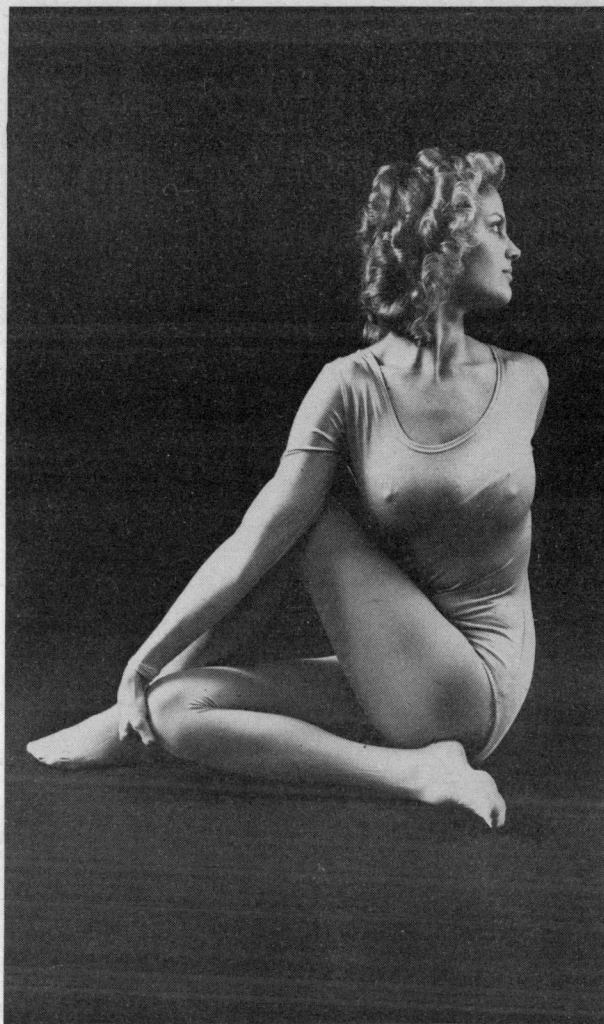

5

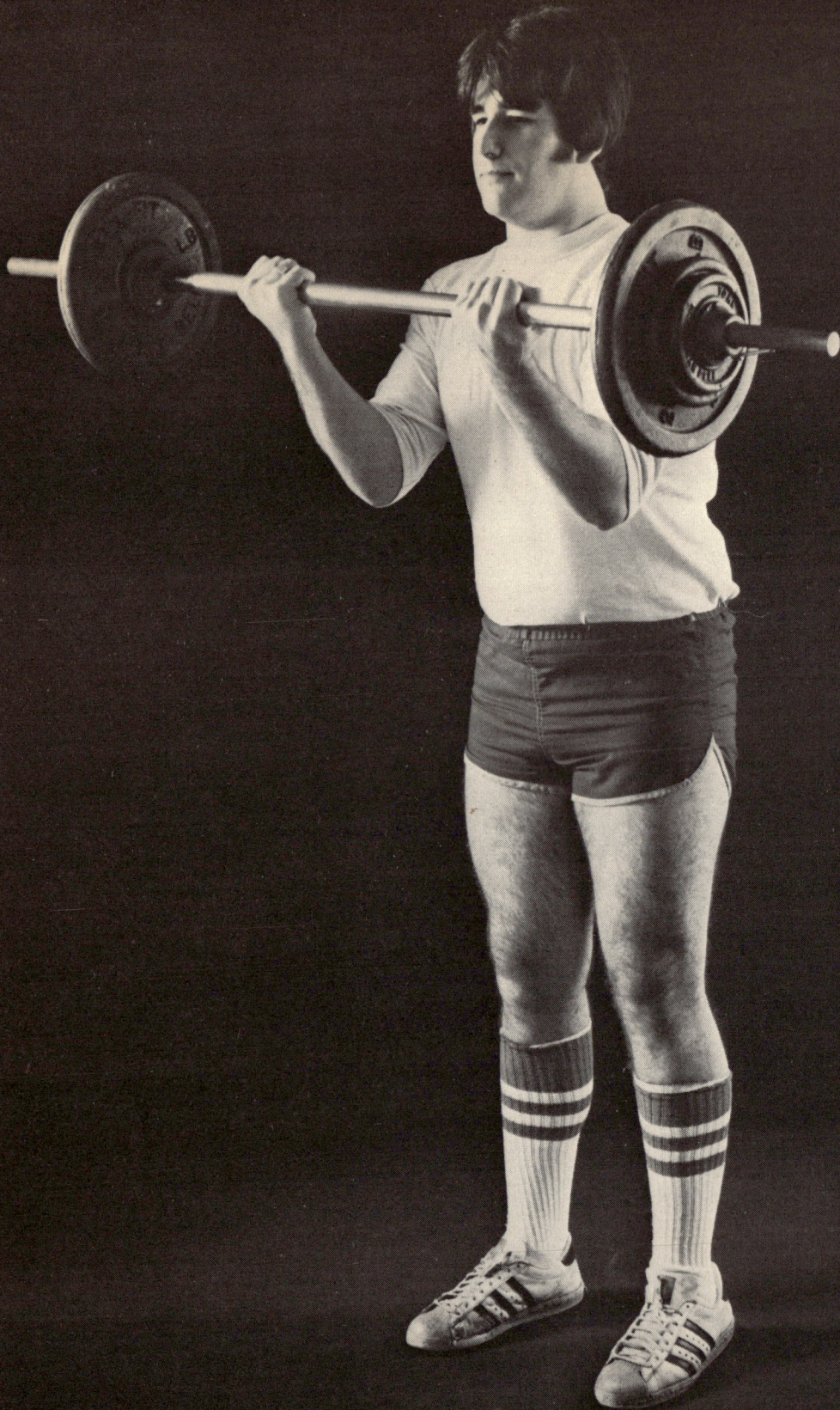

chapter 3

Strength

MUSCULAR STRENGTH IS necessary for any physical accomplishment—from picking up a bag of groceries to developing a strong tennis backhand. Without sufficient strength, your attempts to improve a particular skill—like your tennis backhand—will be hindered and your attempts to improve your flexibility and endurance in a physical fitness program will be limited. Although the fitness elements of flexibility, strength and endurance are all interrelated, it is your muscular system and the demands you put on it that affect development of fitness in the other two elements. If you do not have the abdominal strength to do a situp, you cannot develop endurance in the abdominal muscle group. If you do not have sufficient strength in your lower back muscles, you will find the lower back flexibility exercises difficult if not impossible. Though total physical fitness involves more than strength development, muscular strength is a prerequisite to development of the other conditioning elements.

How much strength you need for everyday tasks and/or participation in a fitness program is difficult to determine. However, a minimum amount of muscle strength is needed to maintain good posture and physique and to efficiently carry out your daily tasks. It's safe to say that if you are not a physically active person—going from home to office and home again with the only exercise being some skiing or football with the kids on the weekends—your strength is at or below minimum. Muscles are meant to be used. When not used or used enough, they begin to deteriorate. This deterioration not only affects your physical appearance—loose, flabby arms, legs and stomach—but also decreases your efficiency. You must use more energy for a given movement or task than a physically fit person. By increasing your strength, you improve your posture and muscle tone, thus your physical appearance. You can perform heavier tasks in less time with less energy and with more body efficiency. In addition, you run less risk of injuring the major joints in your body and reduce minor aches, stiffness and soreness brought on by everyday tasks.

To determine if you have the very minimum strength requirements in your lower back, arm, shoulder and abdominal muscles, go back to the Personal Physical Fitness Evaluation Chart in Chapter 1. If you passed all the Muscular Strength Tests, you possess the *minimum* amount of strength that is considered healthy. If you failed any one or all of the tests, your health could very well be in danger.

EXERCISE METHODS FOR STRENGTH DEVELOPMENT

There are three exercise methods for developing muscle strength—*isometrics, isotonics* and *isokinetics*. Isometric exercise involves muscle contraction with no body movement; isotonic exercise (calisthenics and weight training) refers to muscle contractions with movement; and isokinetic exercise involves muscle contraction with movement and with a controlled resistance. Each of these methods has its advantages and disadvantages.

Isometrics has received much attention largely because strength is developed without any body movement. In performing isometric exercises, a muscle or muscle group is exerted against an immoveable object such as a wall or against another muscle group. The chief advantages are that no equipment is needed to perform the exercises and they can be performed anywhere at anytime—sitting behind the desk at the office, in the commuter train, at the theater or standing at the bus stop. Each exercise only takes 6-8 seconds so that the time invested for significant returns in muscle strength is minimal. The non-body movement and brief exercise time make isometrics ideal for the bedridden or wheelchair-confined person or for those people who must spend many hours of the day sitting.

(Above right and below right) Chinning yourself is one of the best strength producing exercises there is for the upper part of the body. It can be even more effective if the exerciser holds positions on the way up and on the way down.

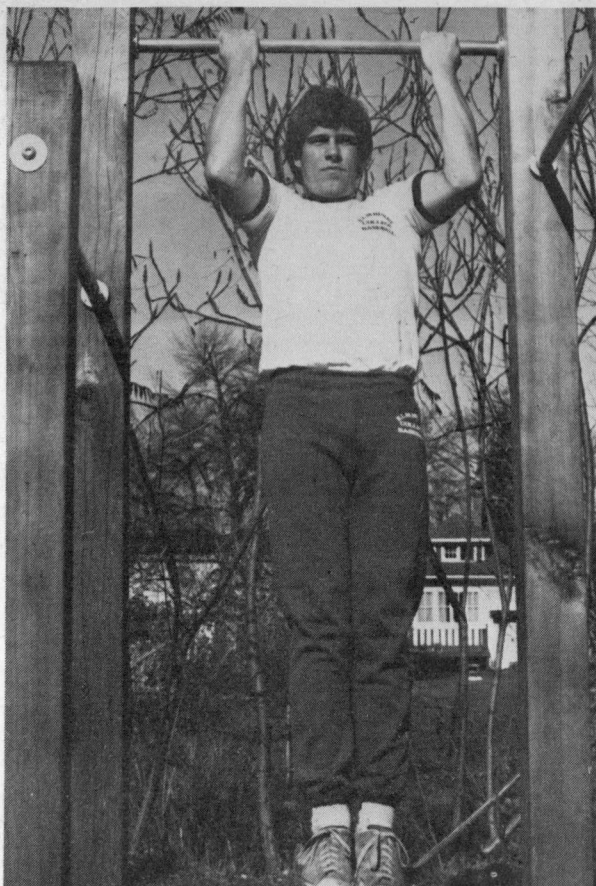

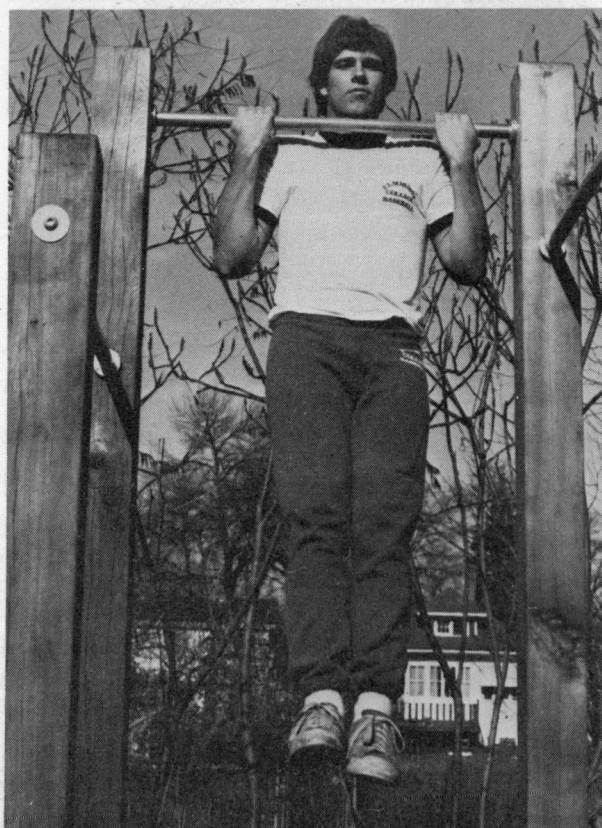

There is also some evidence that isometric exercise is efficient as a spot reducer, especially in the waist, hip and thigh regions.

However, isometric exercises do have their disadvantages. The most glaring is the fact that for an increase in strength, you must exert two-thirds of your maximum force. In doing an isometric exercise, it's difficult to know if you're exerting enough to make an improvement. You have no definite way of knowing whether you're exerting 10 percent, 50 percent or 100 percent of your force. Another problem is the specificity of isometric exercise. Each exercise is for one muscle area. Because of this, you have to exercise each muscle area for any kind of general conditioning. And this brings up another problem—boredom. In performing a battery of isometric exercises designed for improving each body muscle group, it's easy to lose your concentration because of the sameness and lack of move-

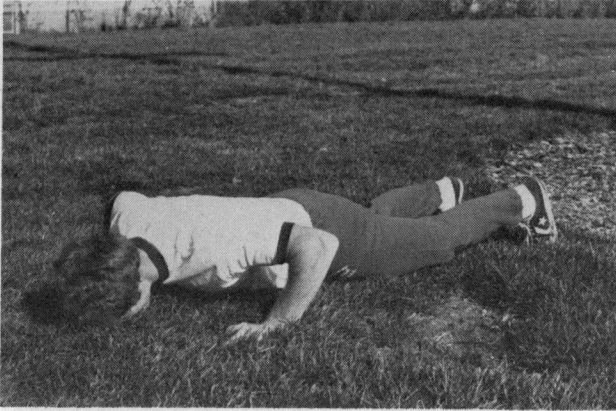

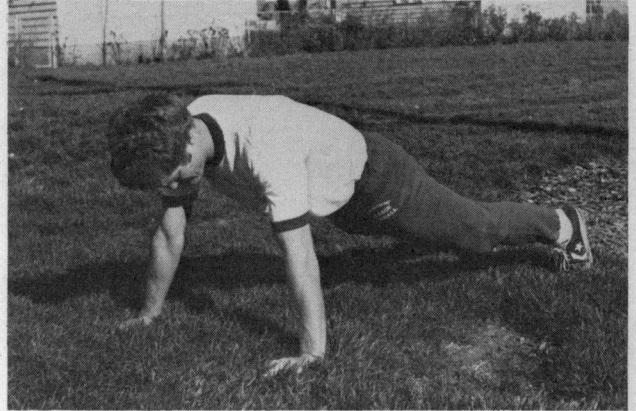

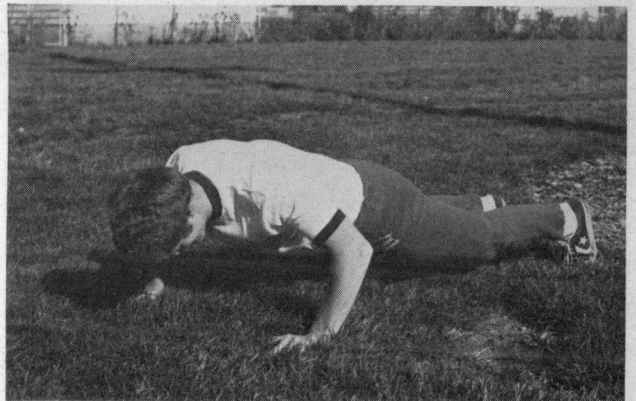

The Pushup is an excellent exercise for developing arm and shoulder strength. To begin, you lie face down with legs together, hands under shoulders with fingers pointing straight ahead (above left). Push body off the ground by extending arms so that your weight rests on your hands and toes (above right). Then lower yourself, keeping your back straight, until your chest touches the ground (right).

ment. Finally, isometric exercises do absolutely *nothing* for muscular endurance or flexibility. In fact, isometrics without supplementary flexibility exercises can actually reduce the range of movement in your joints.

Isotonic exercises are the two types most of use are most familiar with—*calisthenics* and *weight training*. Calisthenic exercises have several advantages. Very little or no equipment is required for doing the exercises; they're easy to learn and perform; vigorous workouts can be done in short periods of time; you can work on specific areas of the body; and last, very little space is needed for performing the exercises. Unfortunately, calisthenics are the least effective of all the methods for rapid increases in muscle strength. However, for the average adult who wants to develop adequate strength and improve muscle tone, calisthenics will fulfill the need.

It is generally agreed that weight training is the fastest and best method for increasing muscle strength. Weight training is a systematic series of resistance exercises using the overload principle. As the capacity of a muscle or group of muscles increases in strength, the intensity, or weight in the case of weight training, is also increased. Using weight training you can precisely control the exercise load and easily single out and work on a specific muscle or muscle group.

However, there are some disadvantages to weight training. First of all is the cost of the equipment and/or finding a gym to work out in that has all the equipment. Secondly, weight training does not improve cardiovascular fitness and at best should be used as a supplement to flexibility and cardiovascular exercises. In fact, some weight lifting exercises, especially those which require only limited movement, can actually reduce the flexibility in your joints if not supplemented. Even though some might think working with heavy weights might be a disadvantage in that you are risking injury, if the proper precautions are taken with respect to proper breathing, doing the exercises correctly and properly adjusting the weight, injury risk is minimal.

Isokinetic exercises are most widely associated with the exercise machines found in health clubs. These machines control the amount of resistance against which the exerciser works. At a slow speed there is very little resistance but as speed is increased, so is the amount of resistance. Since the machines adapt automatically to the amount of effort being exerted, there is little chance of overstressing a muscle or damaging a weak area such as the knee. Isokinetic machines also allow the exerciser to work on isolated muscle groups with a variety of special exercises. This specific body conditioning is of great benefit to the athlete or sports enthusiast who has special sport technique needs.

Once again, isokinetic exercises do not help build cardiovascular endurance or flexibility and should therefore not be used as a total program but merely as a supplement to build strength and muscle endurance. The other disadvantage is finding the machines to work on. Joining a health club can bite into the pocket a bit. If you have a YMCA or YWCA close by, they may have a Nautilus, Apollo Exerciser or Pro Gym. If you don't want to join a health club and/or do not have access to any type of isokinetic machine, it is possible to do isokinetic exercises with the help of a partner. The disadvantage of this method is

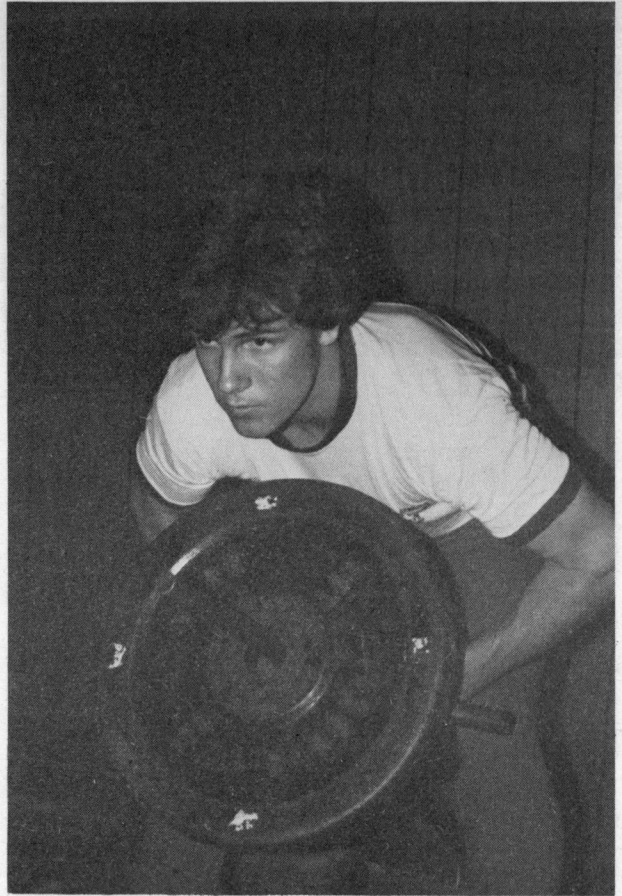

The primary purpose of the Bent-Rowing exercise is to strengthen the muscles that hold the shoulder blades in proper alignment. To do this exercise your upper body must be parallel with the floor, legs slightly spread with knees flexed. Gripping the barbell, you raise it to waist height using only your arm and shoulder muscles. Then lower the barbell to ankle height level and repeat. For stabilization you can utilize a table to rest your forehead upon.

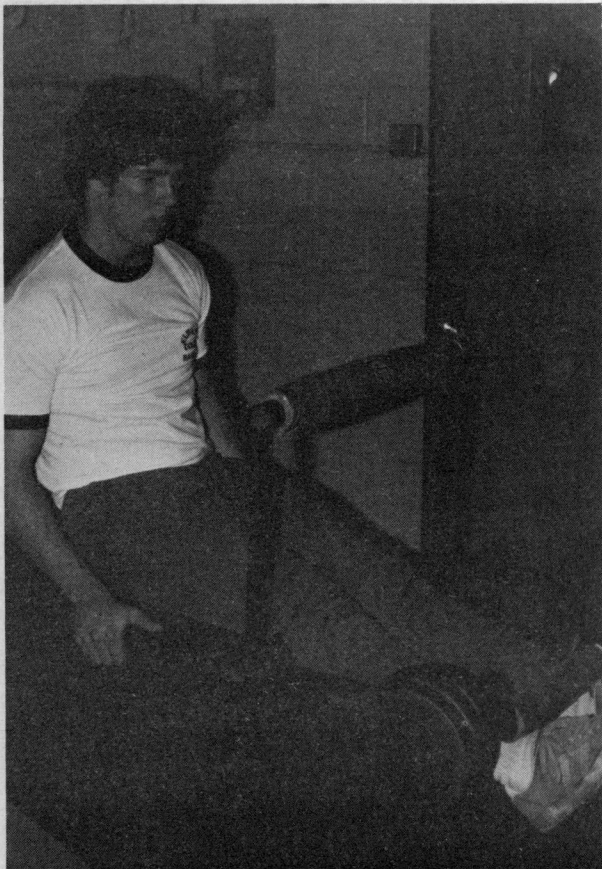

A good exercise for strengthening the legs is illustrated here. If you're doing the exercises at home, the leg exercise can be accomplished without special equipment as used here. Simply put weights in a sack or bag and tie the bag so it hangs down from your ankles.

that the resistance which the partner exerts is not nearly as controlled, but nevertheless can be effective. A discussion of exercise machines can be found later in this chapter. The isokinetic exercises in this chapter will be those which require a partner.

STRENGTH DEVELOPING EXERCISES

How much strength will you develop in doing these exercises? It depends on how much strength you have when you start the exercises. It also depends on your body composition and type. As noted previously, there are notable differences in people's bodies, and some will never acquire the strength or musculature that others will, no matter how diligently they work at it.

The person who is already blessed by good muscular development won't come close to seeing the quick improvement that the underdeveloped exerciser will achieve. In some cases, the well-developed person will soon reach the stage where all he or she accomplishes by strength exercises is strength maintenance.

The beginner, however, whose musculature is relatively undeveloped will see fast and vast improvements, usually in 3 to 4 weeks. In fairness, it should be said that after that first period of development, gains in strength will come more slowly and won't be nearly so pronounced.

Before getting into the various strength developing exercises, it is important to realize the interrelationship of strength and endurance. When doing exercises to improve your development in one, you are going to gain some improvement in the other. However, a minimum amount of strength is needed in order to improve and build up your endurance. All of the calisthenic, weight training and isokinetic exercises in this chapter can be used to build both strength and endurance. It is the way in which you perform the exercise that determines which fitness element you are improving the most.

Strength is the ability of a muscle or muscle group to overcome a maximum resistance in one effort—for example, being able to perform a bicep curl with a 100-pound weight. Endurance, on the other hand, is the ability of a muscle or muscle group to sustain an effort for a period of time—for example, being able to do 50 bicep curls with a 50-pound weight. A strength developing exercise involves *few* repetitions (usually

6-10) with a maximum amount of resistance, while endurance exercises involve *many* repetitions with a lesser amount of resistance. So in doing the following exercises, the object is not how many repetitions you can perform but how much resistance you can progressively overcome.

For building strength, then, you need to overcome progressively increased resistances. For weight training exercises that means simply adding to the amount of weight you are lifting. For calisthenics, since the only resistance is the weight of the body, you can employ the use of a slant board which increases resistance against the force of gravity or do the exercises using some sort of weight. For the isokinetic exercises, using a partner, simply have the partner apply more resistance.

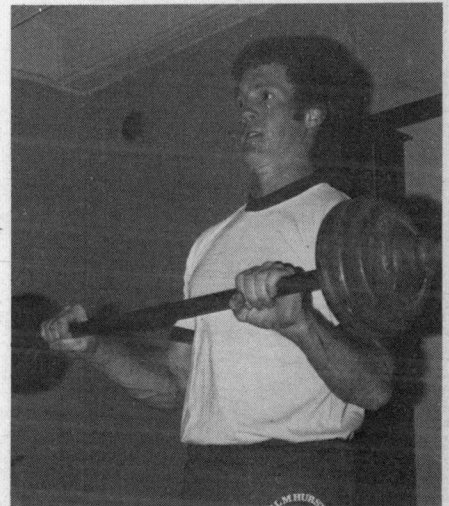

(Above and below) Two stages of a barbell exercise for developing strength in the hands, wrists, arms and shoulders. For maximum results, the movements should be done slowly.

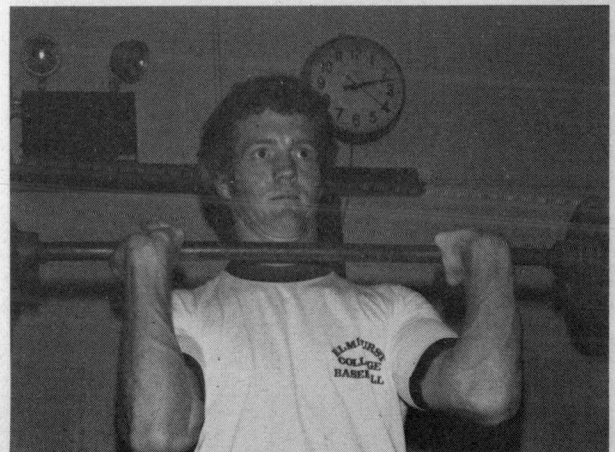

Isometrics

When performing the following isometric exercises use two-thirds of your maximum force—less than that will be of little benefit. Hold each contraction for 6-8 seconds and during the contraction do little breathing—try to only breathe between contractions. There is no set order for doing the following exercises nor do you have to do them all at one time. But to gain the most benefit from isometrics, the exercises should be done three times during the day. Remember that isometric exercises are very specific so that for general body conditioning, you should pick at least one exercise for each muscle group in the body.

Arm and Shoulder Push (arm and chest muscles)

1. Stand in doorway and place hands at shoulder height on either side of doorway.
2. Push outward using two-thirds of your maximum force for 6-8 seconds.

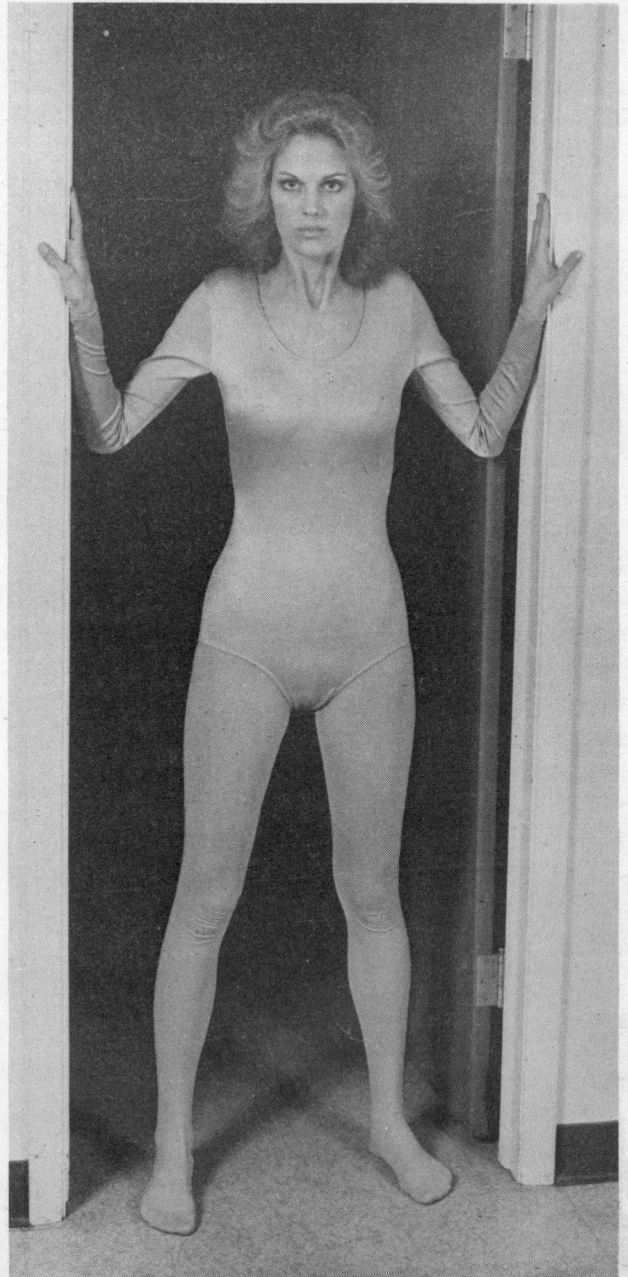

Neck Push (neck muscles)

1. Standing or sitting, place the heel of your right hand on your right temple.
2. Push to the right with your head and push to the left with your hand.
3. Hold for 6-8 seconds using two-thirds of your maximum force.
4. Using left hand against left temple, repeat exercise.
5. With hands clasped, place palms of hands on forehead and repeat exercise.
6. With hands clasped, place palms on back of head and repeat exercise.

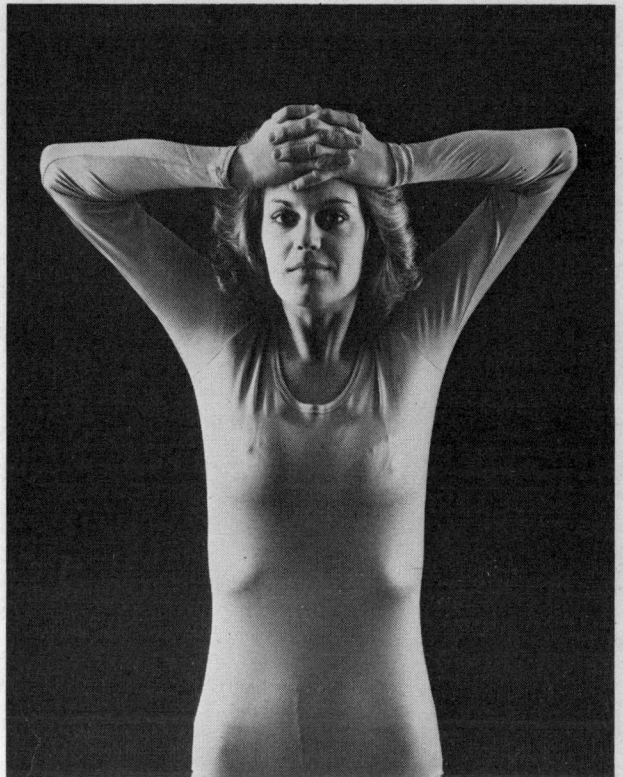

2

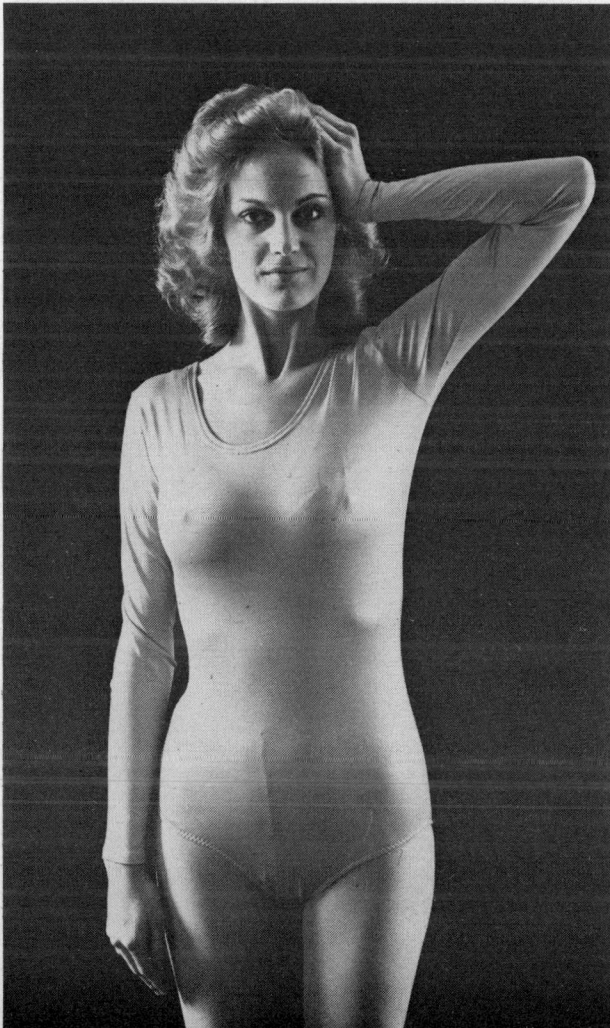

5

6

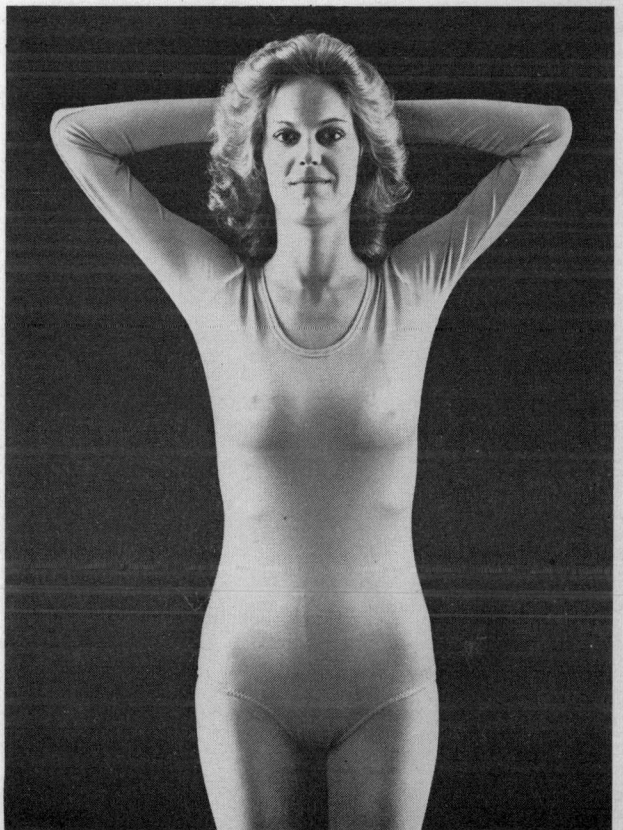

Side Arm Push (shoulder muscles)

1. Stand in doorway, hands at sides, palms toward legs.
2. Press hands outward against doorway, keeping elbows straight, for 6-8 seconds.

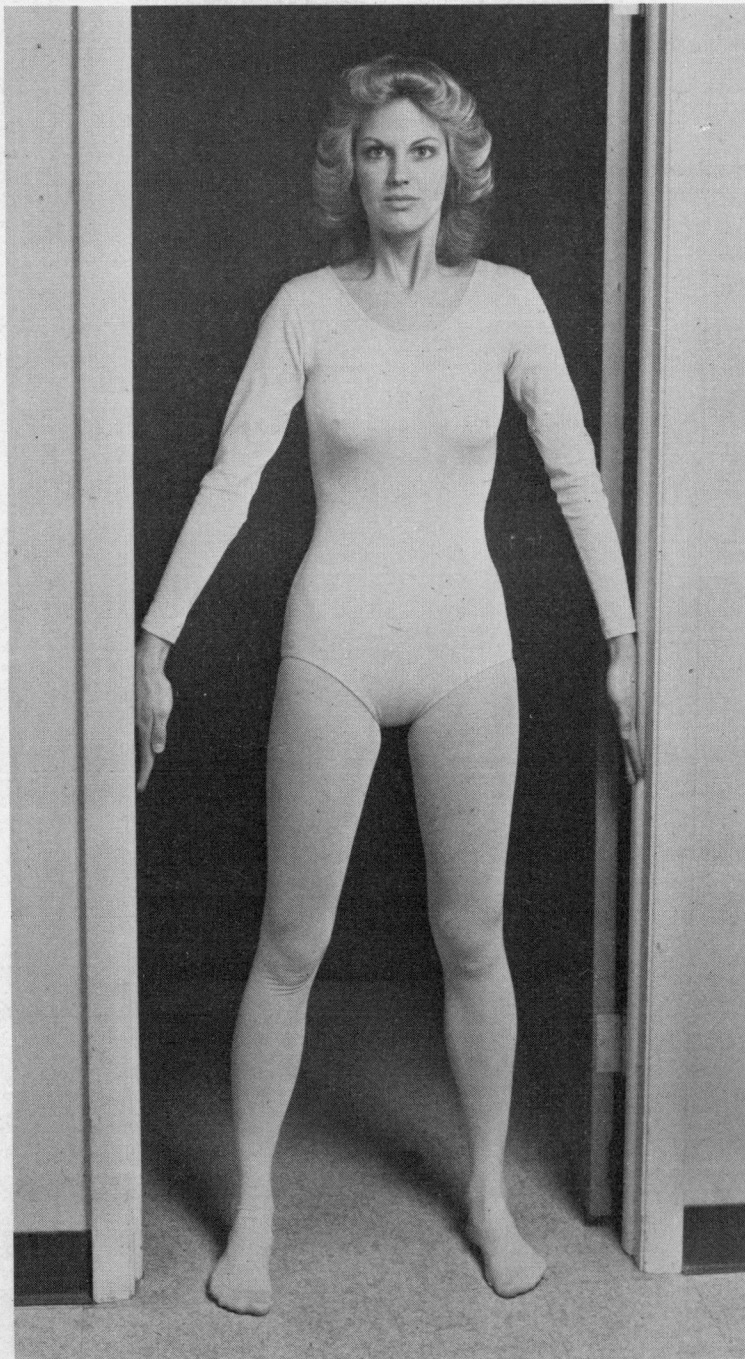

Overhead Push (shoulder, arm and chest muscles)

1. Stand in doorway and place hands overhead on door casing. (If you're not tall enough, stand on a sturdy, hard chair or box.)
2. Push upwards for 6-8 seconds.

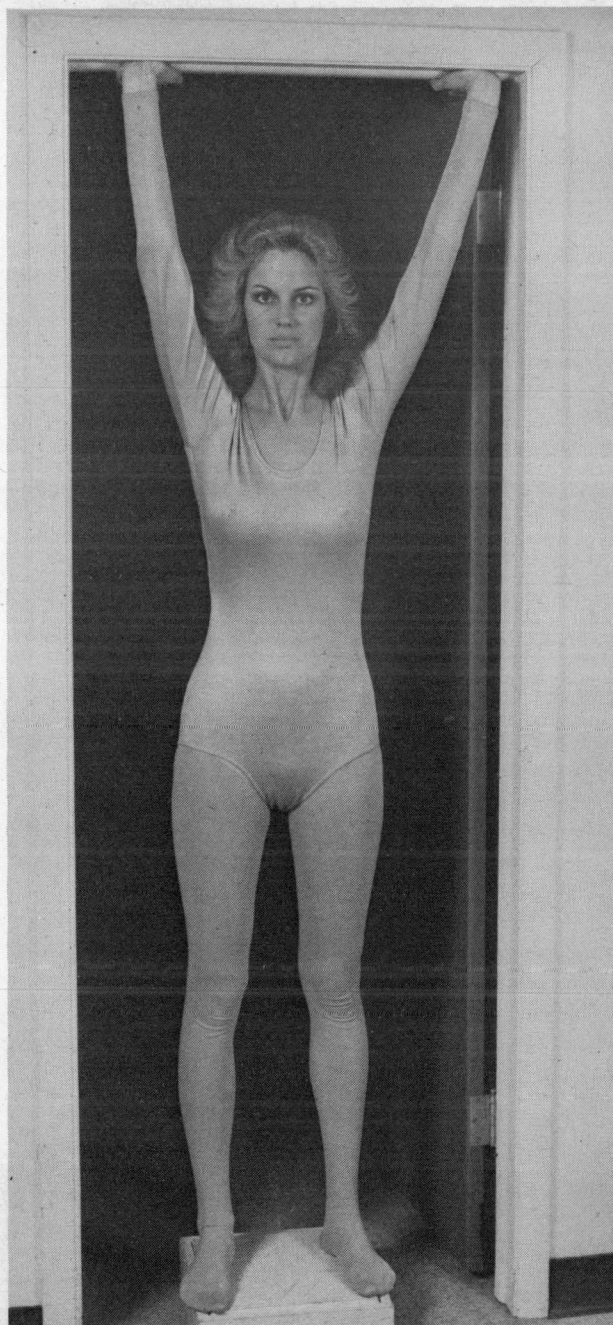

Upper Body Push (chest, shoulder and arm muscles)

1. Stand, back to the wall, hands at sides, palms toward wall.
2. Press hands backward against wall, keeping arms straight for 6-8 seconds.
3. Reverse position with face to wall, hands at sides, palms toward wall.
4. Press hands forward against wall, keeping arms straight, for 6-8 seconds.

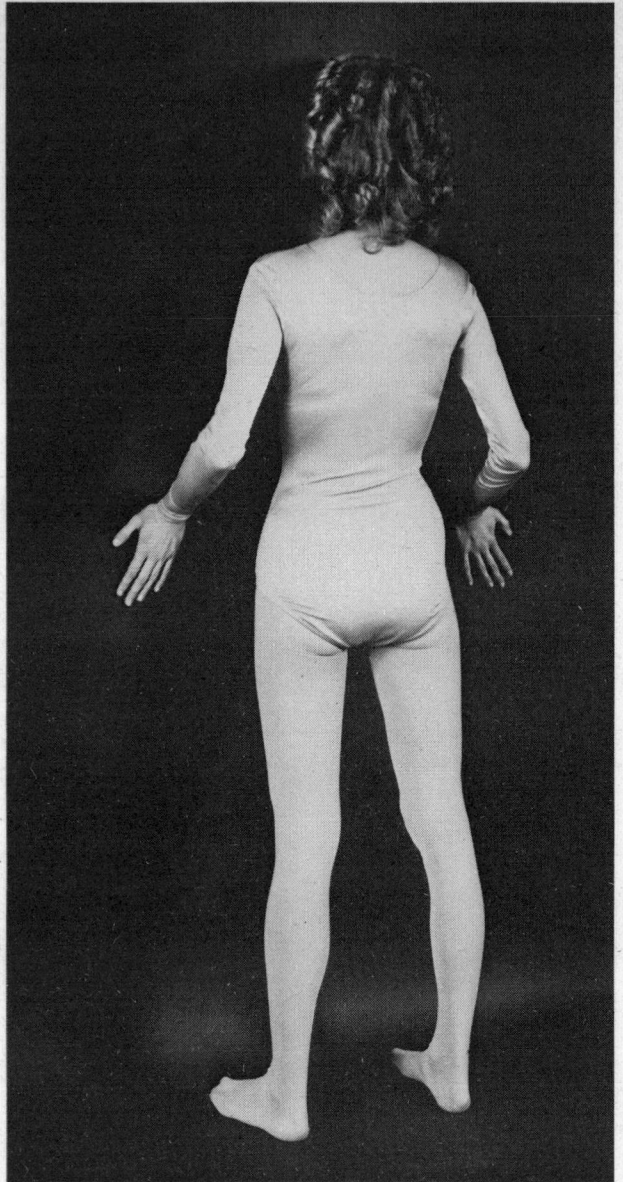

4

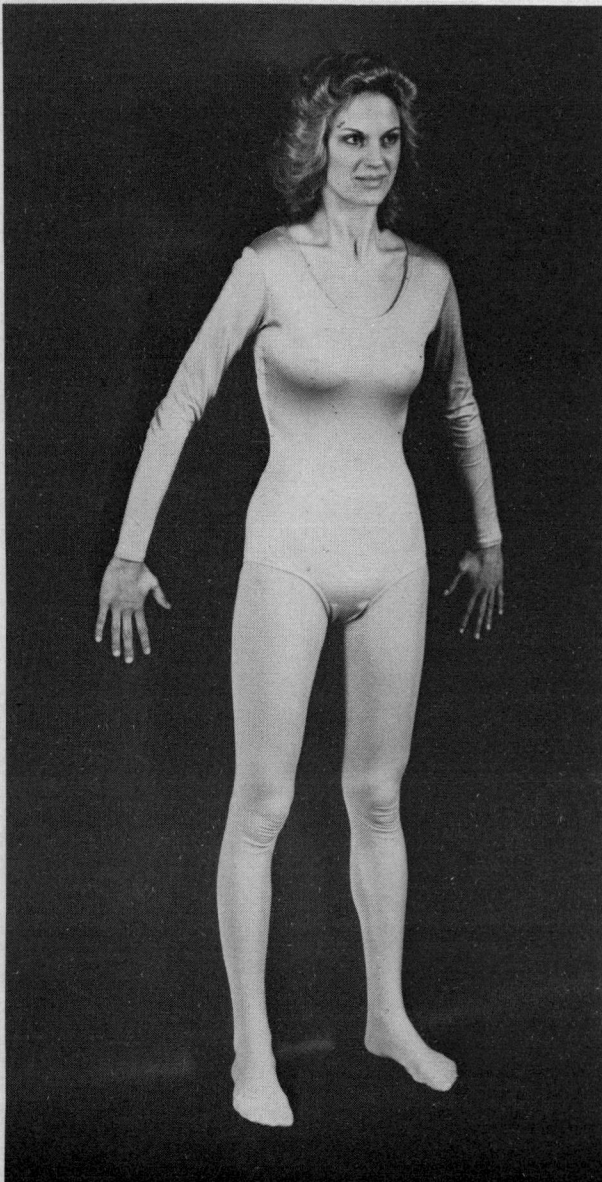

2

Trunk Push and Pull (shoulder, arm and trunk muscles)

1. Stand in doorway, legs comfortably apart, with right hand grasping the front of the door casing and the left hand grasping the back of the door casing.

2. Pull with the right hand and push with the left, as if to twist the body to the right against the pressure. Hold for 6-8 seconds.

3. Reverse hand positions with the left hand grasping front of casing and right hand grasping the back of door casing. Try twisting body to the left against pressure for 6-8 seconds.

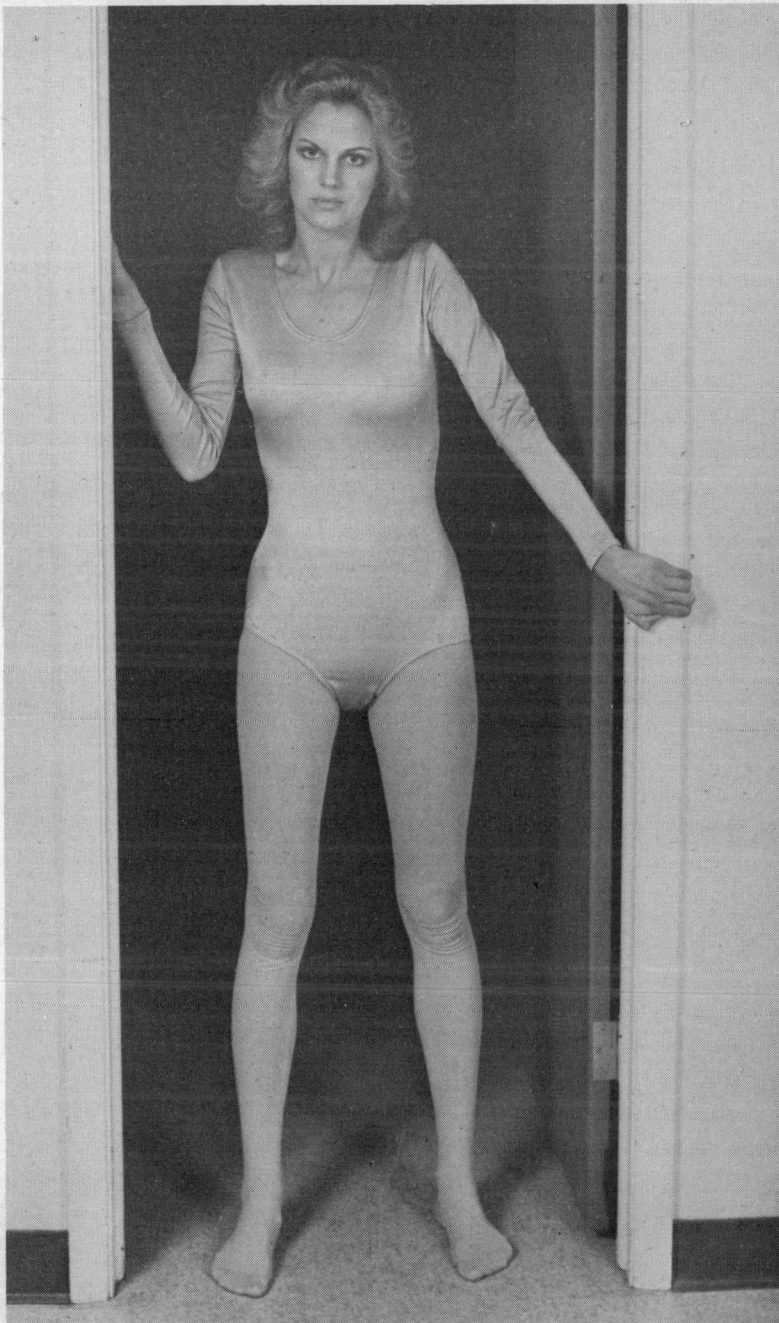

Hand Push (biceps and chest muscles)

1. Stand with feet comfortably spaced, knees slightly flexed. Clasp hands, palms together, close to chest.
2. Press hands together for 6-8 seconds.

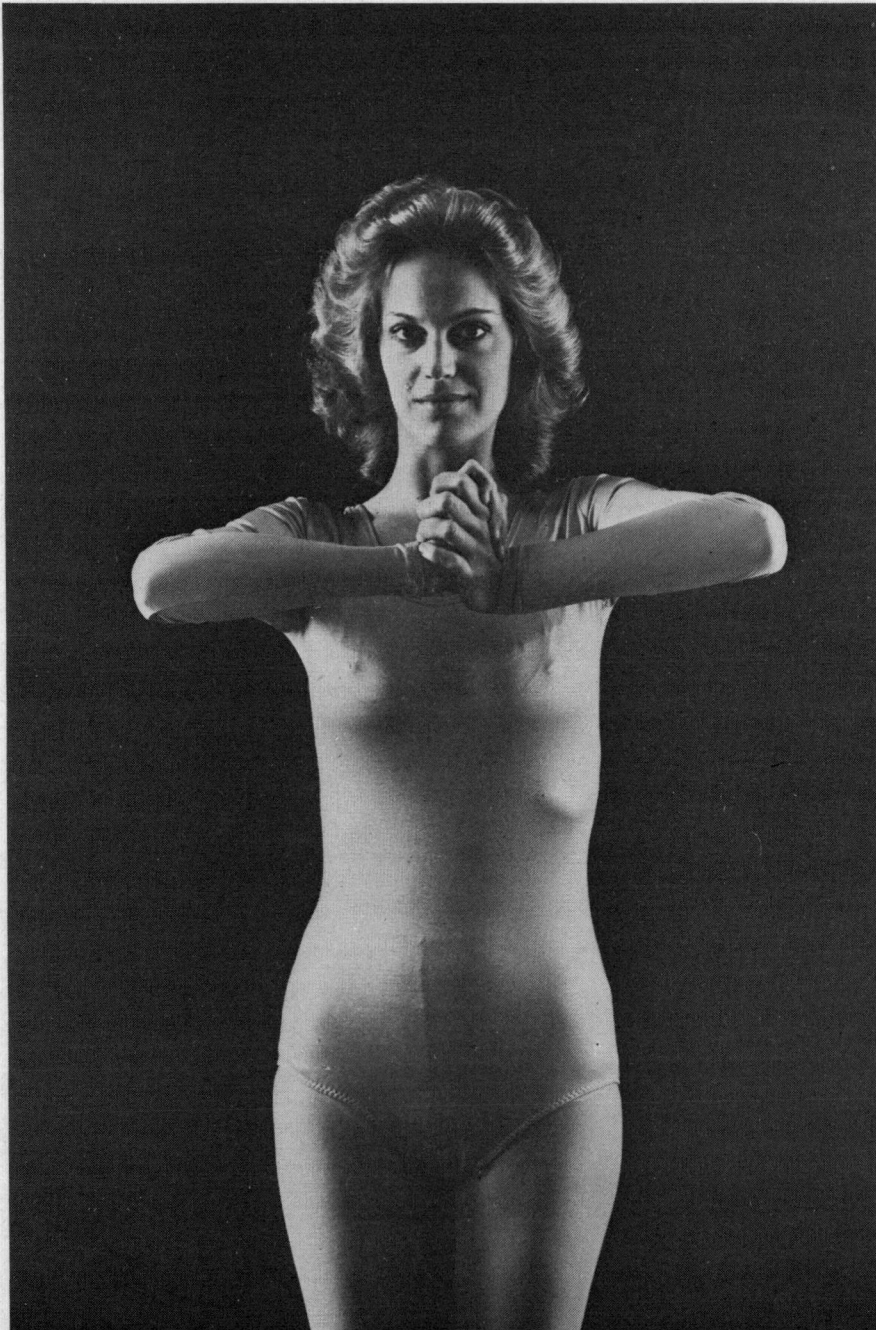

Hand Pull (triceps and chest muscles)

1. Stand with feet comfortably apart, knees slightly flexed. Grip fingers of both hands, arms close to chest.
2. Pull outward with both arms for 6-8 seconds.

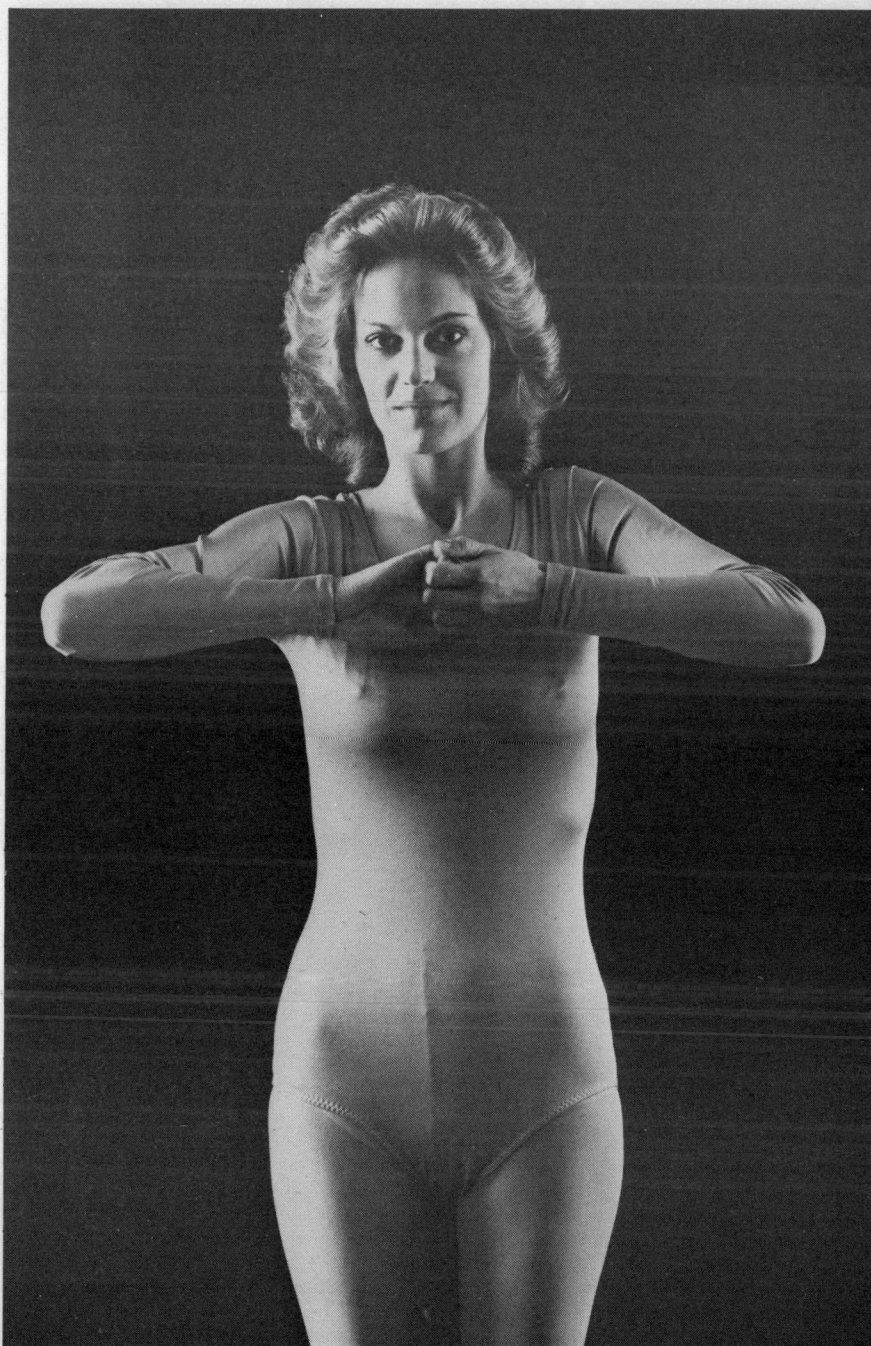

Chair Lift (biceps)

1. Sitting in a chair, feet flat on floor, grip underside of seat with both hands.
2. Pull up for 6-8 seconds.

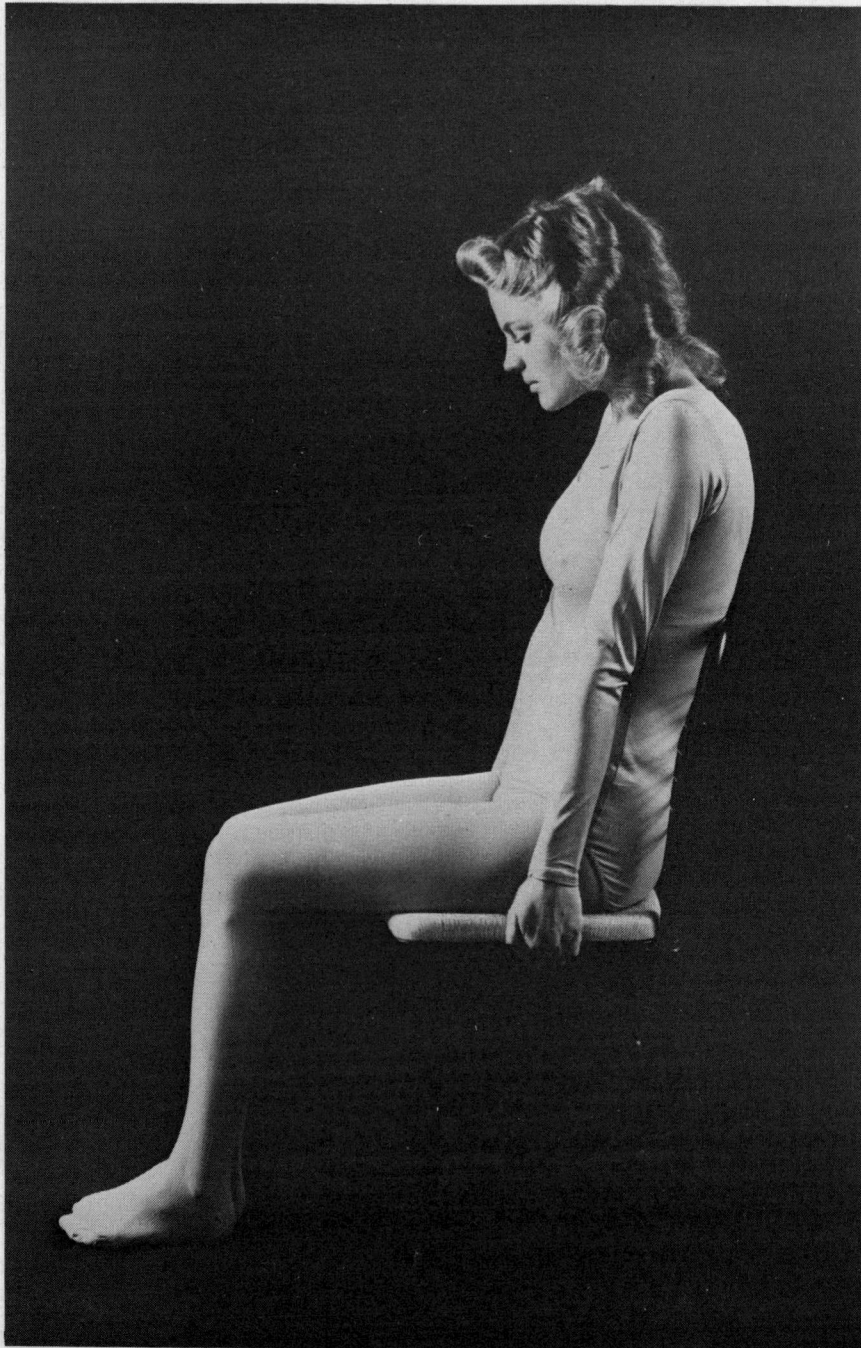

Hand Curl (arm muscles)

1. Stand with feet slightly apart. Flex right elbow, close to body, palm up. Place left hand over right and clasp tightly.
2. Attempt to curl right arm upward toward chest, while giving equally strong resistance with the left hand, for 6-8 seconds.
3. Reverse hand positions and repeat exercise.

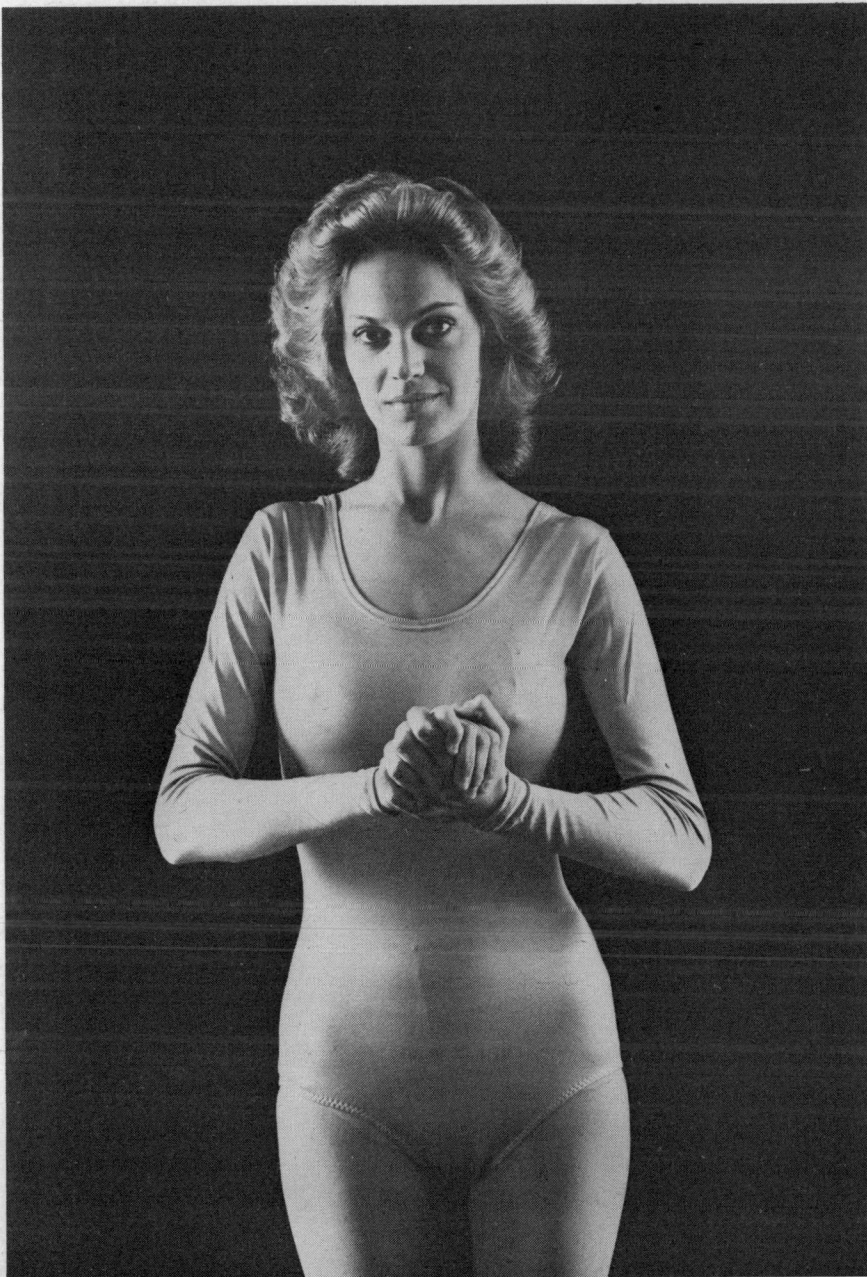

Abdominal Squeeze (abdominal muscles)

1. Stand with knees slightly flexed, hand on knees.
2. Contract abdominal muscles for 6-8 seconds.

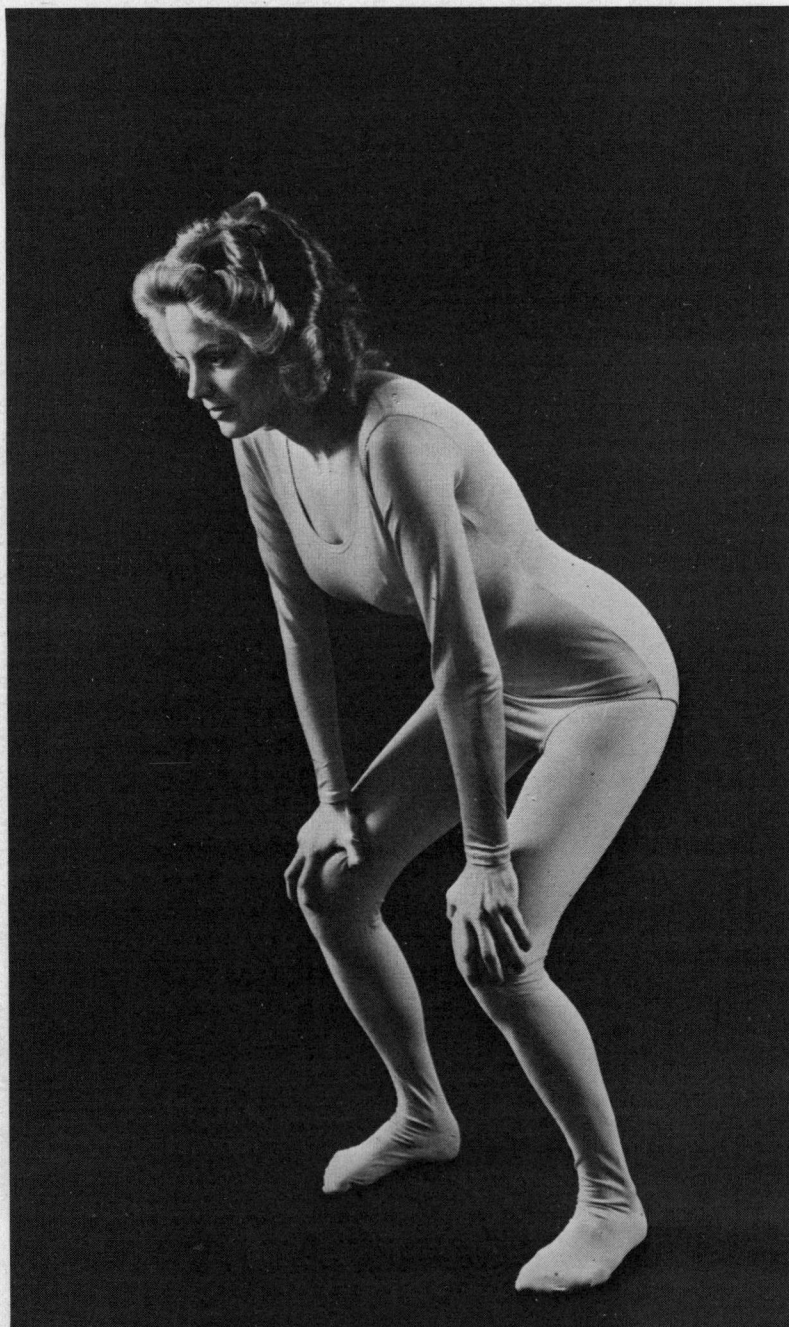

Lower Body Push (lower back, buttock and thigh muscles)

1. Lie face down on floor, arms at sides, palms up, legs placed under table, bed or other heavy object.
2. Keeping hips flat on floor, raise right leg, keeping knee straight so that heel pushes against resistance. Push for 6-8 seconds.
3. Repeat exercise pushing for 6-8 seconds with left leg.

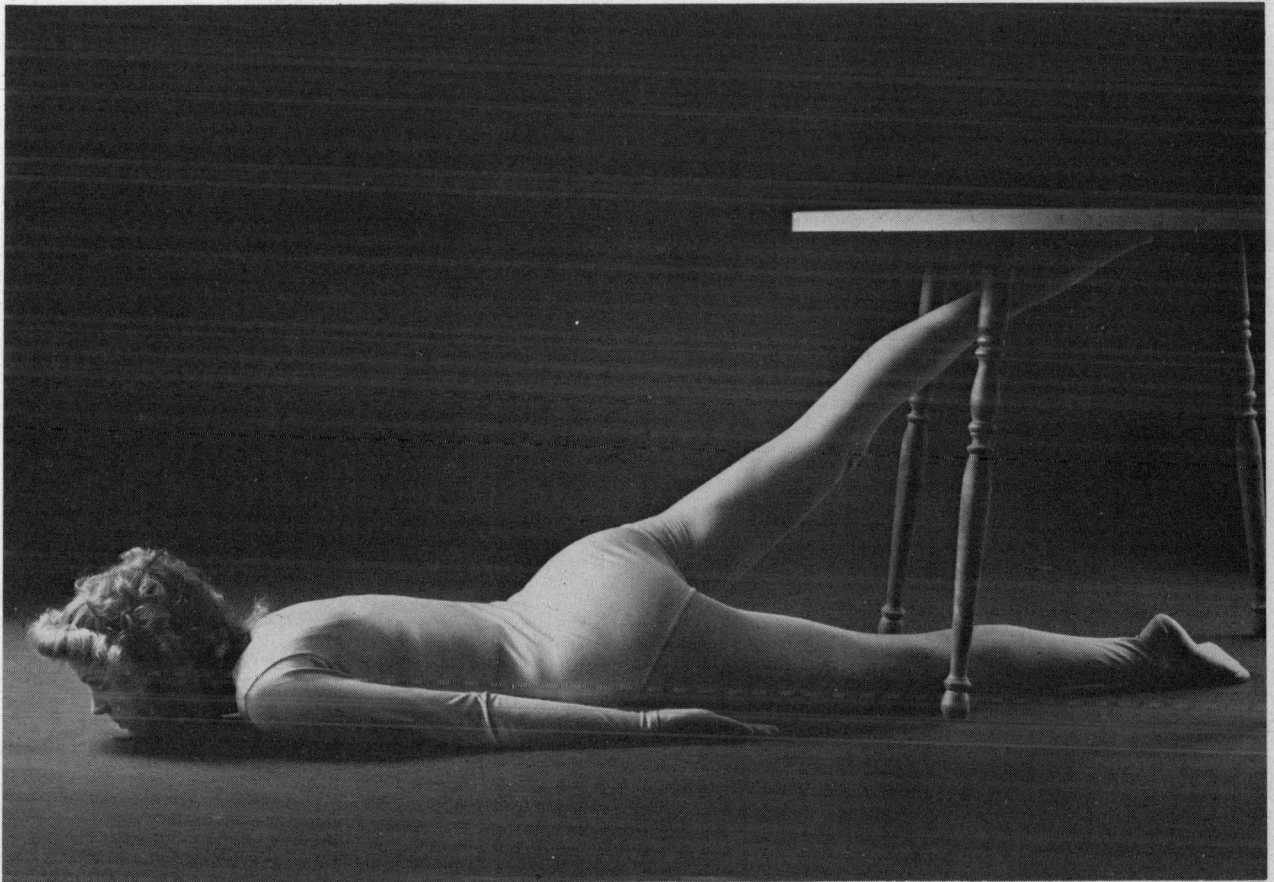

Thigh Push (thigh muscles)

1. Sit in chair with feet flat on floor and hands palm down on thighs.
2. Push downward with arms and push upward with thighs for 6-8 seconds.

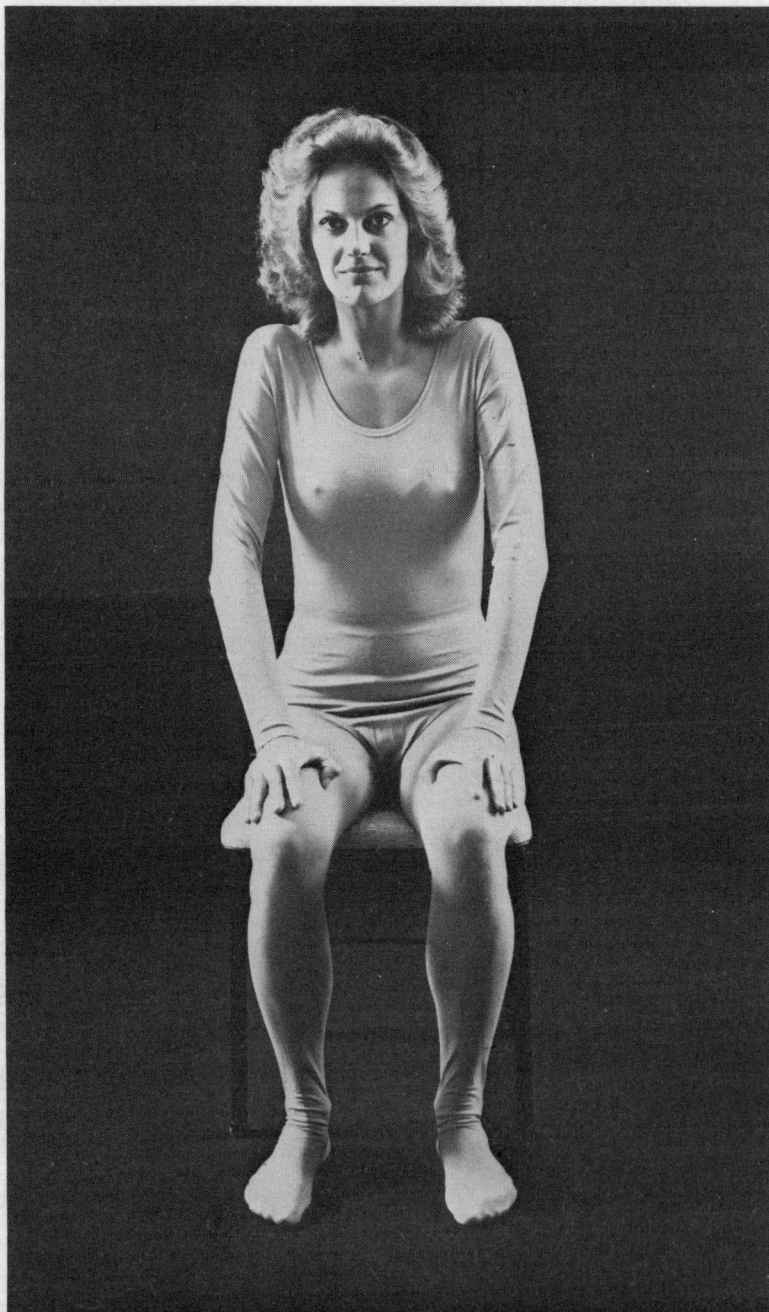

Inner Thigh Squeeze (inner thigh muscles)

1. Sit in chair, arms extended, hands closed in fists and fists placed on inside of each knee.
2. Push outward with arms and push inward with thighs for 6-8 seconds.

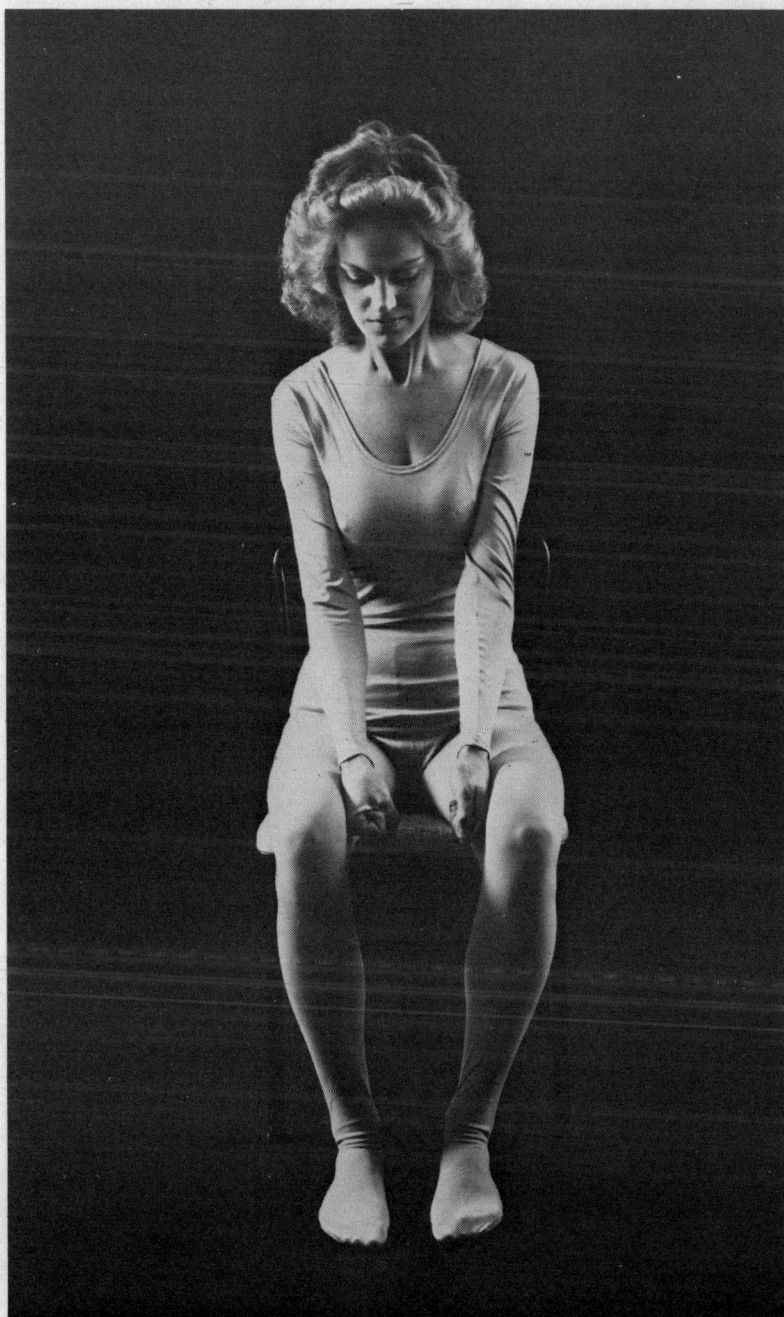

Outer Thigh Push (outer thigh muscles)

1. Sit in chair, legs extended with each ankle pressed against the inside of sturdy chair legs.
2. Keeping legs straight, try to push them outward for 6-8 seconds.

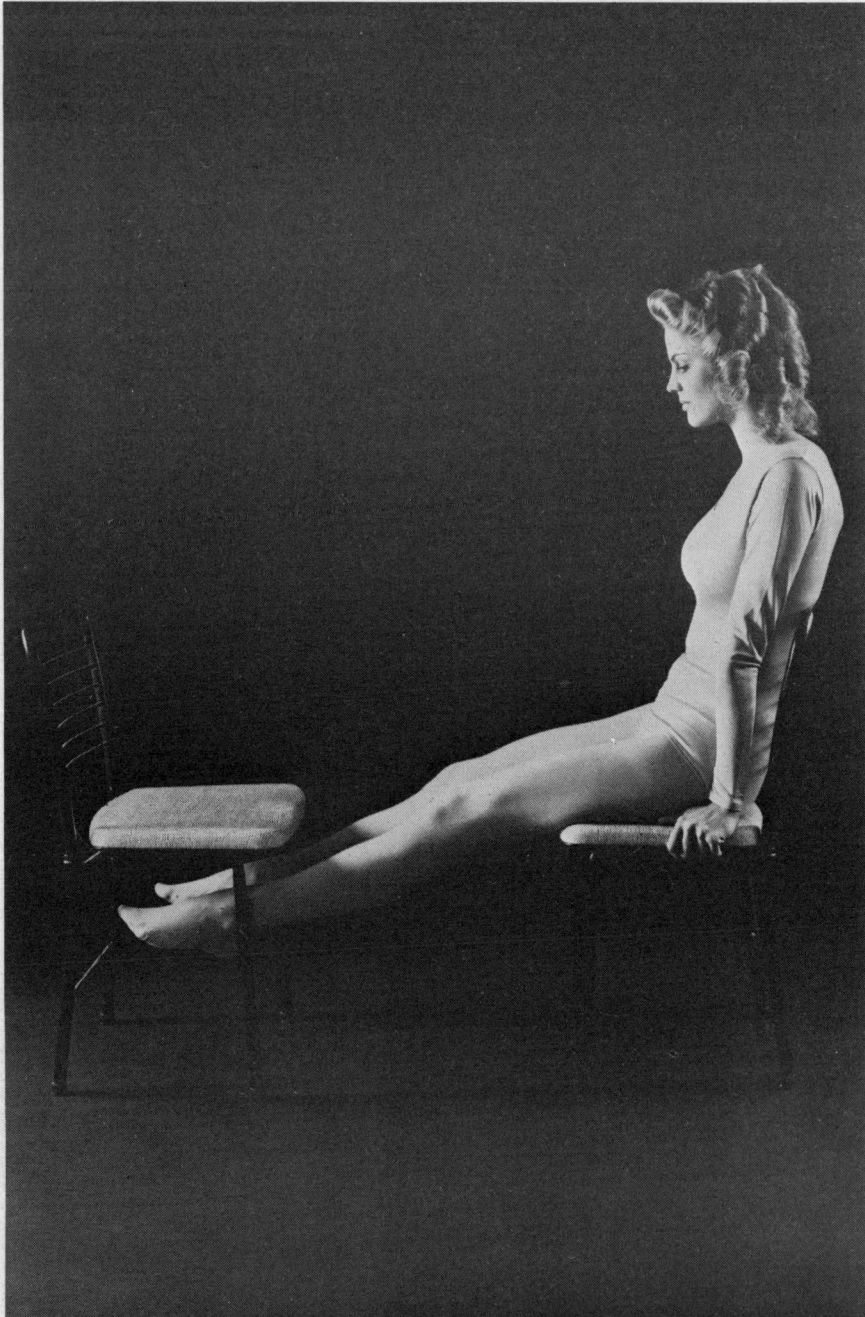

Raised Leg Push (leg muscles)

1. Sit in chair, legs extended straight out, right ankle crossed over left ankle, hands gripping sides of chair.
2. Push down with right leg and push up with equal force with left leg for 6-8 seconds.
3. Repeat exercise with reversed leg positions—the left ankle crossed over the right ankle.

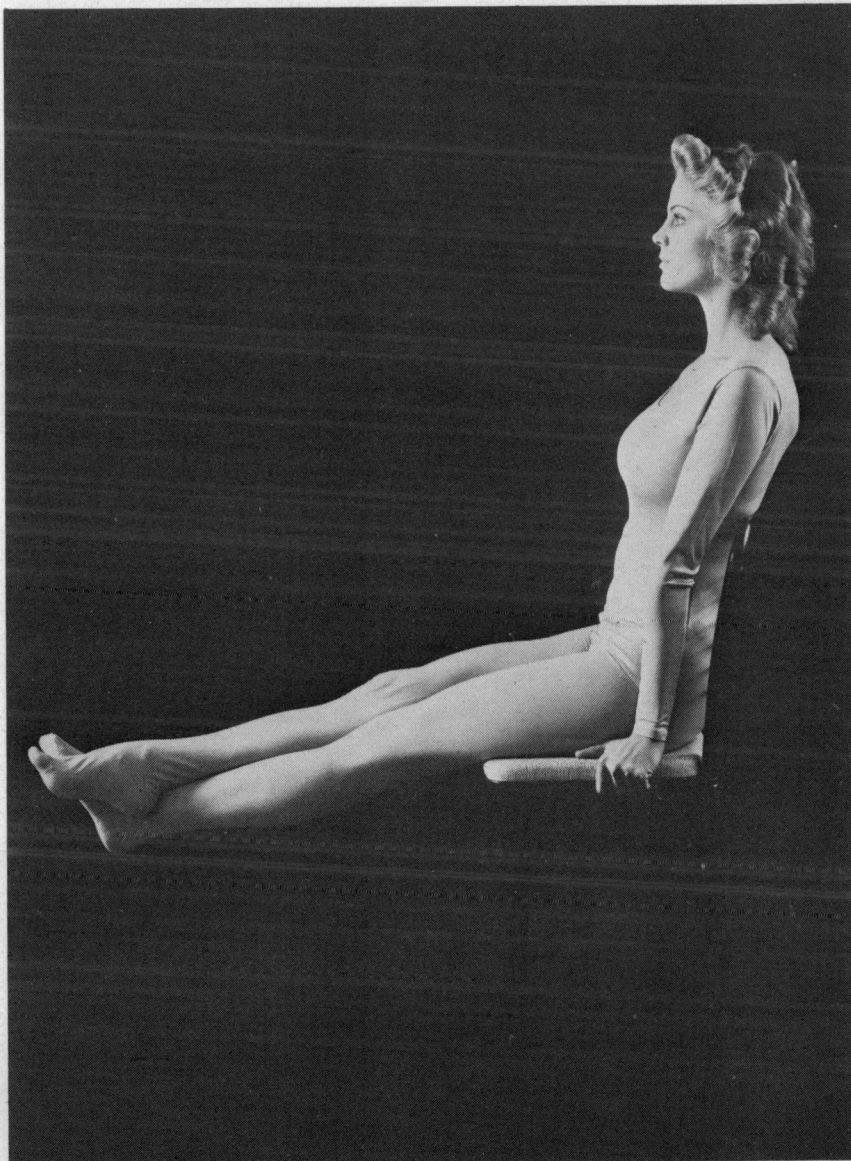

Inner Thigh Push (inner thigh muscles)

1. Sit in chair, legs extended with each ankle pressed against the outside of sturdy chair legs.
2. Keeping legs straight, try to pull them together for 6-8 seconds.

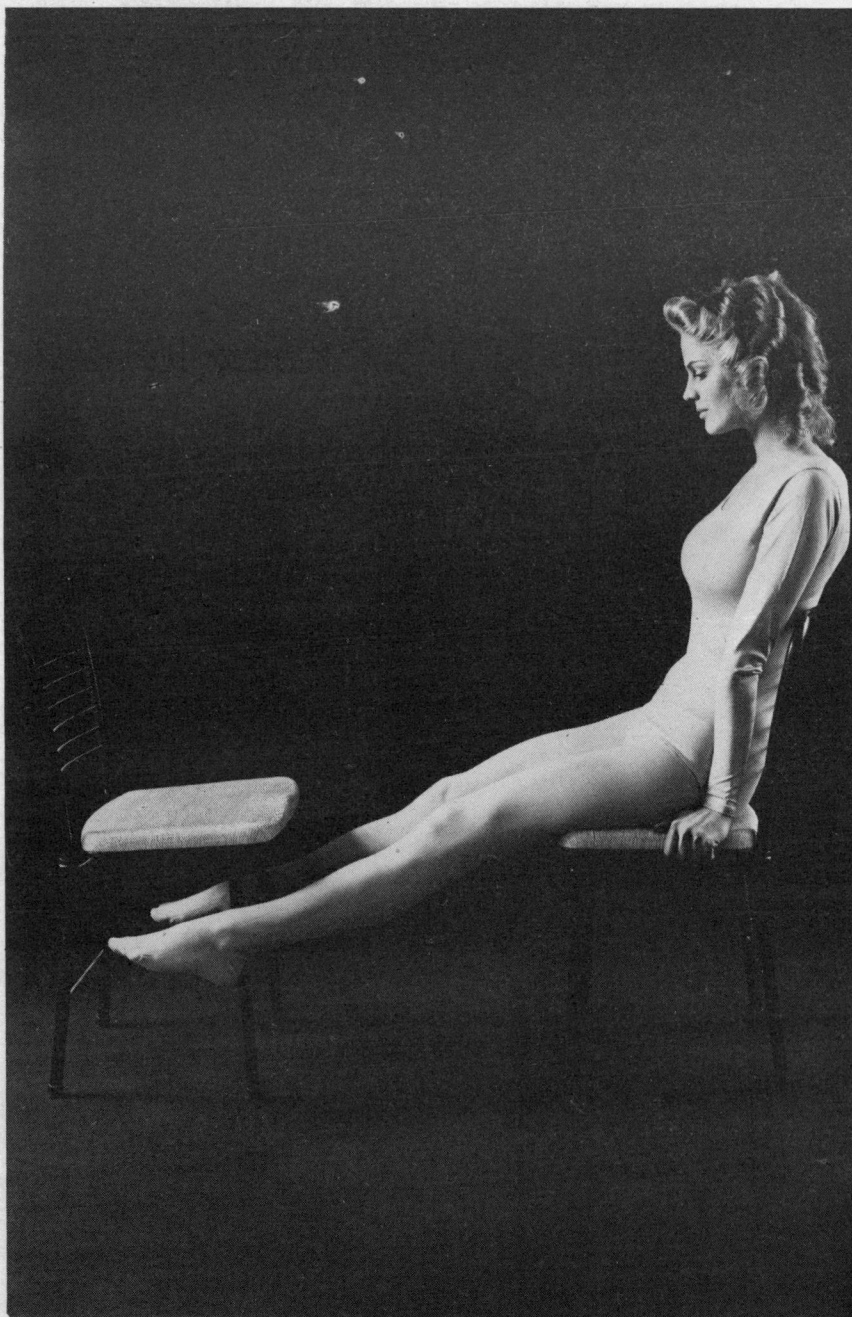

Sitting Leg Push and Pull (leg muscles)

1. Sit in chair with left ankle crossed over right, feet resting on floor, legs bent at 90-degree angle. Hands should be gripping underside of chair.
2. Try to straighten right leg while resisting with left for 6-8 seconds.
3. Reverse leg positions with right ankle crossed over left and repeat exercise.

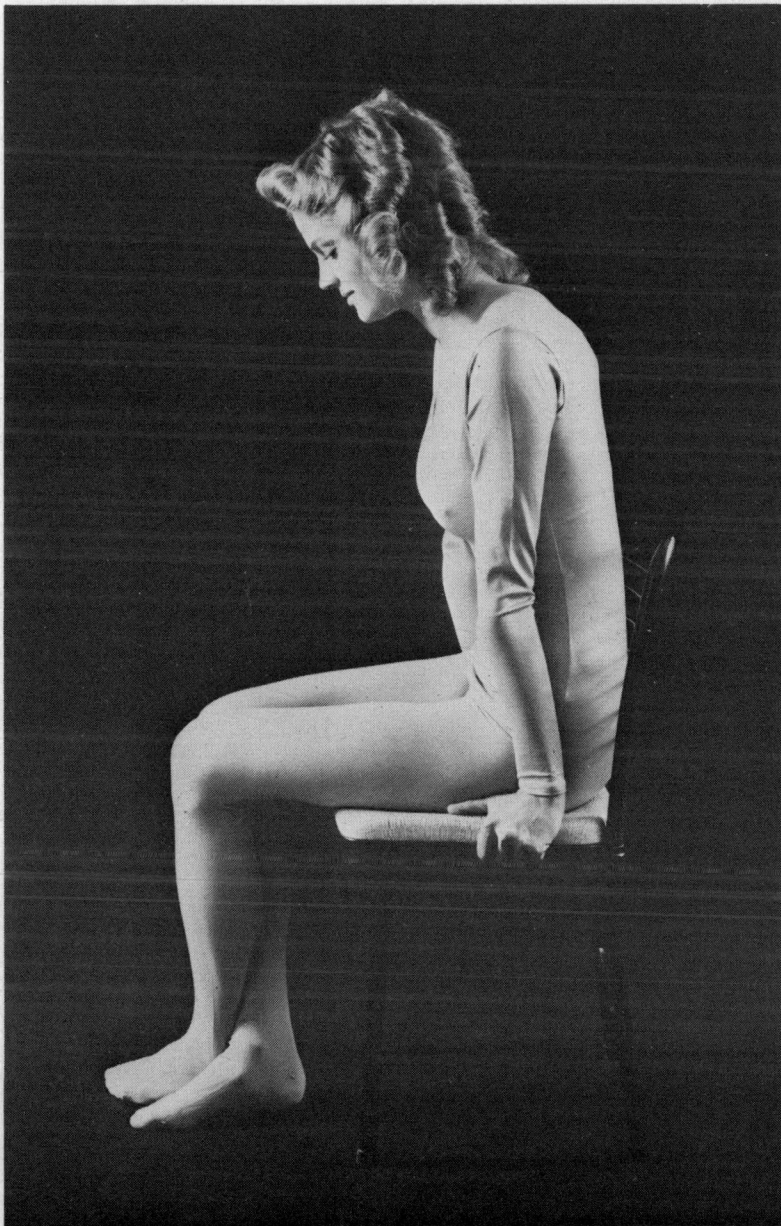

Isotonics *(Calisthenics)*

Perhaps the best approach to building strength using calisthenics is the use of circuit training. With this method you choose a sequence of 6-10 calisthenic exercises for the muscles you wish to strengthen. To begin you determine the maximum number of each exercise that you can do in 1 minute. When you've determined this number, reduce it by one-third for each exercise—e.g., if you can do 21 situps in 1 minute, reduce that number by one-third, which would be 14 situps. Once you've reduced your maximum number for each exercise by one-third, your objective is to complete the "circuit" of exercises in a progessively diminishing amount of time. For example, the first time you try completing all the exercises for the predetermined repetitions, it may take you 7 minutes. The next time you may complete the circuit in 6 minutes, so you add 1 repetition to each exercise. For a good 21-minute workout, you should complete three 7-minute circuits. To impose increased demands, the number of repetitions for each exercise is increased while the time remains the same.

Chinup (arm and shoulder muscles)

1. With chinning bar adjusted to approximately 3 inches beyond extended arm, grasp bar with underhand grip.
2. Flex arms, raising body until chin is over bar.
3. Return to starting position.

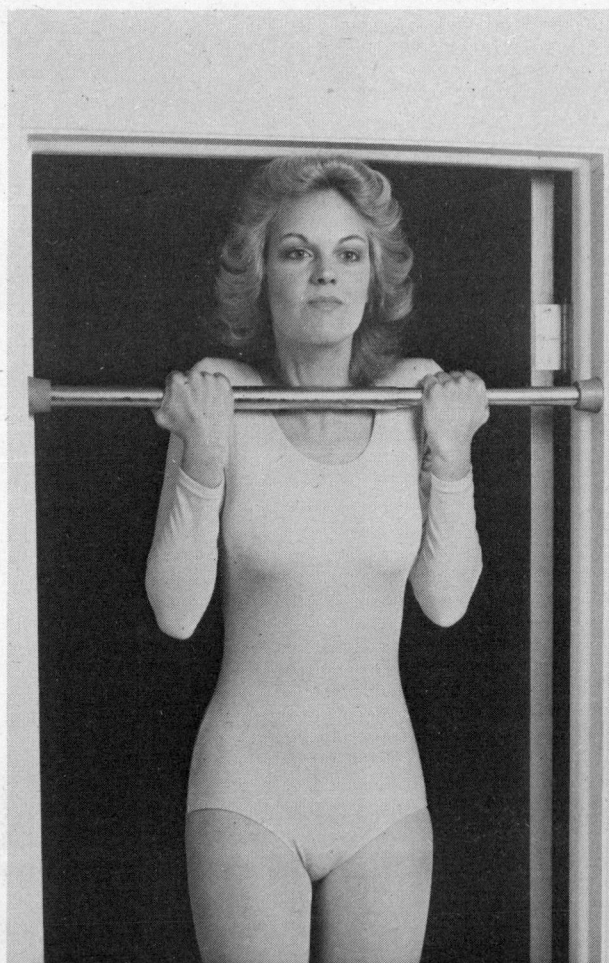

Pushup (arm, shoulder and chest muscles)

1. Lie face down on the floor, legs together, hands on floor under shoulders with fingers pointing straight ahead.
2. Push body off floor by extending arms so that your weight rests on hands and toes.
3. Keeping back straight, lower body until chest touches floor.

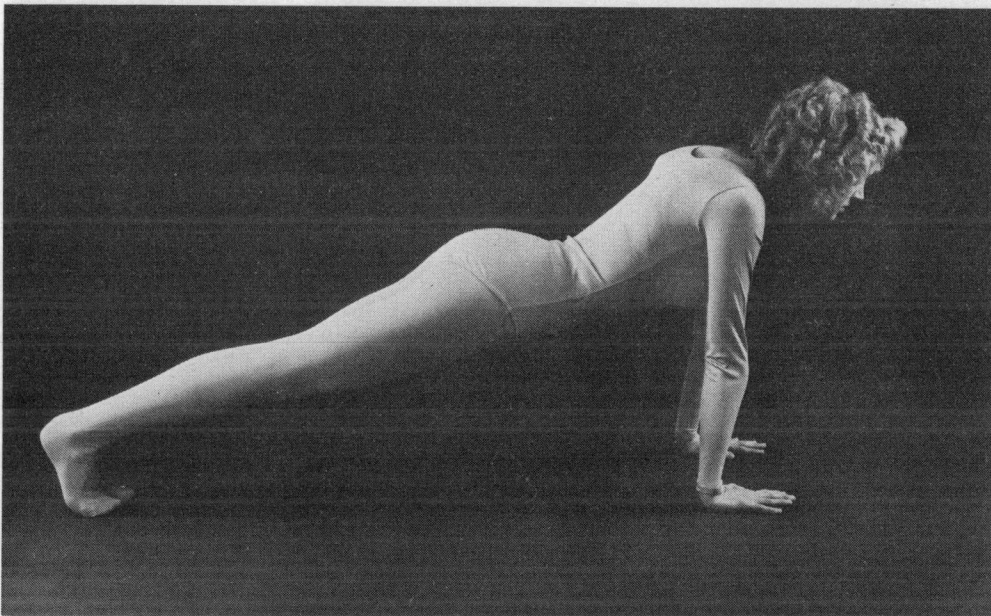

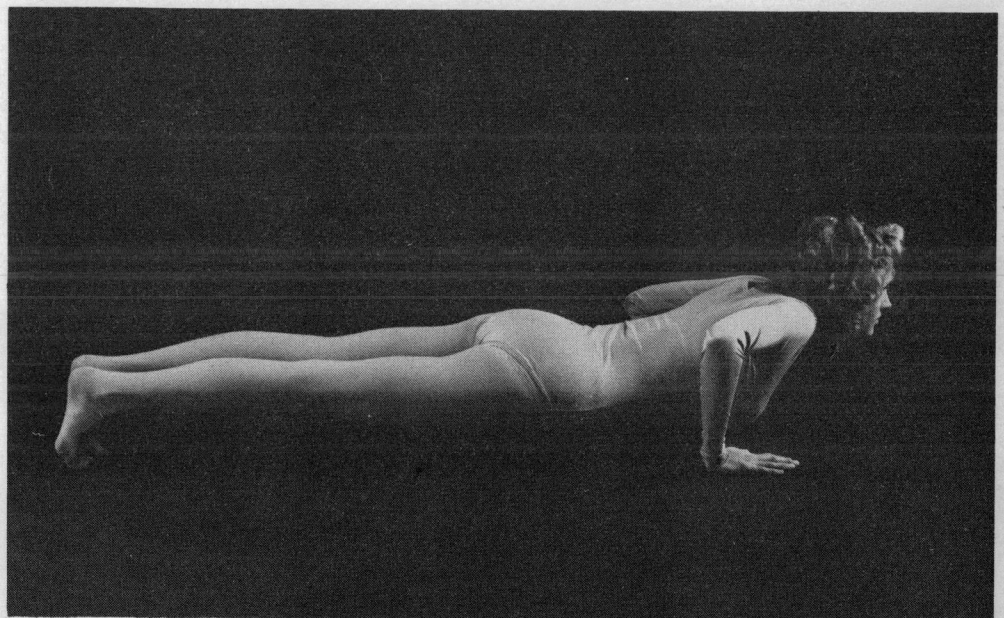

Chair Dip (arm and shoulder muscles)

1. Using a stationary chair, grasp sides of chair, keeping arms straight, sliding feet forward so that your weight rests on your arms.
2. Keeping back straight, lower body as far as possible and return to starting position.

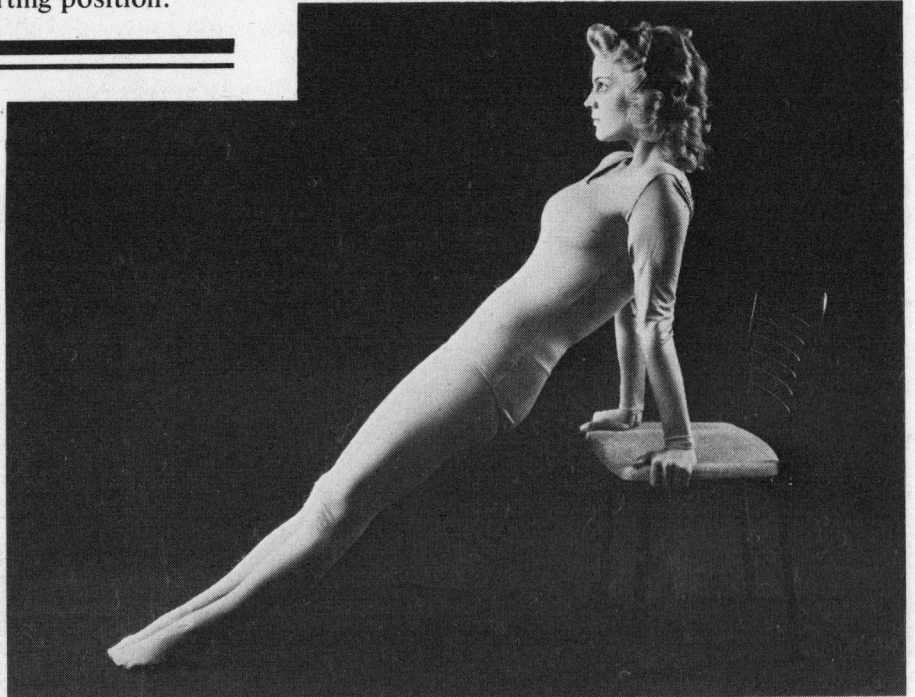

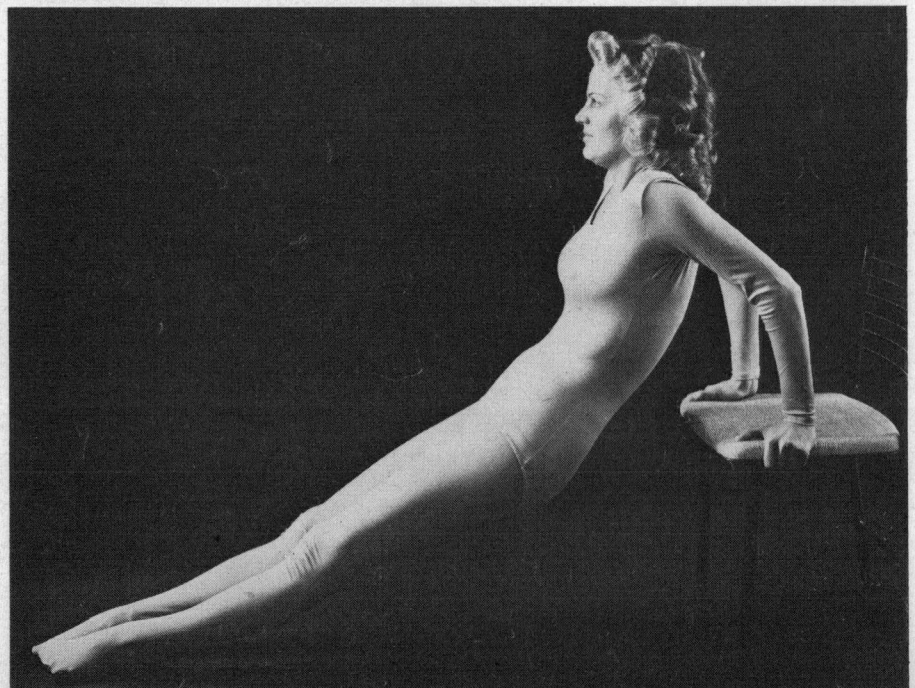

Coffee Grinder (arm, shoulder, lateral trunk muscles)

1. Support body on the floor with extended right hand and right foot with left arm at side.
2. Move feet and body in a circle using right arm as a pivot.
3. Repeat exercise with left arm and foot extended.

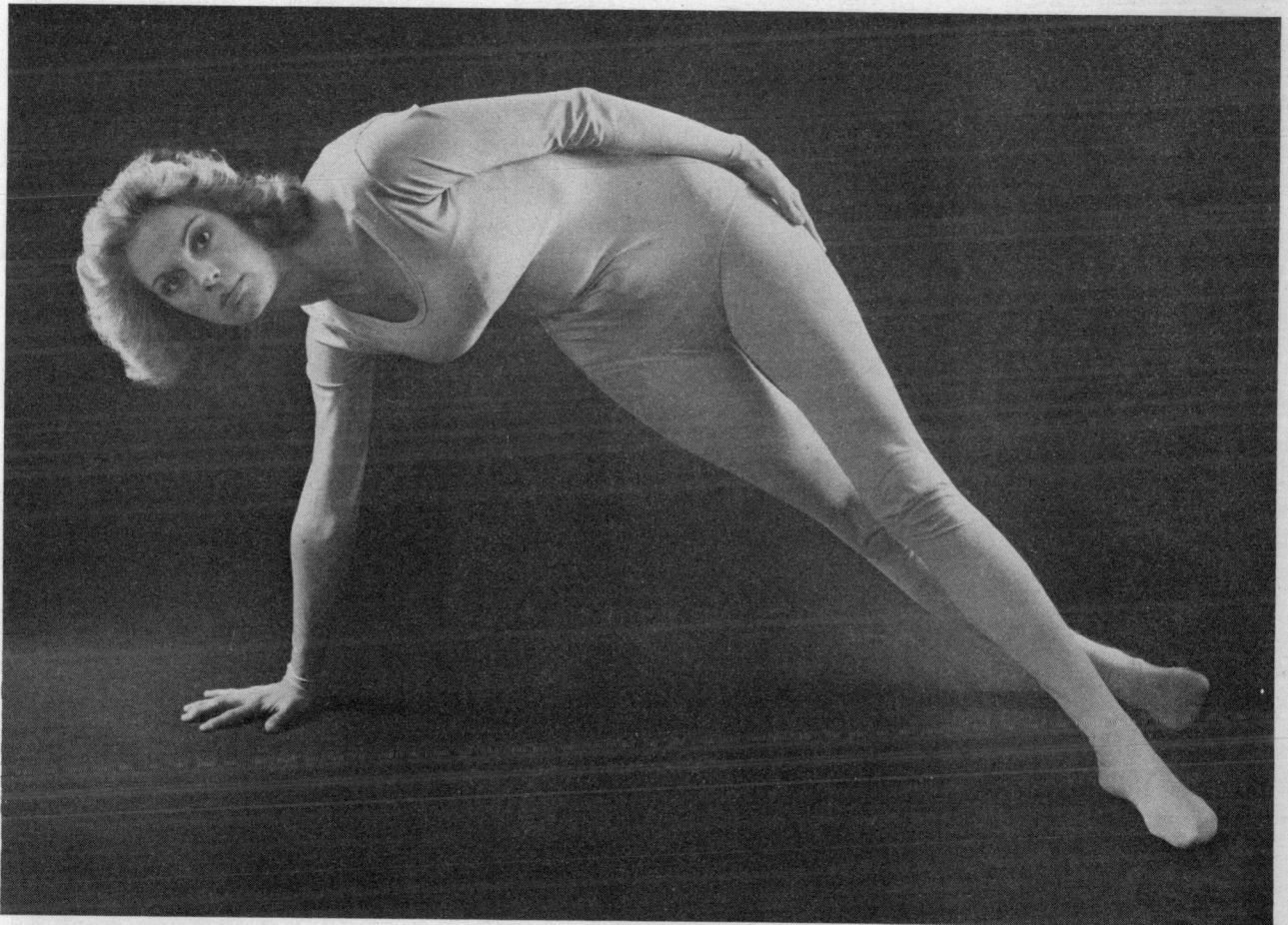

Situp (abdominal muscles)

1. Lie face up on floor with knees bent and fingers laced behind head.
2. Curl up to sitting position, keeping feet flat on floor and touch right elbow to left knee.
3. Return to starting position and repeat, alternating right and left elbow touches.

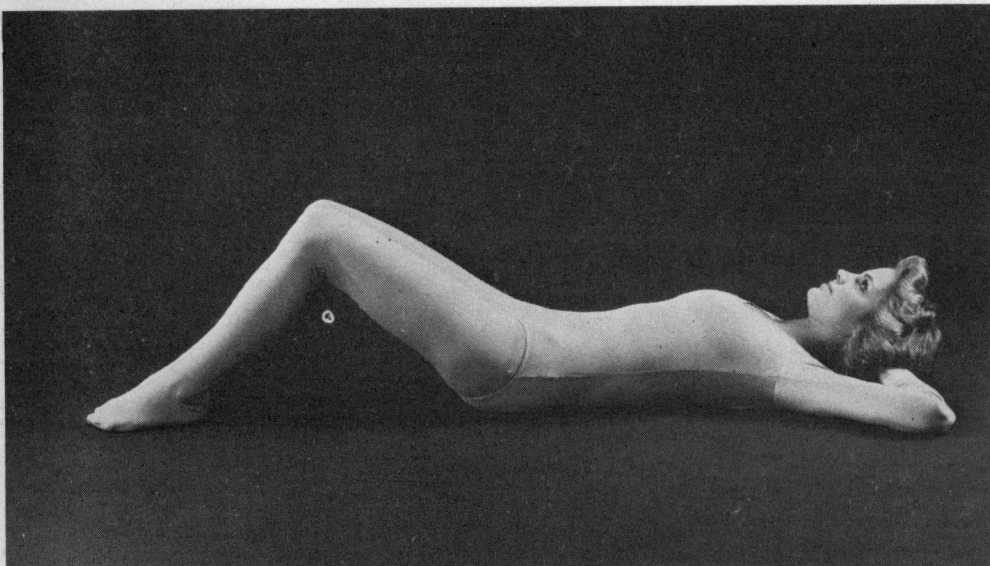

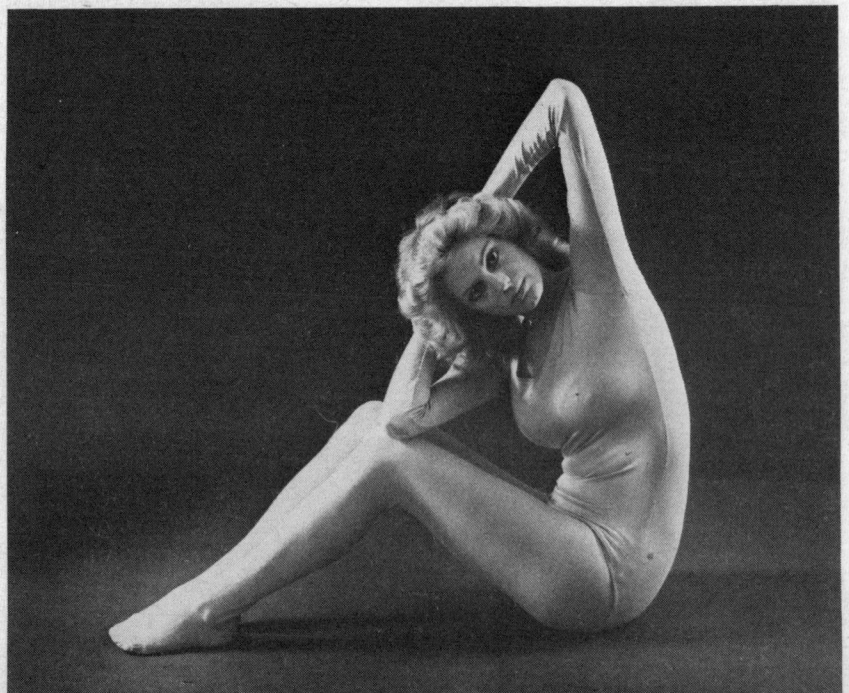

"V" Sit (abdominal muscles)

1. Lie face up on floor, legs straight, arms extended straight behind head.
2. Raise legs and arms up and forward so body forms a "V."
3. Return to starting position.

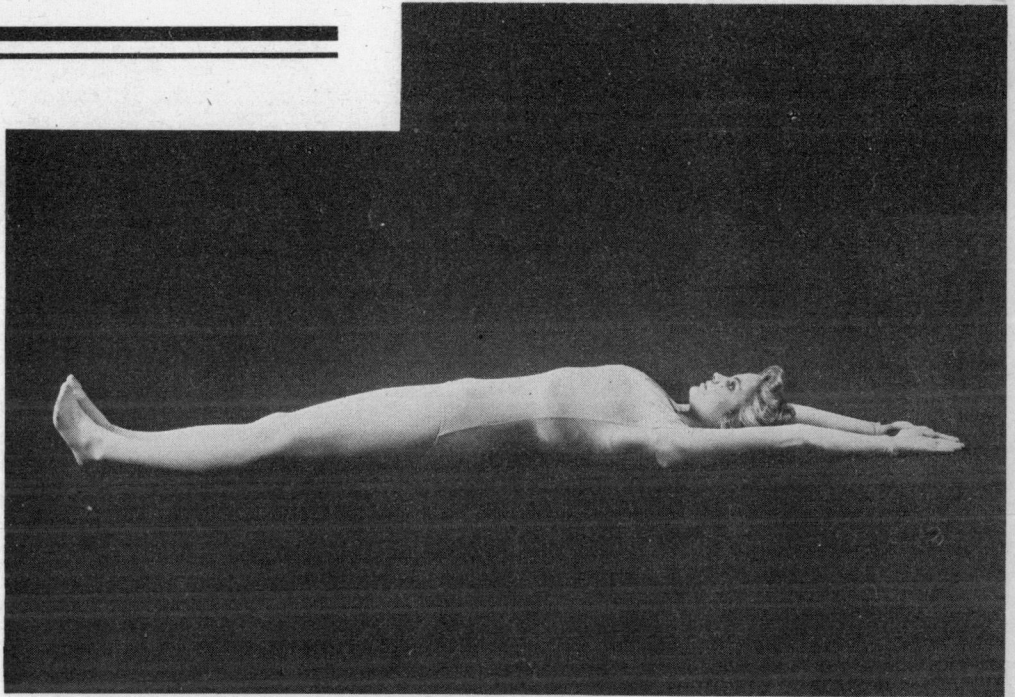

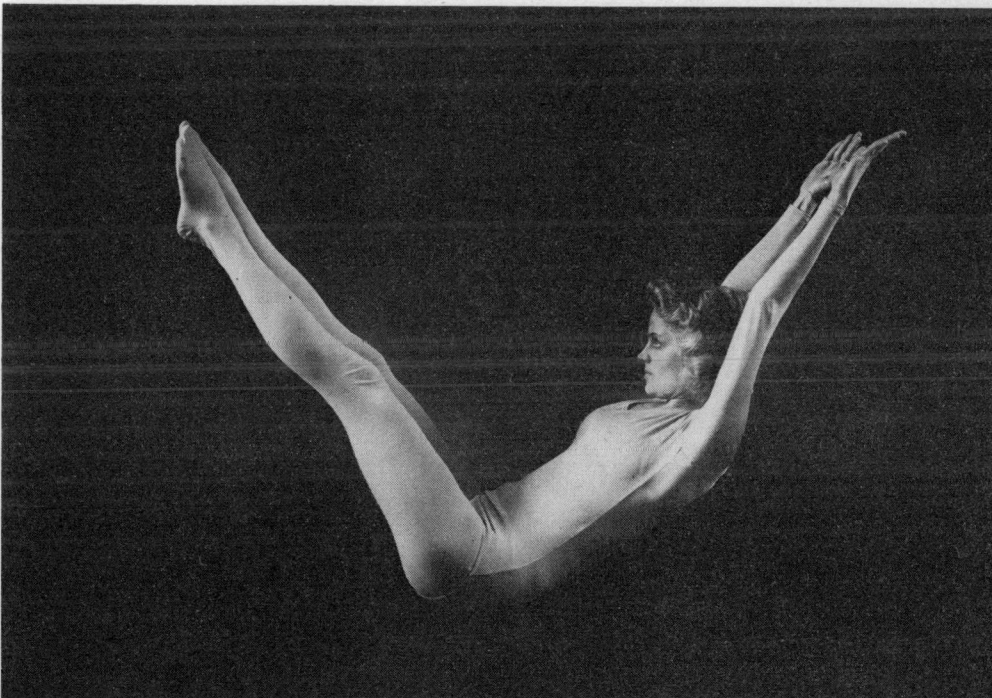

Prone Arch (back muscles)

1. Lie face down on the floor, legs straight, fingers laced behind neck.
2. Arch back, lifting legs and chest off the floor.
3. Extend arms fully forward.
4. Return hands to back of neck.
5. Flatten body to floor.

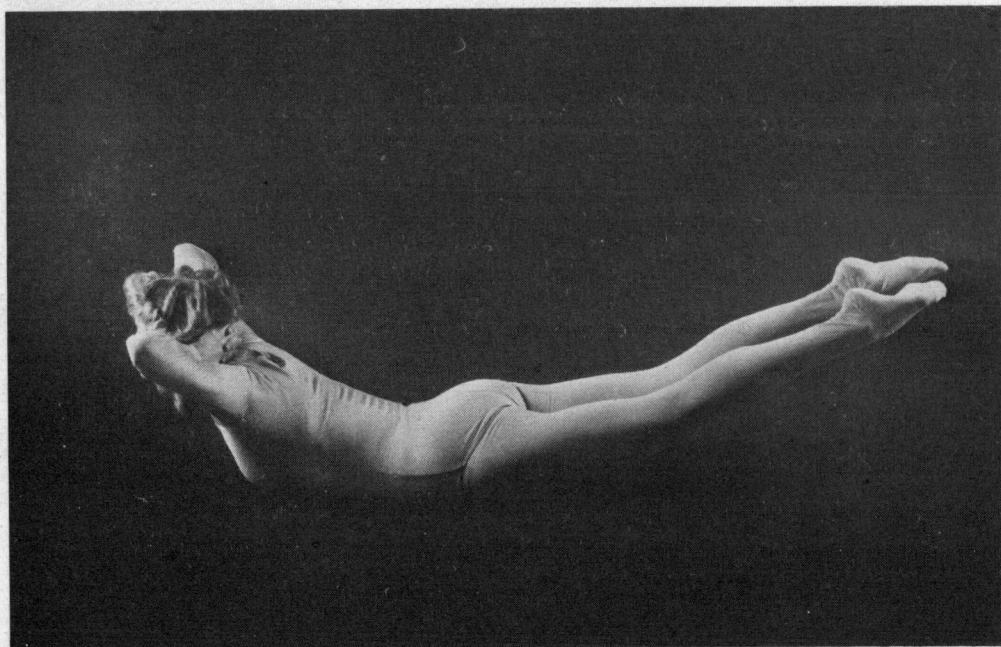

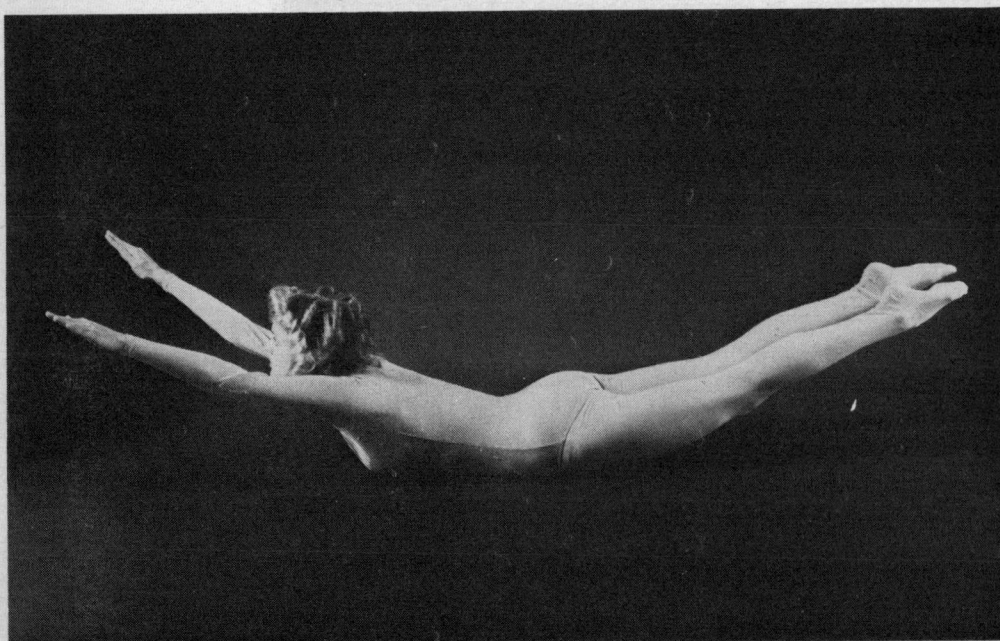

Back Lift (back muscles)

1. Lie face down on the floor, legs tucked under sofa or heavy chair, fingers laced behind neck.
2. Arch back, lifting chest as high off the floor as possible.
3. Return to starting position.

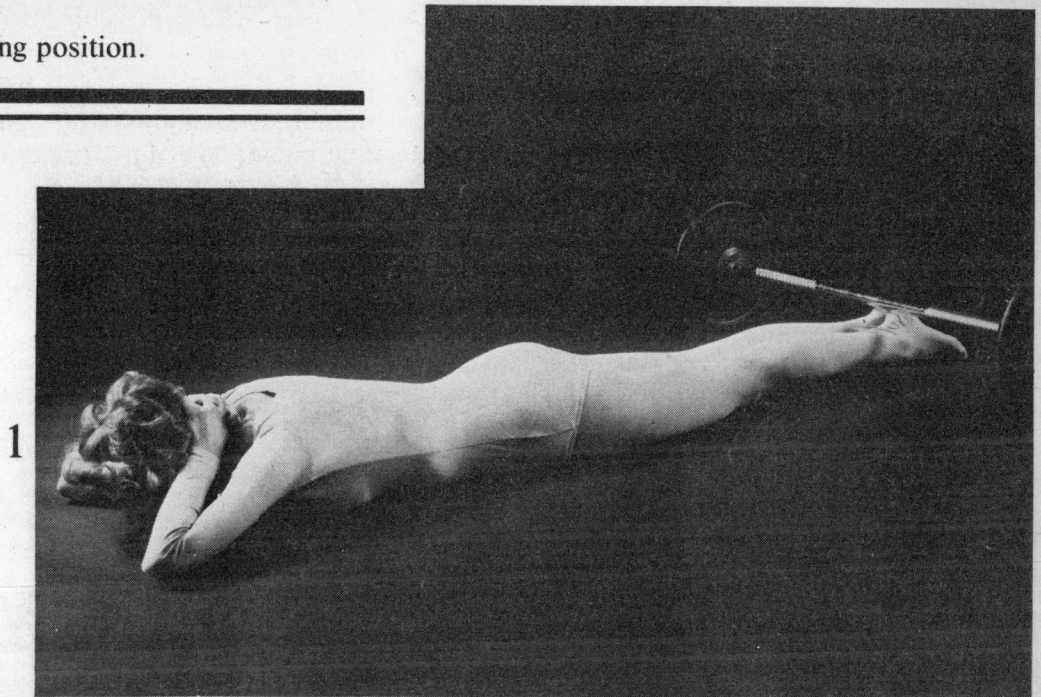

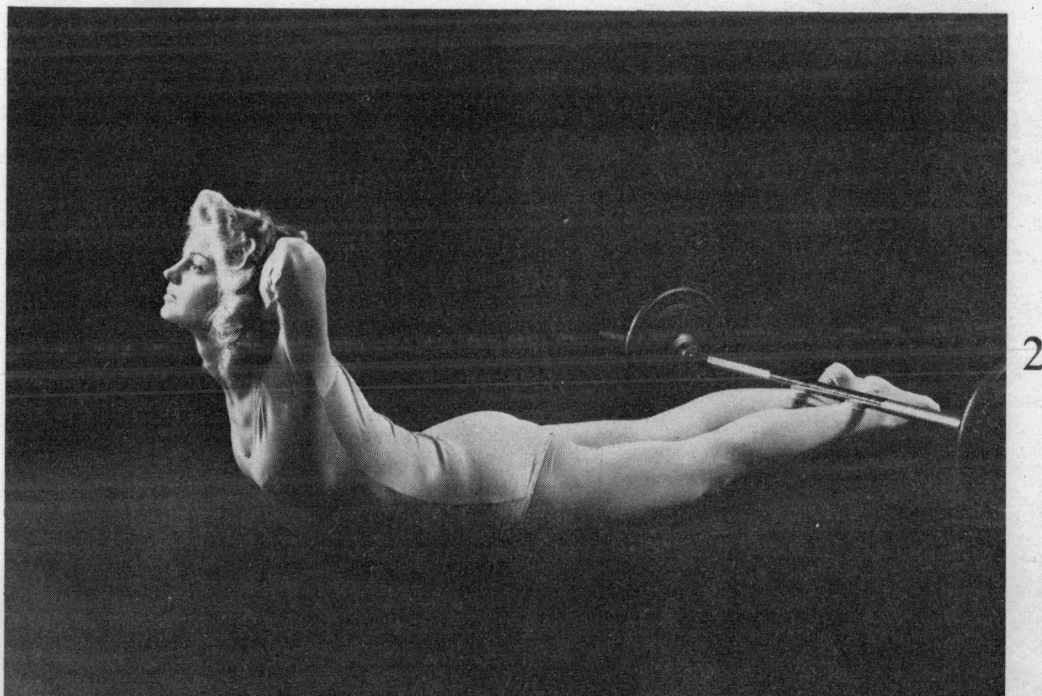

Weight Training

Weight *lifting* is the term used to describe the competitive sport. Weight *training* is a more precise name for exercises used for physical development and conditioning. It is the use of weights combined with the "overload" principle, in which intensity, load and repetition vary according to the individual program. In weight training, a participant never tries to see how much he can lift. Resistance progession is the procedure.

Equipment for weight training exercises includes the use of a weight rack, weight bench, slant board, barbells, dumbbells and a set of variable progressive weights. Barbells are probably the most familiar to us since they are used by weight lifters in weight lifting competition. Barbells vary in length from 4-6 feet with weighted plates weighing 1¼, 2½, 5, 10, 25, 50 and 100 pounds. A sturdy bench has many uses in a weight training program. It should be 6 feet long, 10 inches wide and 20 inches high with an attached weight rack. Though available commercially, the bench can be easily constructed using 2x4's and 3/4-inch plywood with some sort of thick rubber matting for padding the top of the bench. The slant board is also available commercially but can also be constructed easily.

Note: Where possible, two exercises for the same muscle or muscle group are given—one exercise utilizing the barbell, the other dumbbells. In this way, both sets of weight equipment are not necessary to perform the exercises in this section.

Weight Loads — Determining the amount of weight you should start training with is a job of trial and error. One rule of thumb is to start with

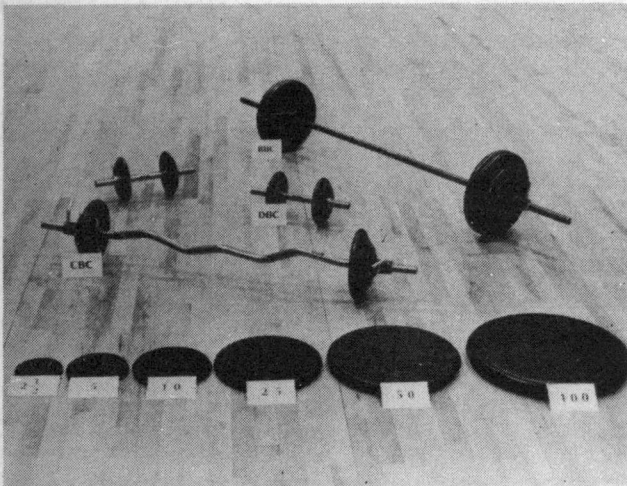

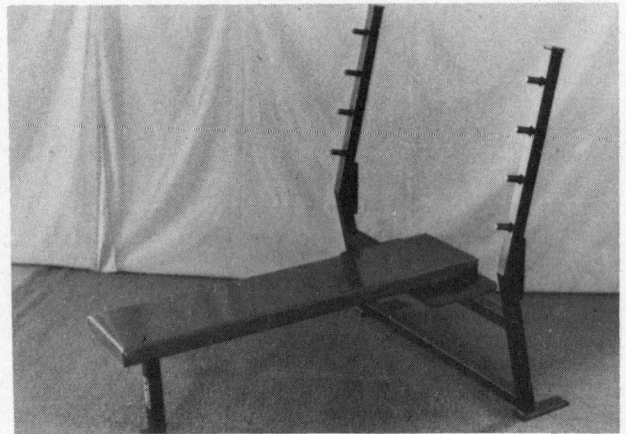

For the weight training exercises you will need some basic equipment. A bench press bench (above) has many uses. The bench should be of heavy-duty construction and approximately 6 feet long, 10 inches wide and 20 inches high. The angled pegs provide support for the barbell with "spotter's" footplates as an additional safety feature. If you can't afford a bench such as this you can easily construct one using 2x4's and ¾-inch plywood with thick rubber matting for padding the bench. (Photos courtesy of Pro-Gym.)

Either a barbell or dumbbells with varied weighted plates (top left) are needed for weight training exercises. Barbells are usually 4 to 6 feet long and together with collars weigh 15 pounds. Standard cast iron weight plates range from 2½ pounds to 100 pounds. Dumbbells with collars weigh approximately 5 pounds each and use weight plates of 1¼, 2½, 5 and 10 pounds.

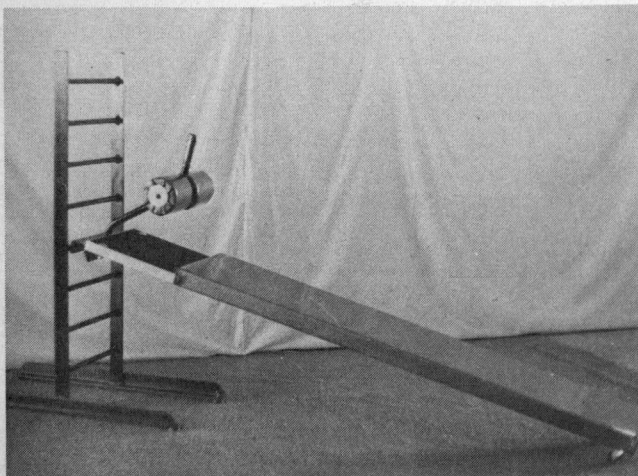

An abdominal board and ladder stand (left) can be used with both the weight training exercises or the calisthenic exercises to increase resistance.

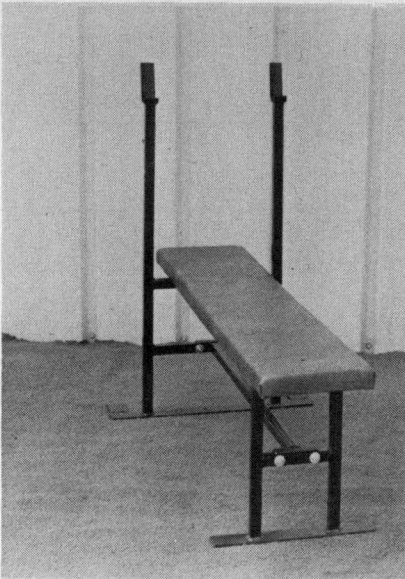

This small weight bench was primarily designed for home use. It comes from Professional Gym, Inc. as four, bolt together, pieces plus the top and has a 250-pound maximum bar and weight plate limit.

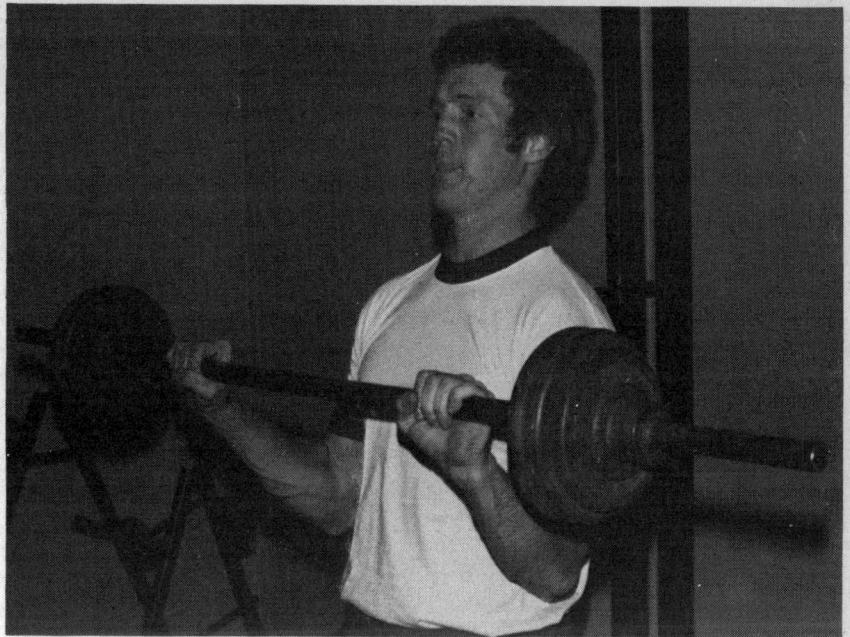

A well chosen sequence of weight exercises, pursued regularly over a period of time, can bring about significant improvement in strength and endurance. Physical condition, posture and appearance can be improved, body measurements reapportioned and sagging body contours firmed up. Weight training is particularly worthwhile in helping the physically underdeveloped person because the regimen and goals can be easily adapted to individual needs and capacities. Even the weakest and smallest individual can be challenged to improve. Progress is obvious in a relatively short time and is satisfying and stimulating to further effort.

10 pounds less than you think you can lift. A better way is to systematically test each muscle group by the trial and error method. As mentioned previously, for maximum strength gain, no less than six and no more than 10 repetitions should be done for each exercise. To determine the correct weight load to start out with, you must experiment for each muscle group to find out the amount of weight which allows the repetitions to remain within that range. For example, to test your biceps, you attempt to do six to 10 bicep curls with a 50-pound weight. If you can complete only five curls, you must reduce the weight by 20 percent or 10 pounds and try the test again. If, on the second test, you completed eight curls, then that is the weight you should start out with. If, for the first test, you could do 12 bicep curls with the 50-pound weight, then the weight is too light and should be increased by 20 percent or 10 pounds. Although this may seem time consuming, resist the temptation to "see how much I can lift." This trial and error method will allow you to determine *safely* the amount of weight that will afford you the greatest gains in strength development and will keep you safe from muscle or joint strains which could result from lifting more than your body can handle. Remember that each joint and muscle group in your body has its own specific weight tolerances—so a weight amount for one muscle group is not applicable to another.

Principles and Safety Factors — The following principles and safety factors should be implemented in any weight training program.

1. Never hold your breath during a lift. This can cause an increase in blood pressure, overwork the heart and restrict the return of blood to the heart and arteries. Exhale during the lift and inhale as the weight is lowered.
2. When lifting heavy weight loads, work with a companion or "spotter" who is ready to assist in case anything should go wrong.

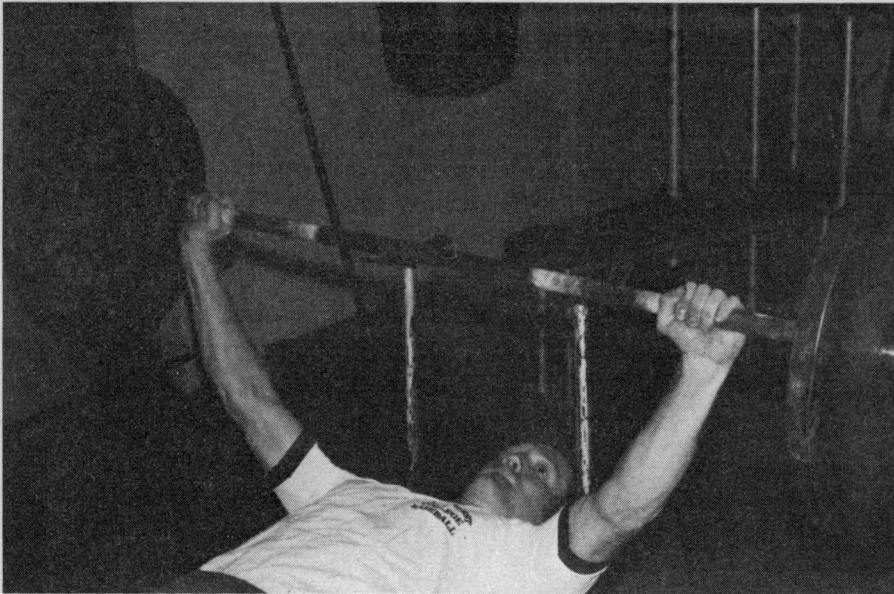

The Bench Press strengthens the muscles of the arms and chest. Before you assume this position, the barbell should be placed on the weight bench racks. With the barbell in the racks, you lie face up on the weight bench with feet on the floor astride the bench. Using the overhand grip, grasp the bar wider than shoulder width apart. Raise barbell by fully extending arms and then lower bar to your chest. Press bar back up to starting position. You should inhale when lowering and exhale while pressing the weight.

3. The starting poundage should not cause any undue strain. As previously advised, use the trial and error system for determining starting weight loads and progress to heavier loads.

4. Each exercise should be performed rhythmically and through the full range of joint motion for the joint being exercised. (For some of the weight lifting exercises, it is not possible to perform the exercise through the full range of joint motion. Flexibility exercises should be done to maintain mobility in the joint.) Performing exercises with weights in a jerky fashion can be dangerous, resulting in joint or muscle injury.

5. A weight training session should be preceded by a warm-up and followed by a cooling-off period.

6. Check your equipment before lifting. A loose collar could result in weight plates falling off and injury to the lifter.

7. *NEVER* attempt to dead lift weights off the floor with knees locked in the extended position and the trunk of your body at a 90-degree angle to the floor. This is almost certain injury to your back. The proper stance is with feet parallel and shoulder width apart, your toes as close to the bar as possible, your hips lowered by flexing the knees, the head looking straight forward, and your back straight.

8. If you want to develop power, you do it by reducing the total weight and increasing the speed of the full motion of an exercise. You develop endurance by reducing the total weight and doing the exercise more times at a slower speed.

9. An alternate day, 3-day-a-week weight training program is all that is necessary for strength development.

Weight Training for Women — One myth surrounding weight training is that a woman who lifts weights for strength development and physique improvement will acquire the large musculature of a man. This is simply not true. It is physically impossible for a woman to develop muscle masses comparable to those of a man. First of all, women lack enough of the hormone androgen, which is the primary factor responsible for the male's muscles' massive response to weight training. Secondly, a woman's muscles are surrounded by much more adipose tissue (fat) than those of a man. When a man trains with weights, the amount of fat between the skin and the muscle rapidly disappears with the skin stretched tightly, exposing the large muscle. When a woman trains with weights, a small percentage of this same adipose disappears but enough remains so the muscle is not exposed. Finally, a woman's muscles are much smaller than a man's, thus no amount of weight training is going to make a woman muscle-bound. So women who were going to skip over this portion of the book—don't. Working with weights will do wonders for your muscle tone and body shape.

Situp (abdominal muscles)
   Equipment: dumbbell or weight plate

1. Lie face up on the floor, feet tucked under a couch or heavy chair, knees flexed, hands holding a dumbbell or weight plate behind neck.
2. Curl up into sitting position, touching elbows to knees.
3. Return to starting position to repeat.
Note: For increased resistance without weight change, do this same exercise on a slant board with toes strapped to top of board and head at bottom.

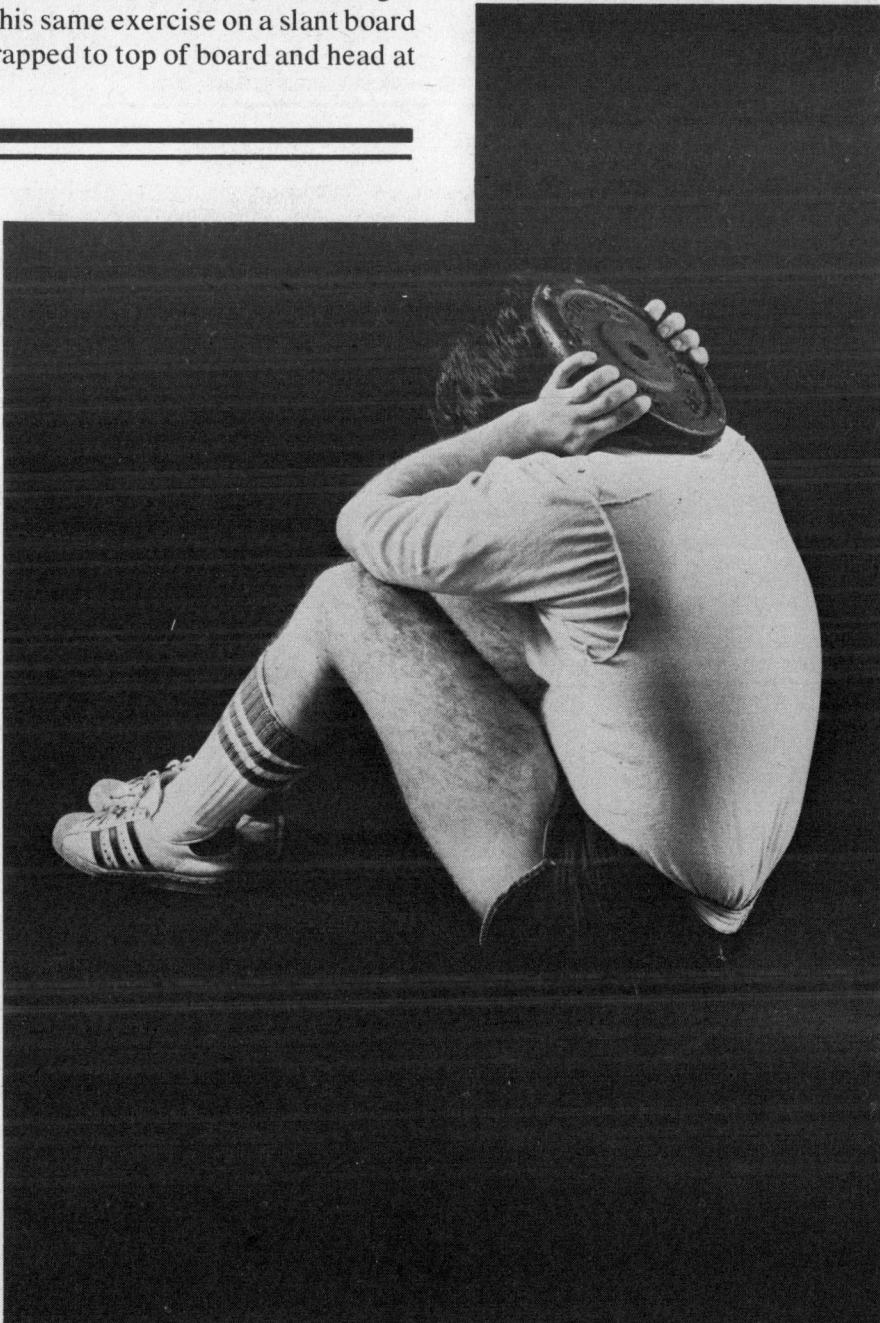

Trunk Raise (lower back, hip and thigh muscles)
Equipment: dumbbell or weight plate and weight bench or table.

1. Lie face down on the bench or table with upper torso extending over the end of the bench, head toward floor. Strap ankles to bench. Hands hold the dumbbell or weight plate behind the neck.
2. Lift upper body to parallel position with the floor but no higher.
3. Return to starting position to repeat.

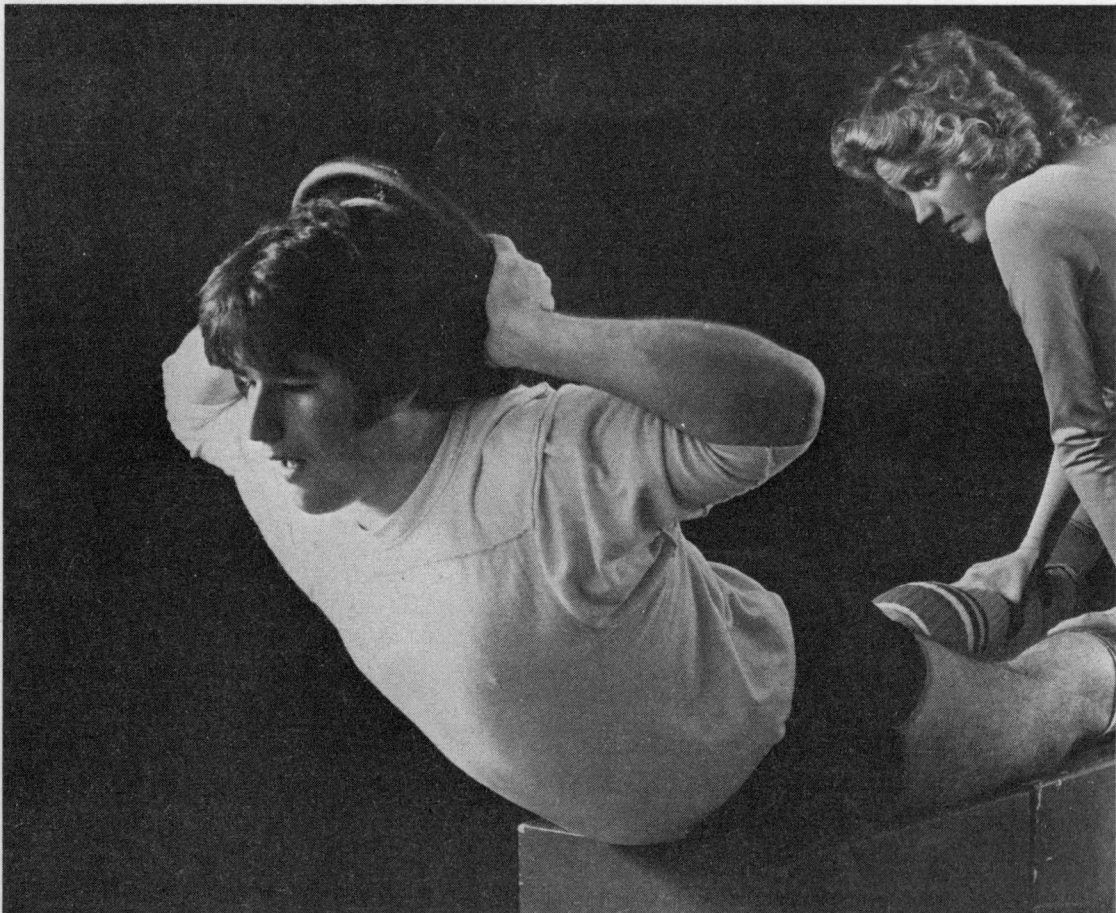

Heel Raise (calf muscles)

> Equipment: barbell with towel wrapped around bar, block of wood 2 inches thick, barbell racks or spotter.

1. Stand with toweled portion of barbell against back of neck, hands gripping bar in overhand grip, knees flexed, feet 6-10 inches apart, toes on block of wood.
2. Straighten knees and lift heels as high as possible above block of wood.
3. Return heels to floor.

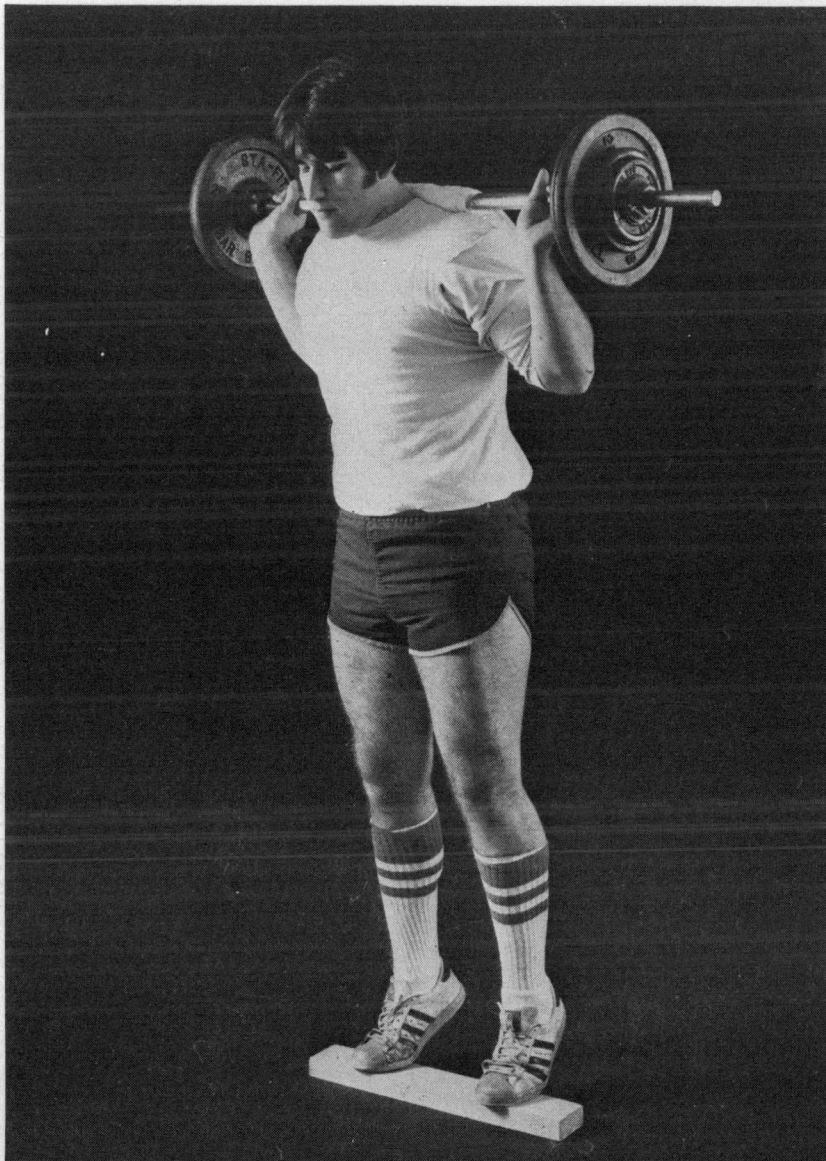

Half Knee Bends (hip, ankle and thigh muscles)
Equipment: barbell with towel wrapped around bar, block of wood 2 inches thick, barbell racks or spotter

1. Stand with toweled portion of barbell against back of neck, hands gripping bar in overhand grip, knees flexed, feet 8-10 inches apart, toes on floor, heels on block of wood.
2. Squat slightly as shown but no further because of possible injury to knee joint.
3. Return to starting position to repeat.

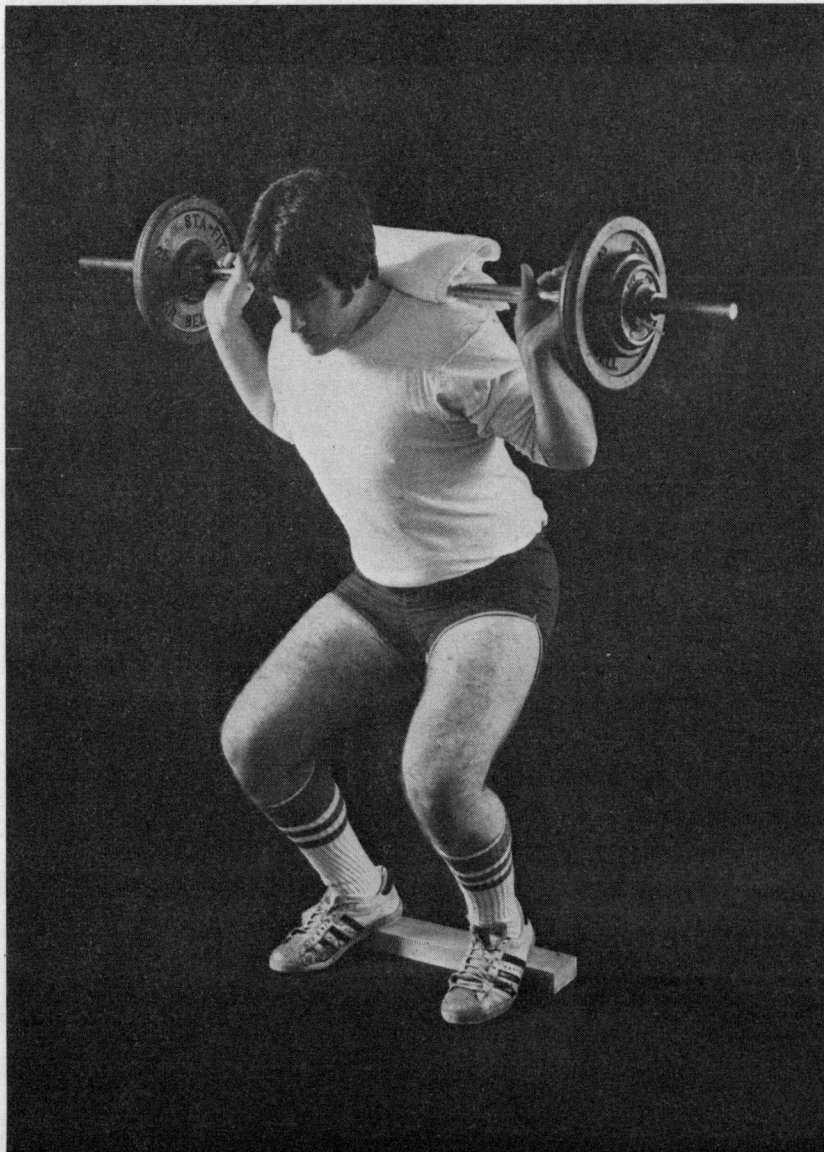

Squat Stand (hip, ankle and thigh muscles)
   Equipment: barbell

1. Stand straddling barbell with barbell at 90-degree angle to body.
2. Bend at knees and waist, keeping back straight and grip barbell with one hand at rear and the other at front.
3. Straighten knees slowly until fully extended, lifting weight off floor.
4. Bend at the knees to lower barbell but do not let it touch the floor to repeat.

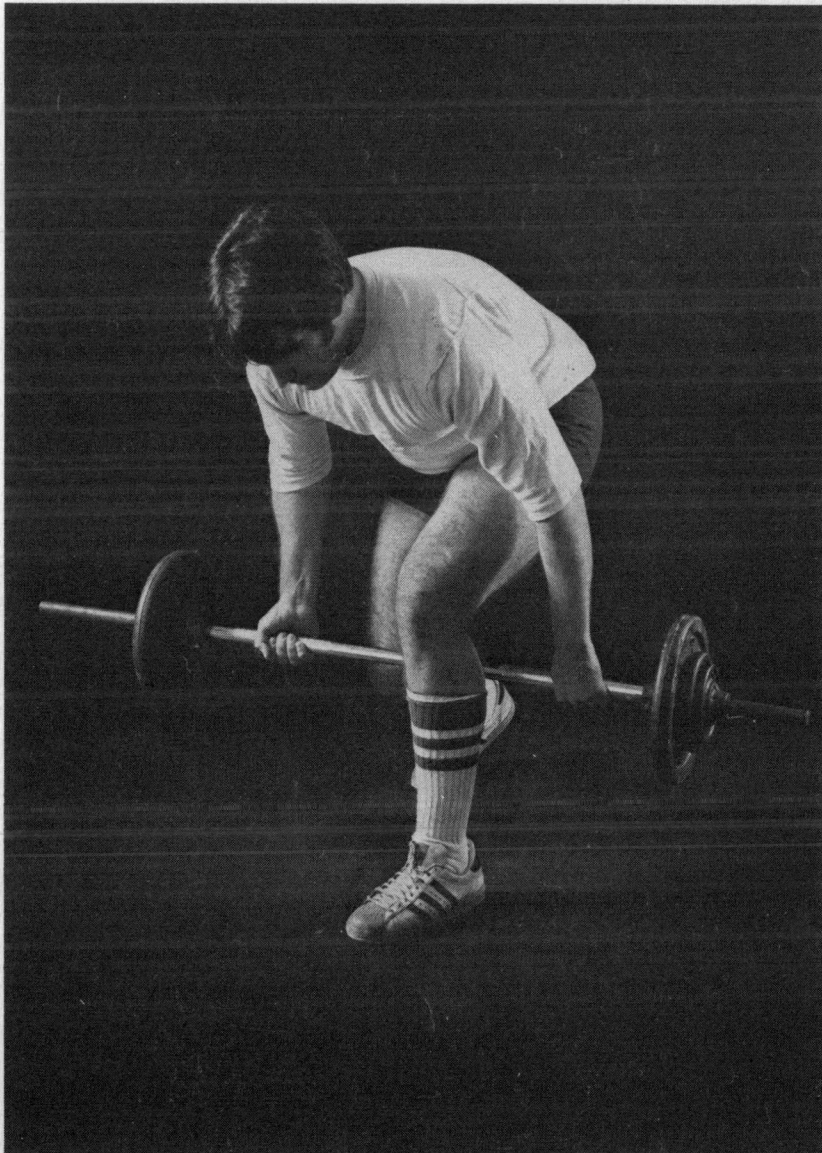

Arm Raise (arm [biceps and deltoids] and chest muscles)

Equipment: weight bench and dumbbells

1. Lie face up on bench with knees over end of bench, feet flat on floor, arms fully extended above body, each hand gripping a dumbbell.
2. Slowly lower arms toward floor as far as possible. (It may be necessary to bend elbows slightly to stabilize elbow joint.)
3. Raise arms slowly to starting position.

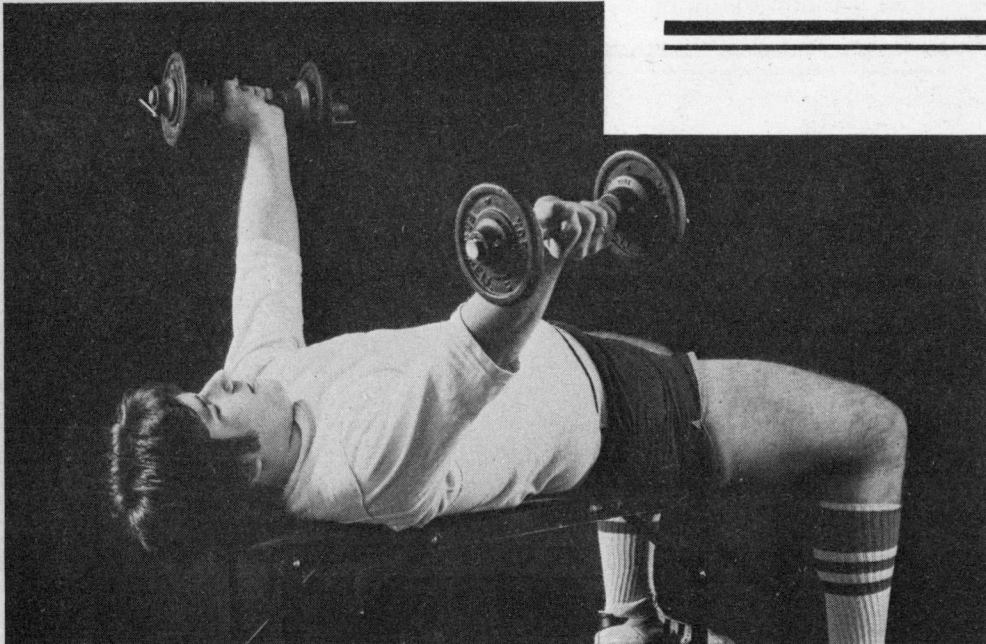

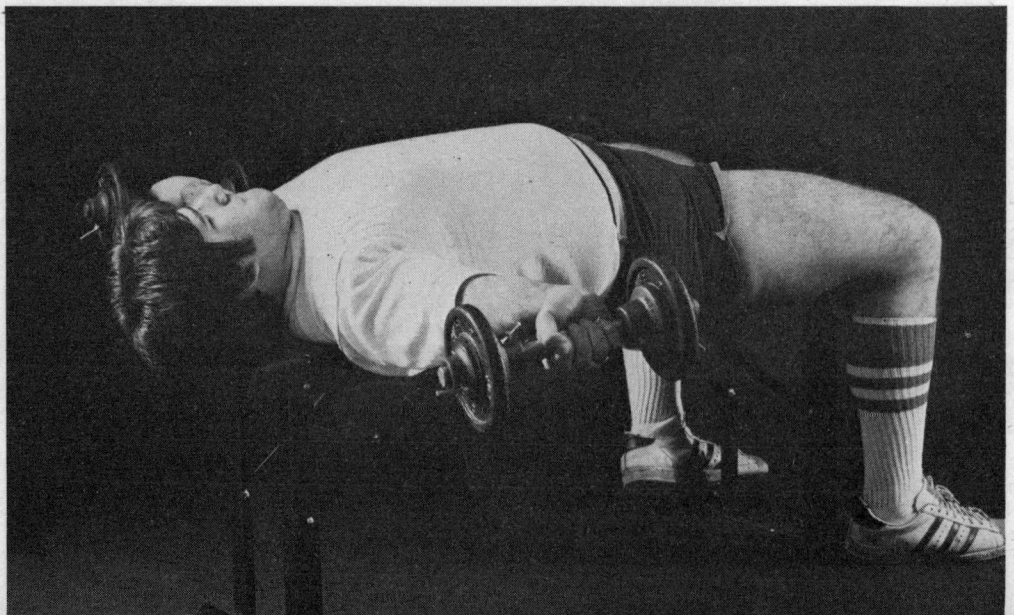

Wing Spreader (upper back muscles)
  Equipment: weight bench and dumbbells

1. Lie face down on bench, hands gripping dumbbells on floor.
2. Raise dumbbells to shoulder height.
3. Lower dumbbells to floor.

Note: This exercise can be done in standing position with feet slightly apart and upper trunk parallel to floor. See picture below.

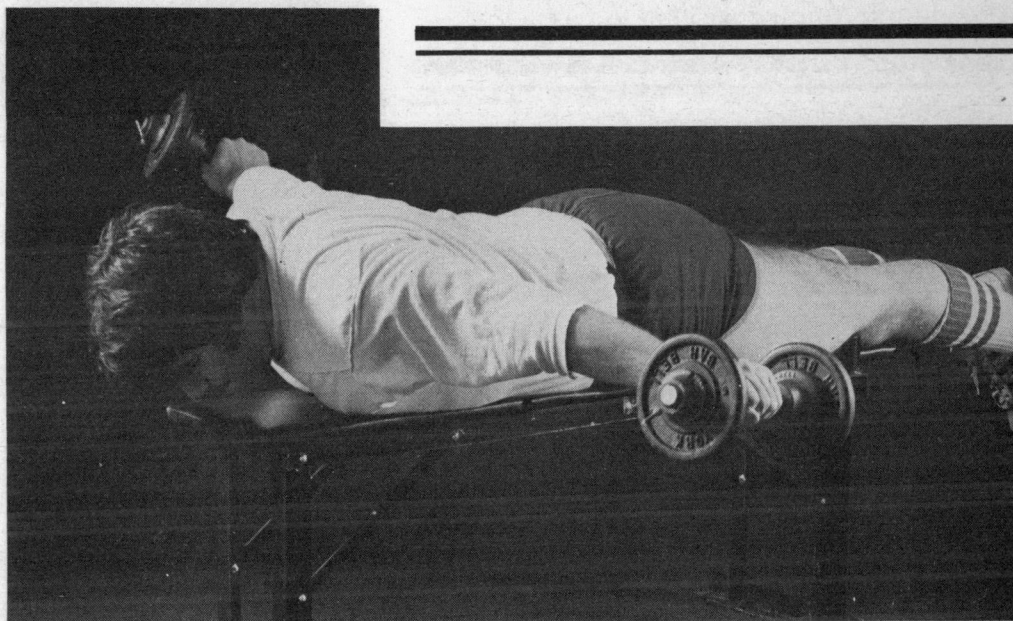

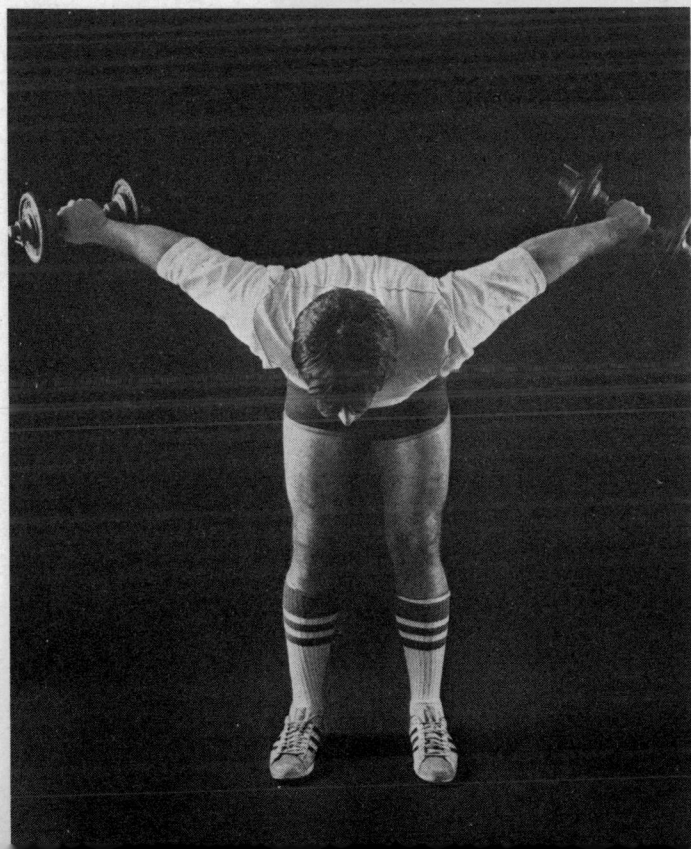

Biceps Curl (bicep muscles)
  Equipment: barbell

1. Stand erect, feet comfortably apart, knees slightly flexed. With arms slightly flexed at elbows, hold barbell in front of you with underhand grip, hands shoulder width apart.
2. Flex elbows fully, lifting bar to chest, keeping elbows close to sides. (*Don't* lean backward or "bounce" bar with leg motion.)
3. Return to starting position to repeat.

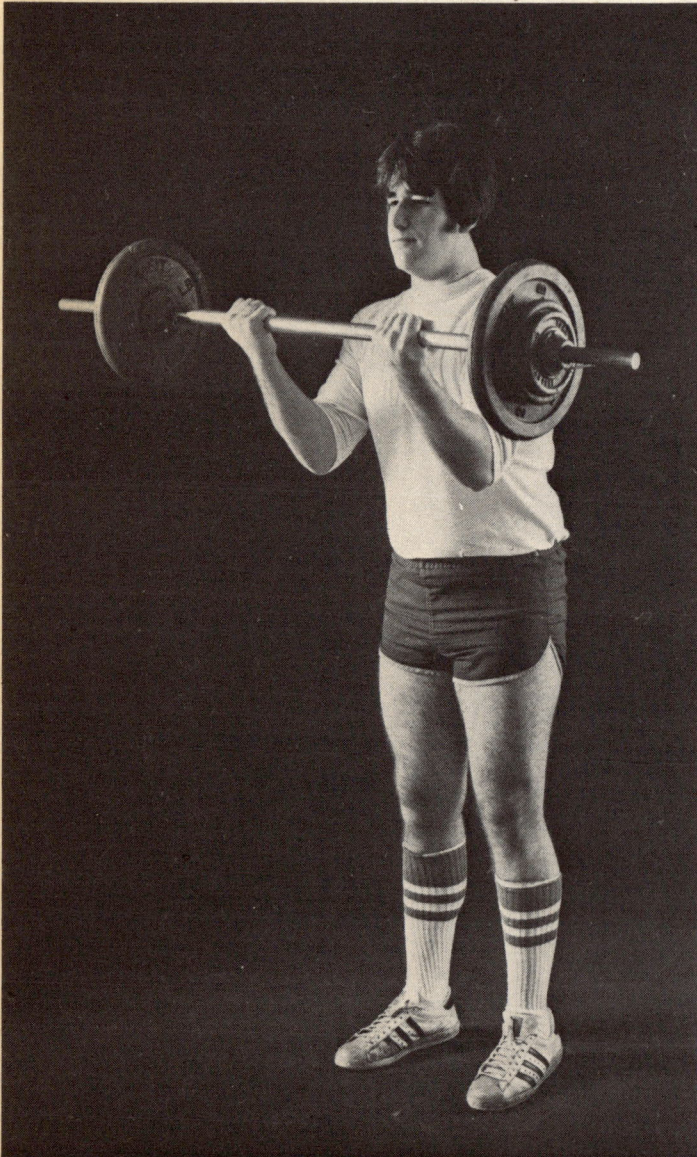

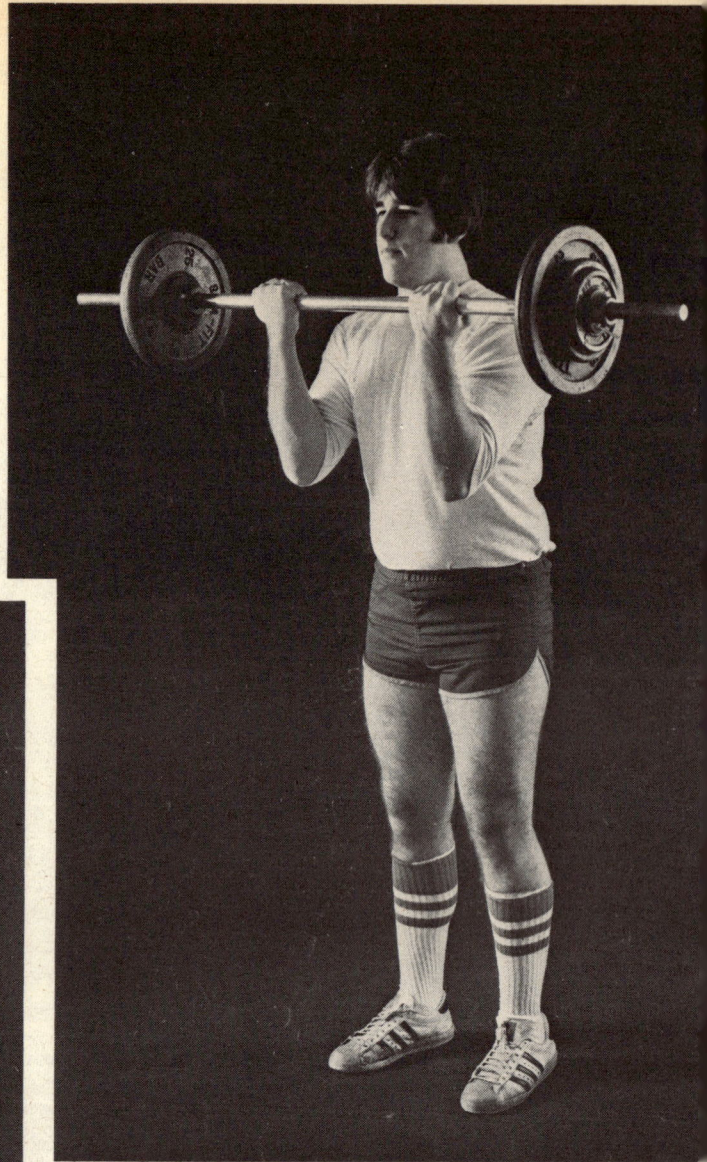

2

1

Triceps Extension (tricep muscles)
  Equipment: weight bench and barbells

1. Sit astride bench with back straight, hands gripping bar in overhand grip.
2. Raise bar to full arm extension above head.
3. Lower bar behind head, by bending elbows.
4. Raise arms to full arm extension to repeat.

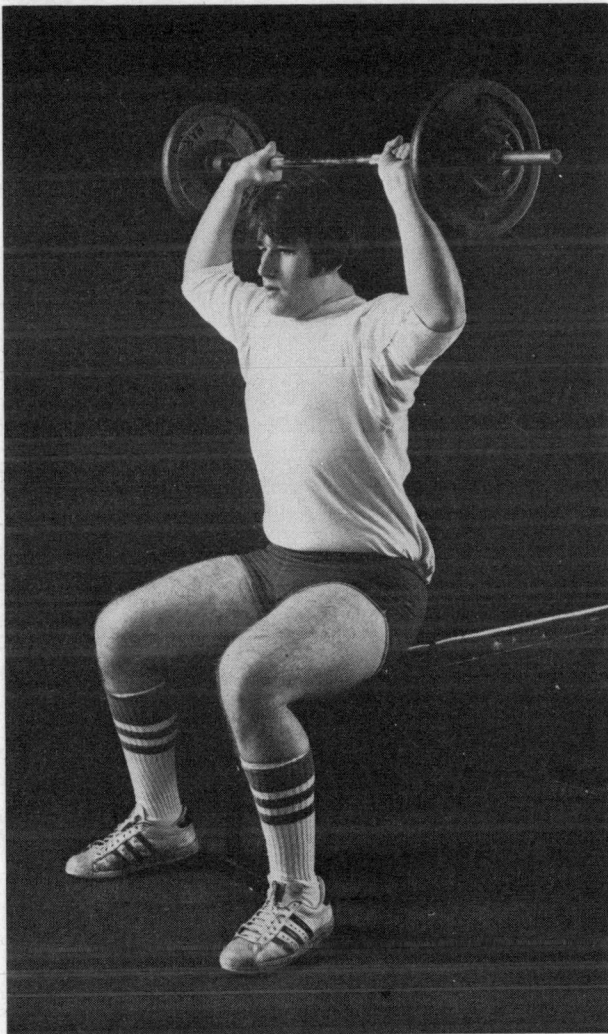

3

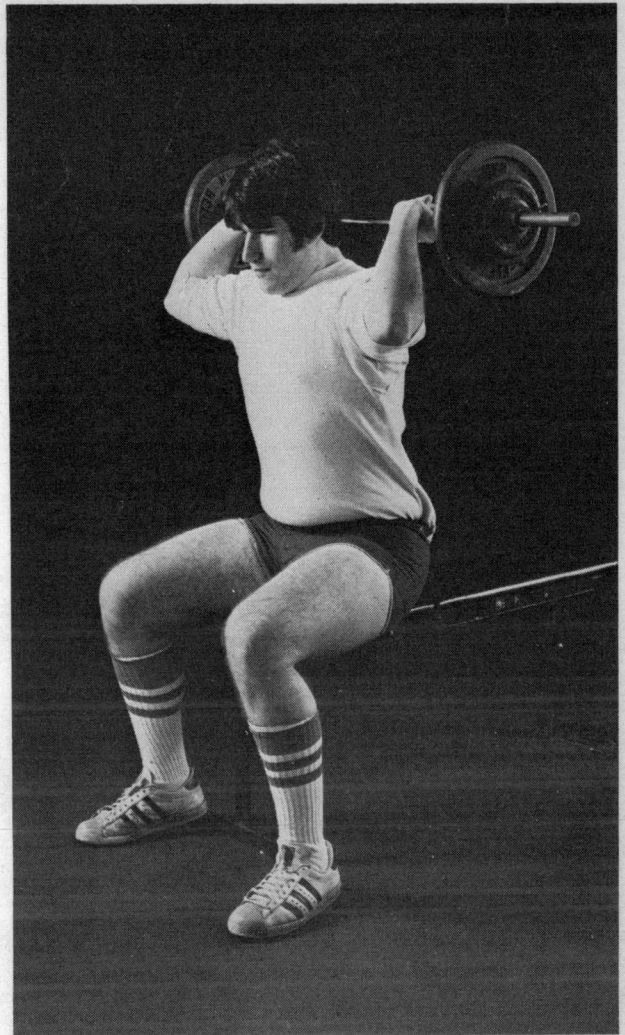

2

Overhead Arm Raise (tricep muscles)
  Equipment: dumbbells

1. Stand erect, feet comfortably apart, arm straight overhead, gripping dumbbell.
2. Lower forearm by bending elbow behind head, keeping upper arm stationary.
3. Raise arm to full extension to repeat.
4. Repeat exercise with opposite arm.

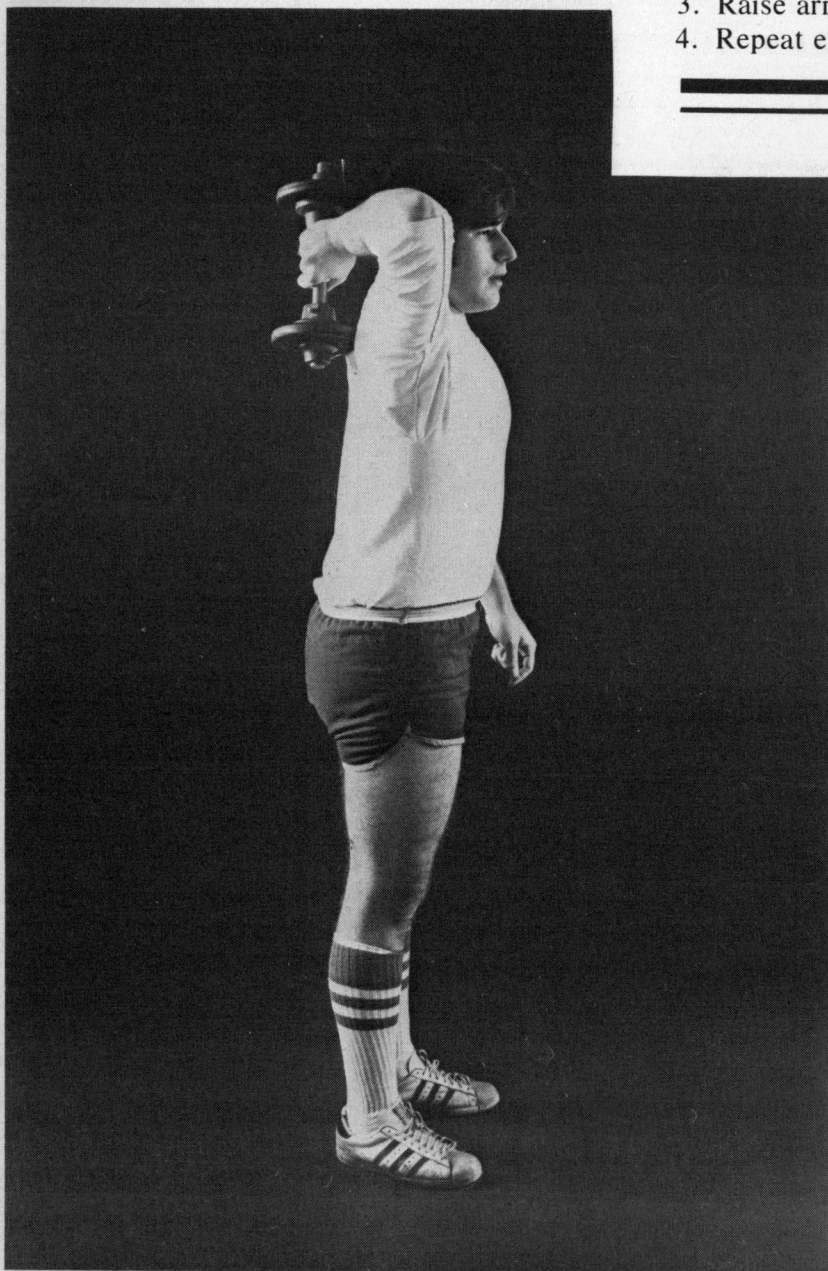

High Pull (shoulder muscles)
   Equipment: barbell

1. Stand erect, feet comfortably apart, hands 2 inches apart gripping barbell in overhand grip, the weight held just below waist.
2. Bend elbows and raise weight straight up to chin level.
3. Return to starting position to repeat.

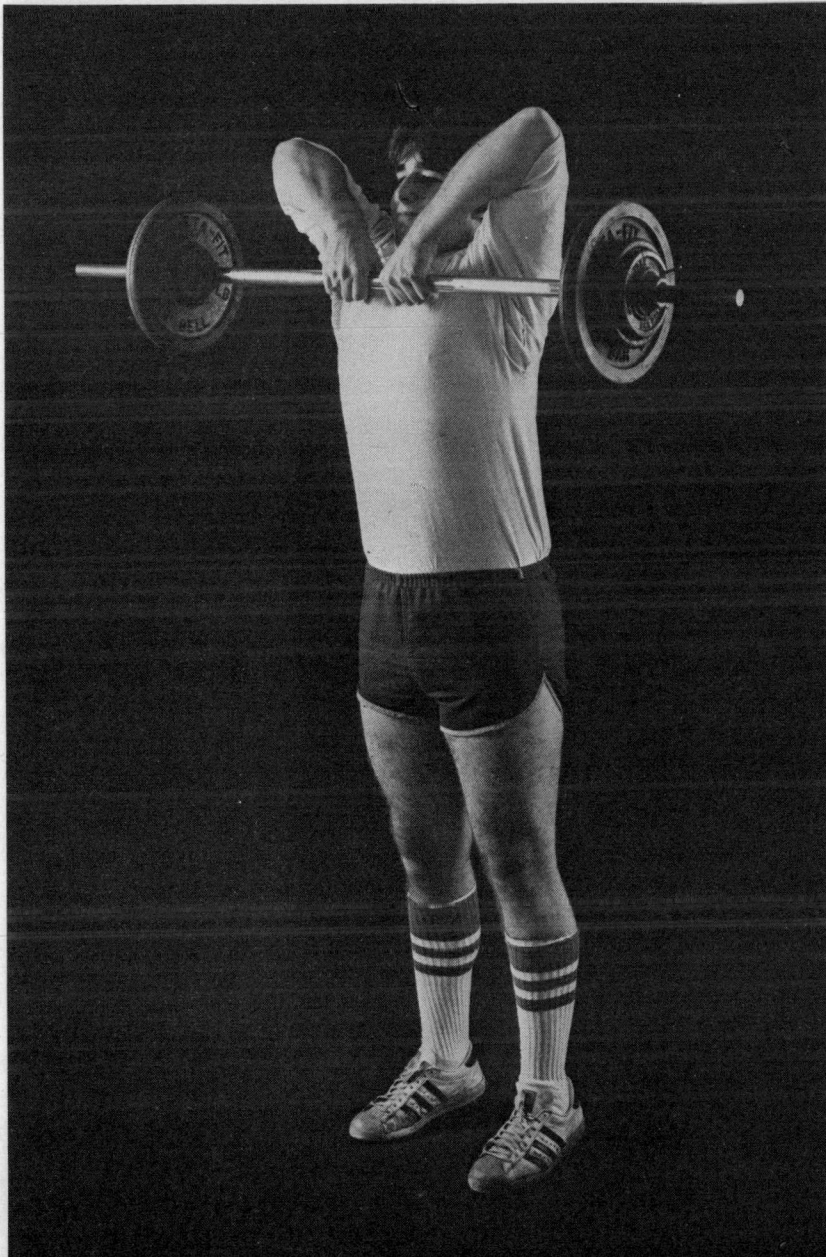

Side Arm Raise (shoulder muscles)
    Equipment: dumbbell

1. Stand erect, feet comfortably apart, hands at sides, each gripping dumbbell in overhand grip.
2. Raise arms laterally to shoulder height, keeping elbows straight.
3. Return to starting position to repeat.

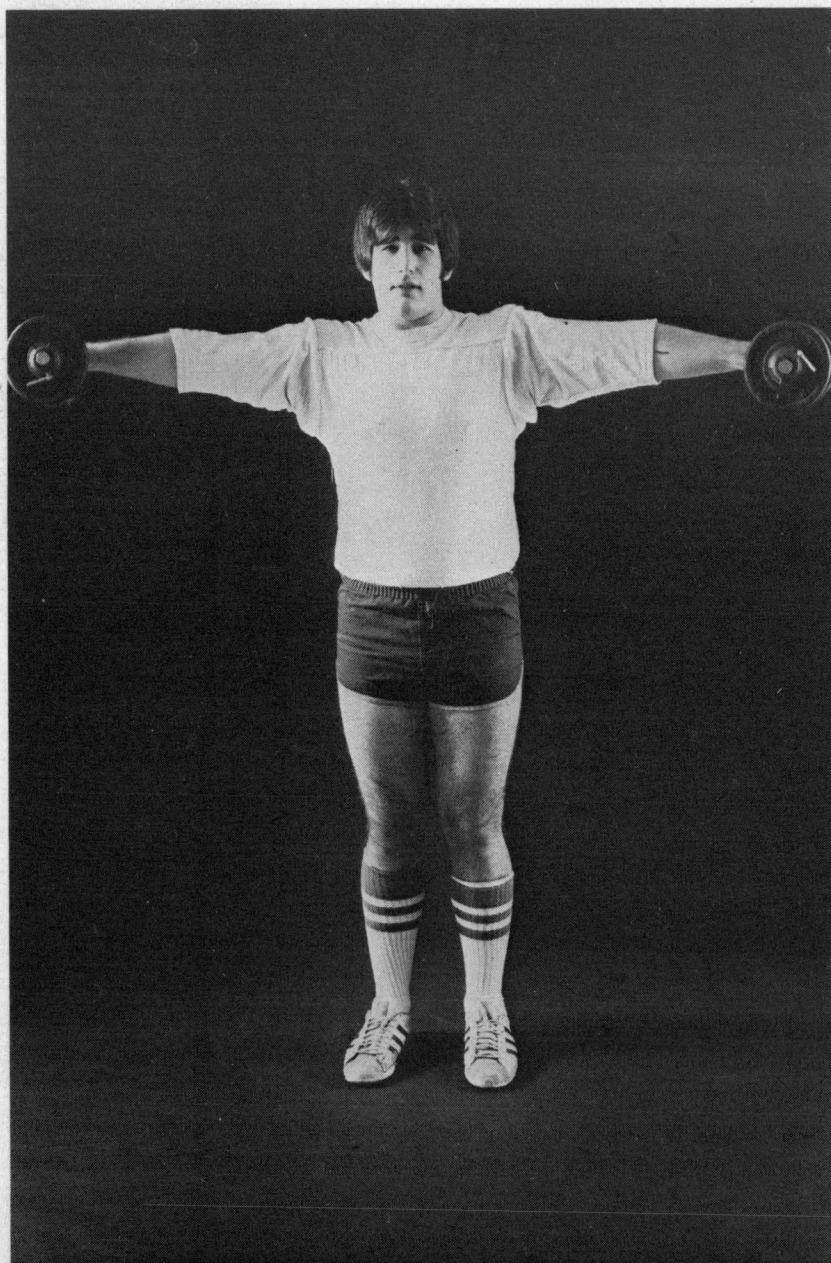

Wrist Curls (forearm muscles)
   Equipment: barbell

1. Sit astride end of weight bench with forearms resting on thighs, hands gripping barbell in underhand grip.
2. Curl wrists upward as far as possible.
3. Extend wrists downward as far as possible.
4. Return to starting position to repeat.

Note: This exercise can be done with dumbbells with each hand gripping dumbbell.

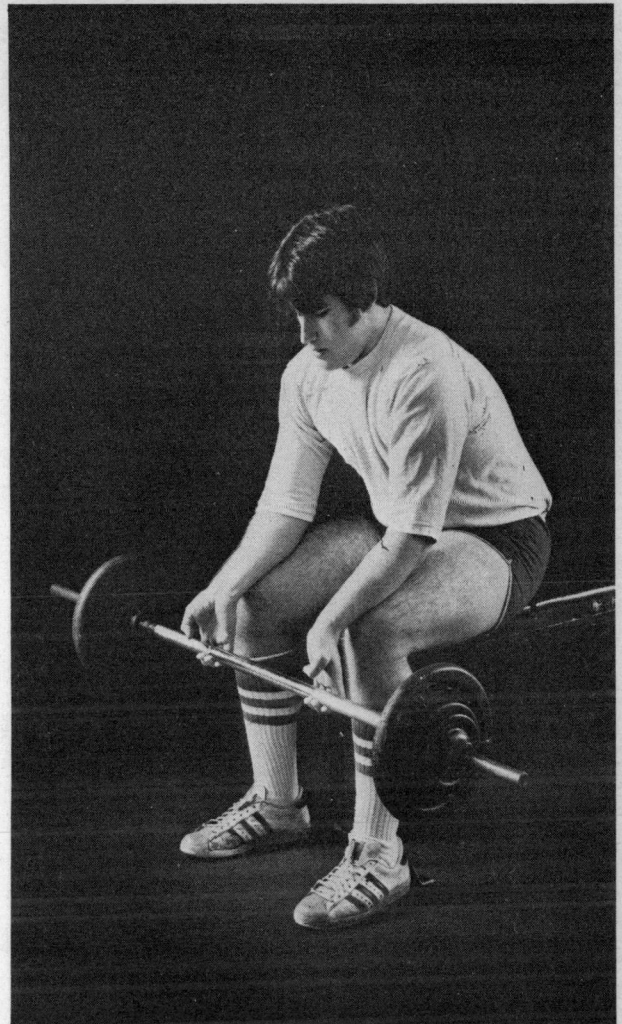

3

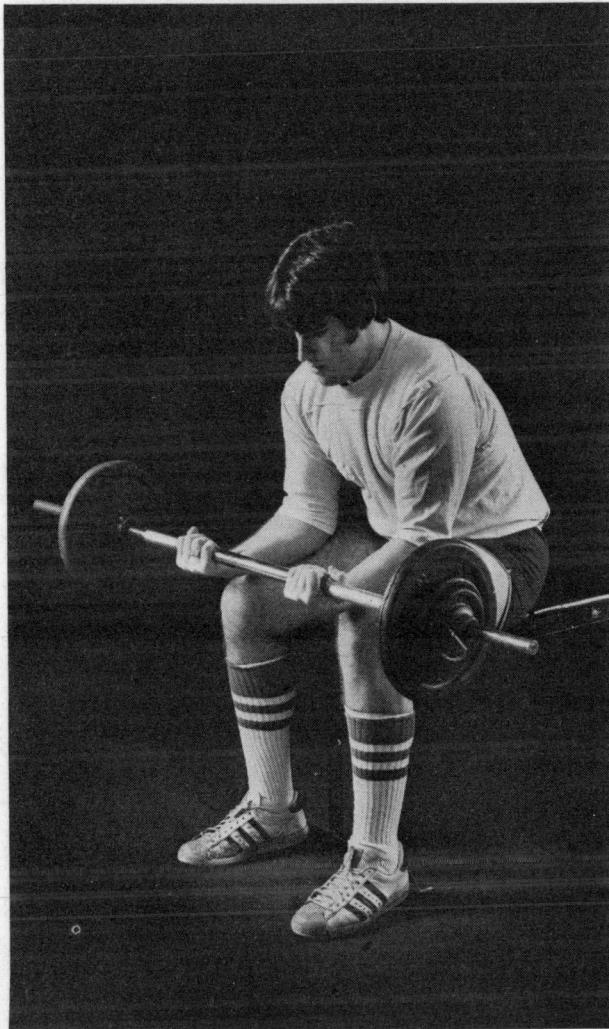

2

Forearm Raise (thumb side muscles of forearm)
   Equipment: dumbbell with only one end
            weighted

1. Stand erect, hands at sides, one hand gripping
   unweighted end of dumbbell in thumb-up grip
   with weight pointing forward.
2. Raise dumbbell as far as possible without
   moving forearm.
3. Return to starting position to repeat.
4. Repeat exercise with other arm.

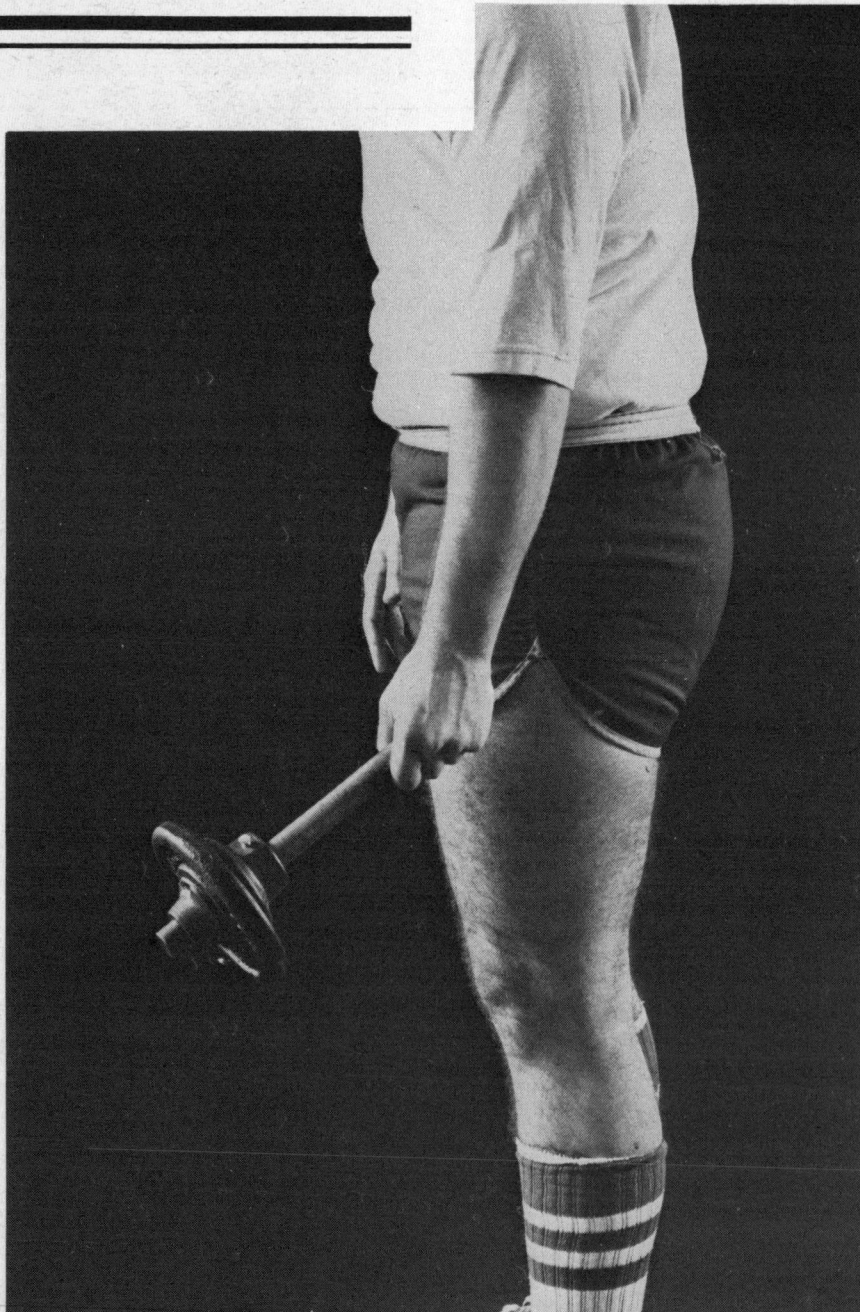

Back Arm Raise (little finger side muscles of forearm)

   Equipment: dumbbell with only one end weighted

1. Stand erect, hands at sides, one hand gripping unweighted end of dumbbell in thumb-down grip with weight pointing backward.
2. Raise dumbbell as far as possible without moving forearm.
3. Return to starting position to repeat.
4. Repeat exercise with other arm.

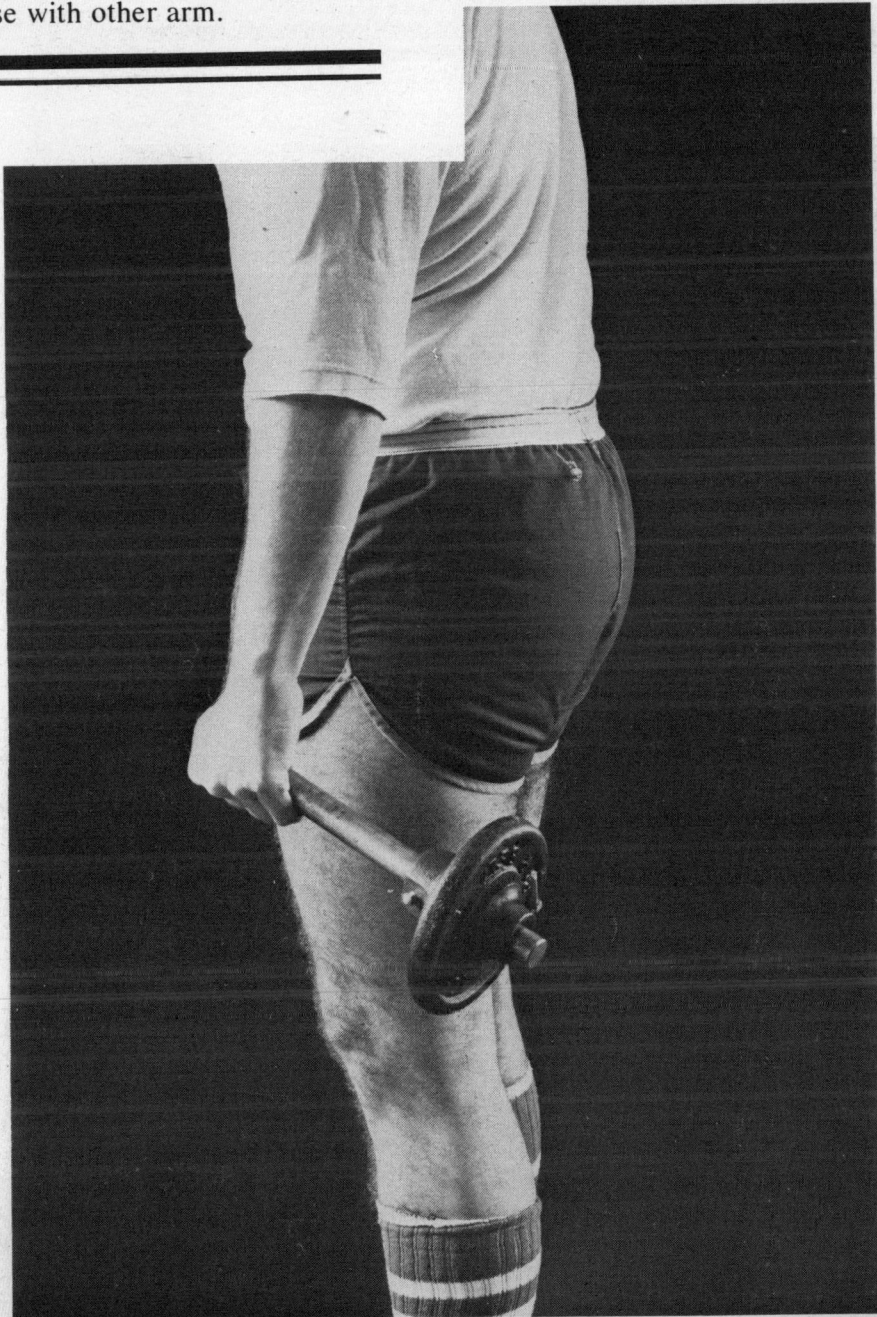

Neck Raise (neck muscles)
   Equipment: weight plate, weight bench and towel

1. Lie face up on bench with head hanging over the end of the bench.
2. Place folded towel on forehead and place weight on top of towel.
3. Raise head as far as possible holding weight stable with hands.
4. Return to starting position to repeat.

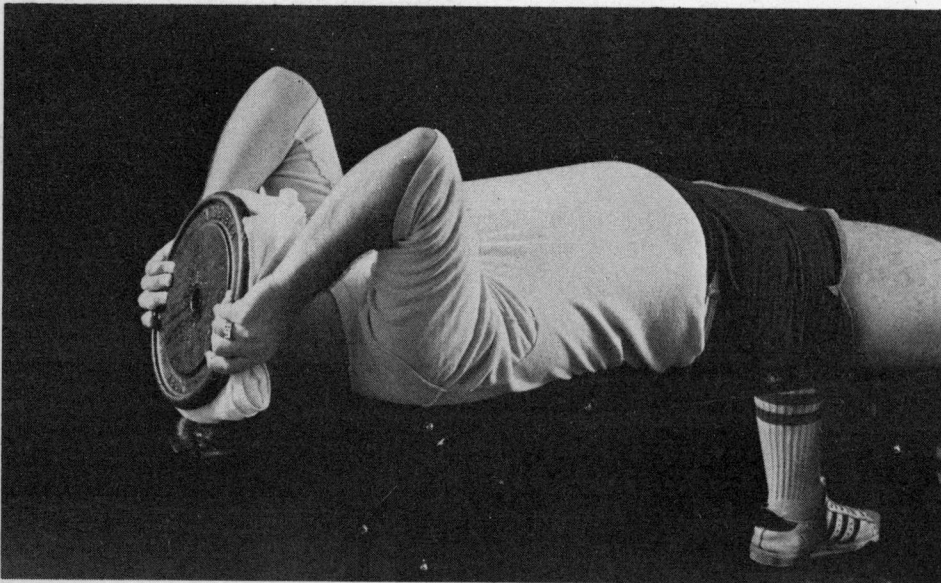

1 & 2

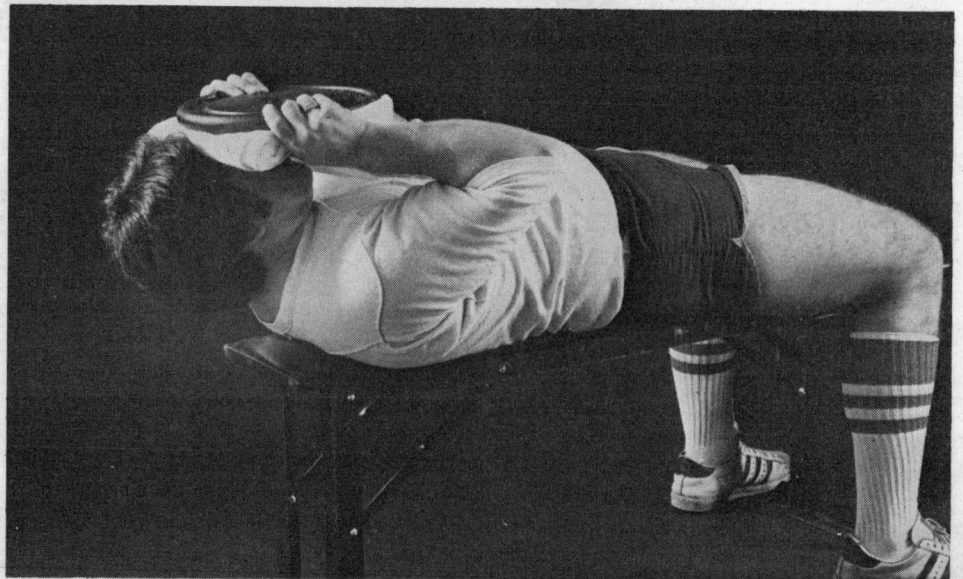

3

Isokinetics

The isokinetic exercises presented here are ones that can be done with a partner. For those of you who don't want to spend the money on weights but can easily find a workout partner, these exercises are ideal. Each exercise should be done slowly and smoothly with no jerky movement. Through trial and error, you and your partner can work out the amount of resistance that is required.

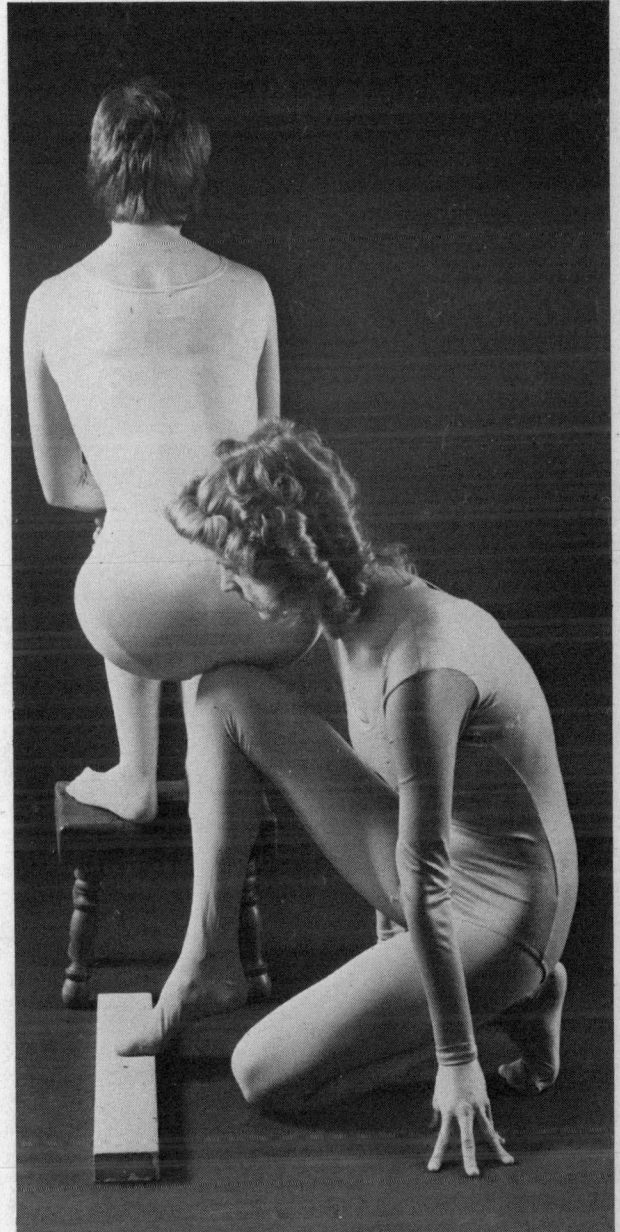

Heel Raises (calf muscles)

1. The exerciser kneels on one leg while one toe of other leg rests on 2-inch thick block of wood with heel on floor. Partner sits on knee with feet resting on a bench, couch or similar structure.
2. Exerciser raises heel as far up as possible.
3. Return to starting position to repeat.
4. Repeat exercise with opposite leg.

Leg Curl (hamstring muscles)

1. Lie face down on the floor, knees bent at 90-degree angle to body, feet together, hands at sides.
2. Partner grips your ankles and provides resistance while you curl your heels back toward your back.
3. Return to starting position.

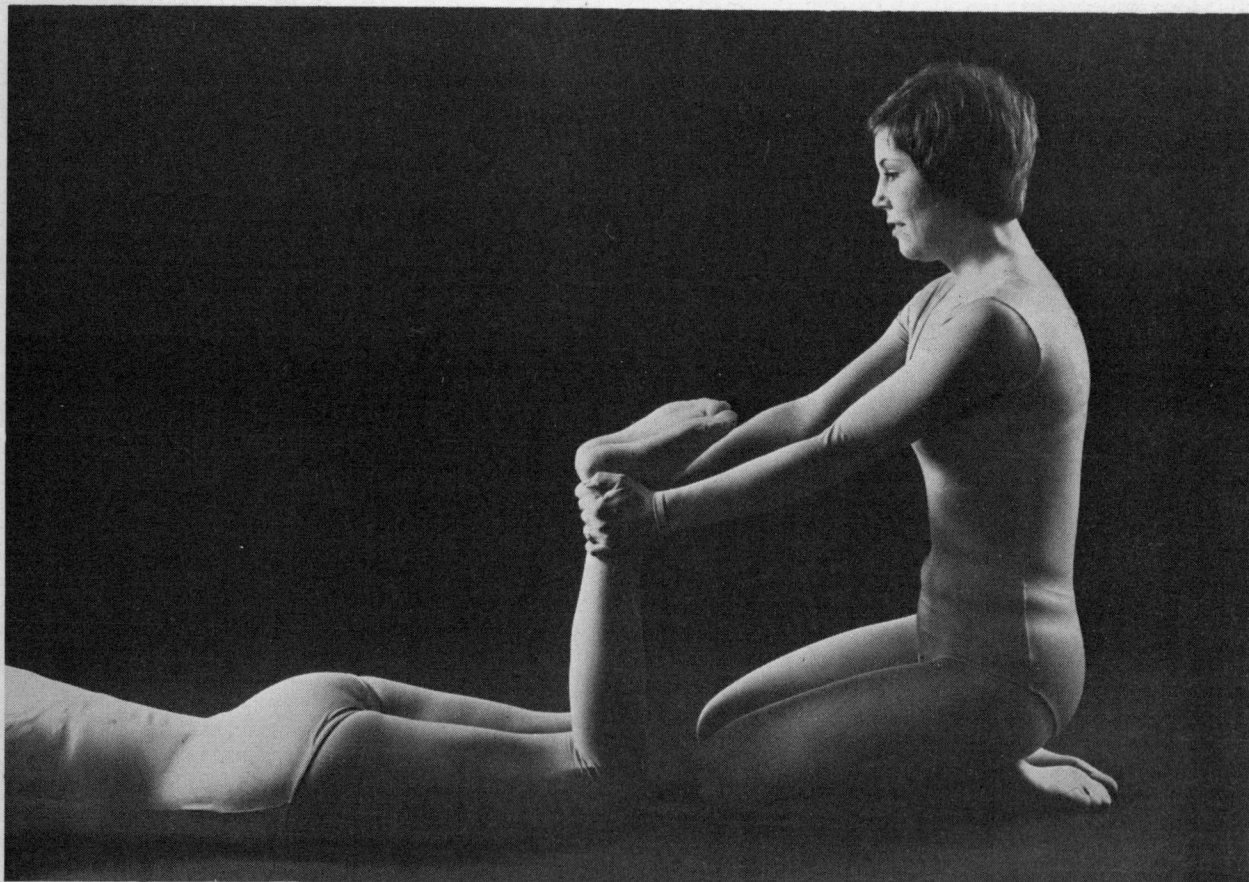

Leg Raise (buttock muscles)

1. Get down on hands and knees and raise left leg parallel to floor.
2. While partner provides resistance, raise left leg above parallel position to the floor.
3. Return to starting position and raise right leg parallel to floor.
4. Repeat exercise with right leg.

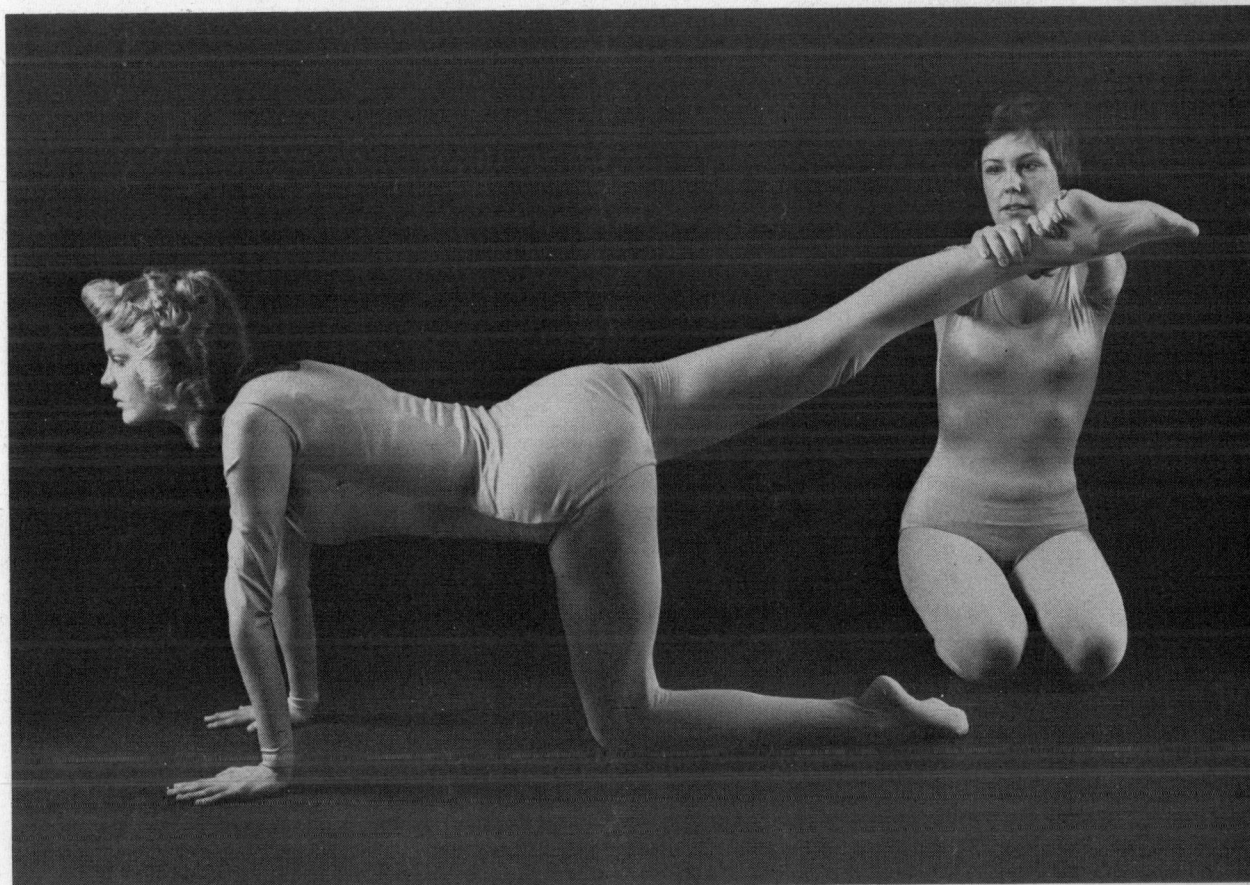

Side Bend (trunk muscles)

1. Stand with feet comfortably apart, trunk bent sideways to the right as far as possible, right arm gripped by partner's hands and left arm bent over your head.
2. While your partner provides resistance, try to straighten to upright position.
3. Reverse position to left side and repeat exercise.

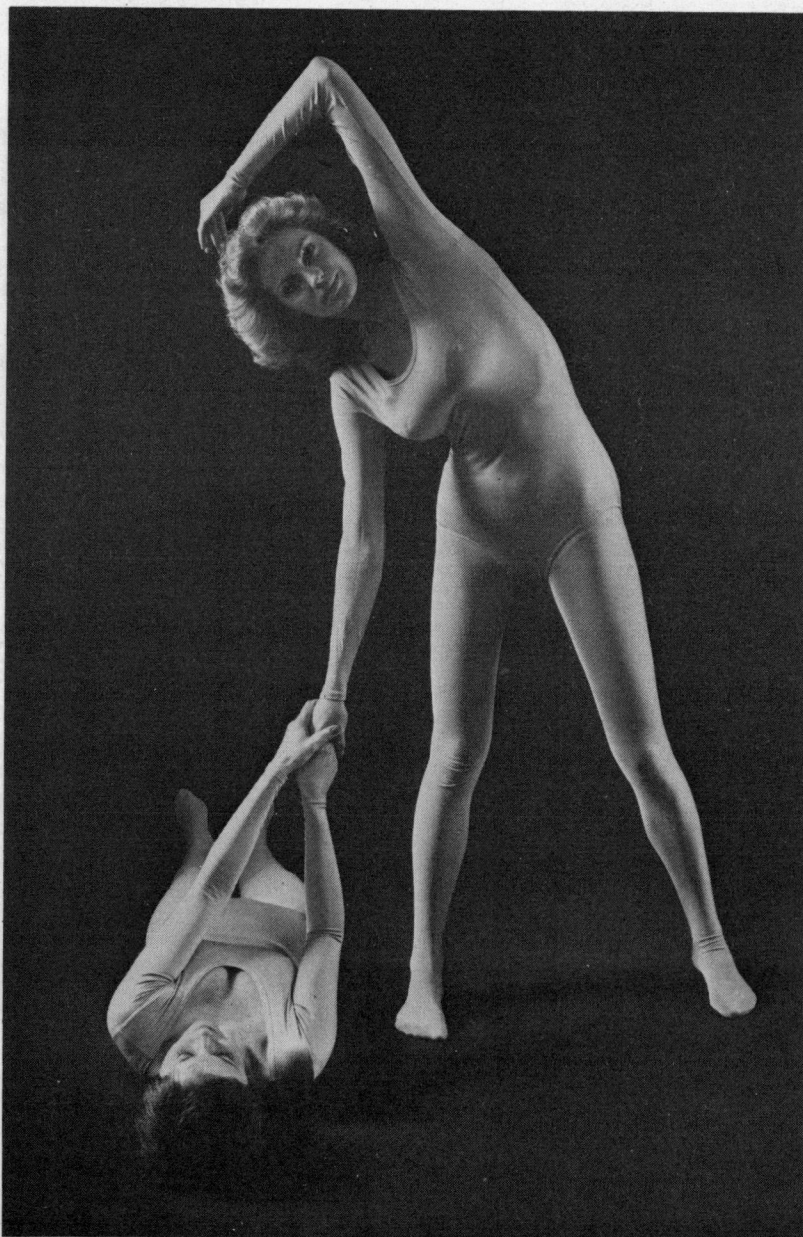

Pec Popper (chest muscles)

1. Lie face up on floor, left arm at side, right arm extended laterally.
2. While partner provides resistance, raise arm in an arc with your shoulder as the axis point. Bend your elbow only slightly and keep arm moving until your fist is above opposite shoulder.
3. Repeat exercise with left arm.

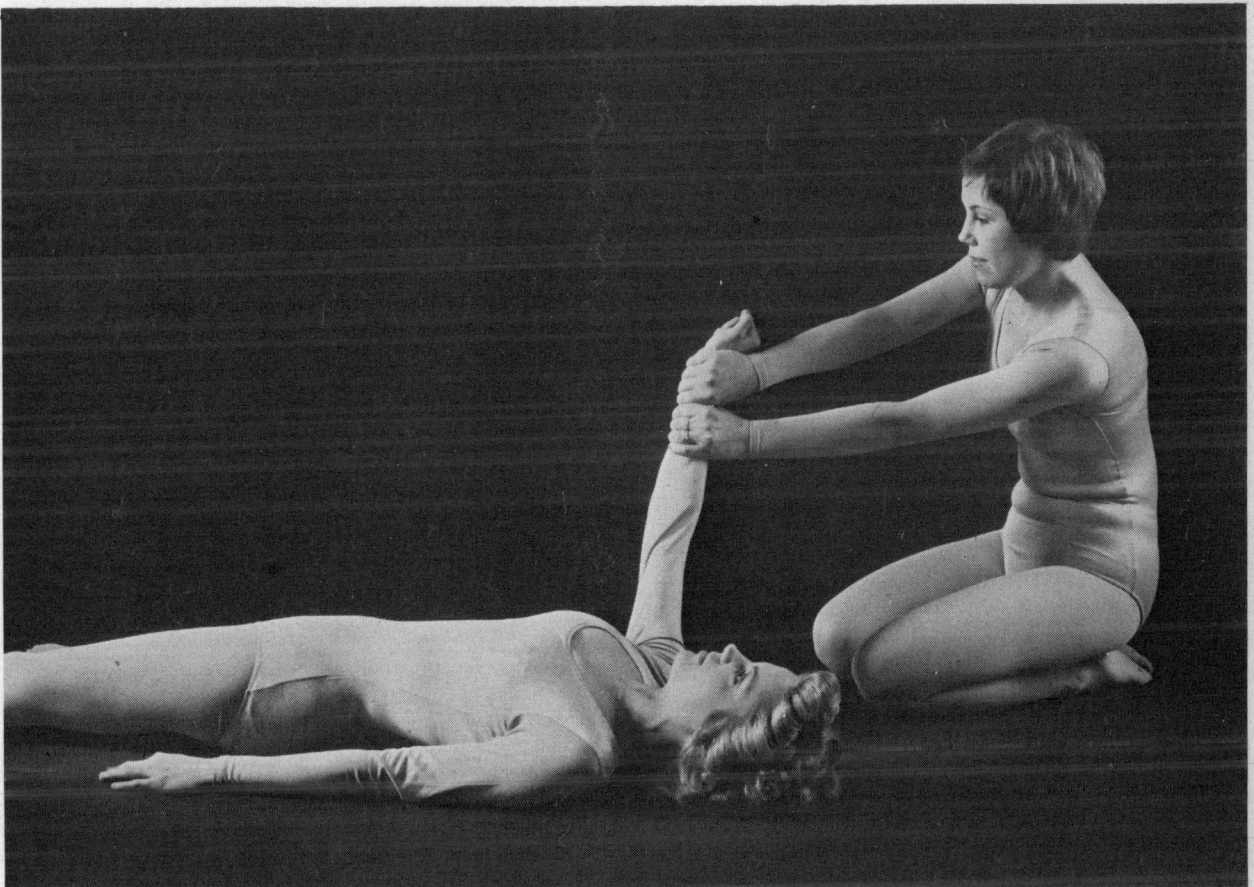

Side Arm Raise (shoulder muscles)

1. Stand erect, feet spread comfortably apart, hands at sides.
2. While partner provides resistance, raise one arm out to the side and up over head, bending elbow only slightly.
3. Repeat exercise with other arm.

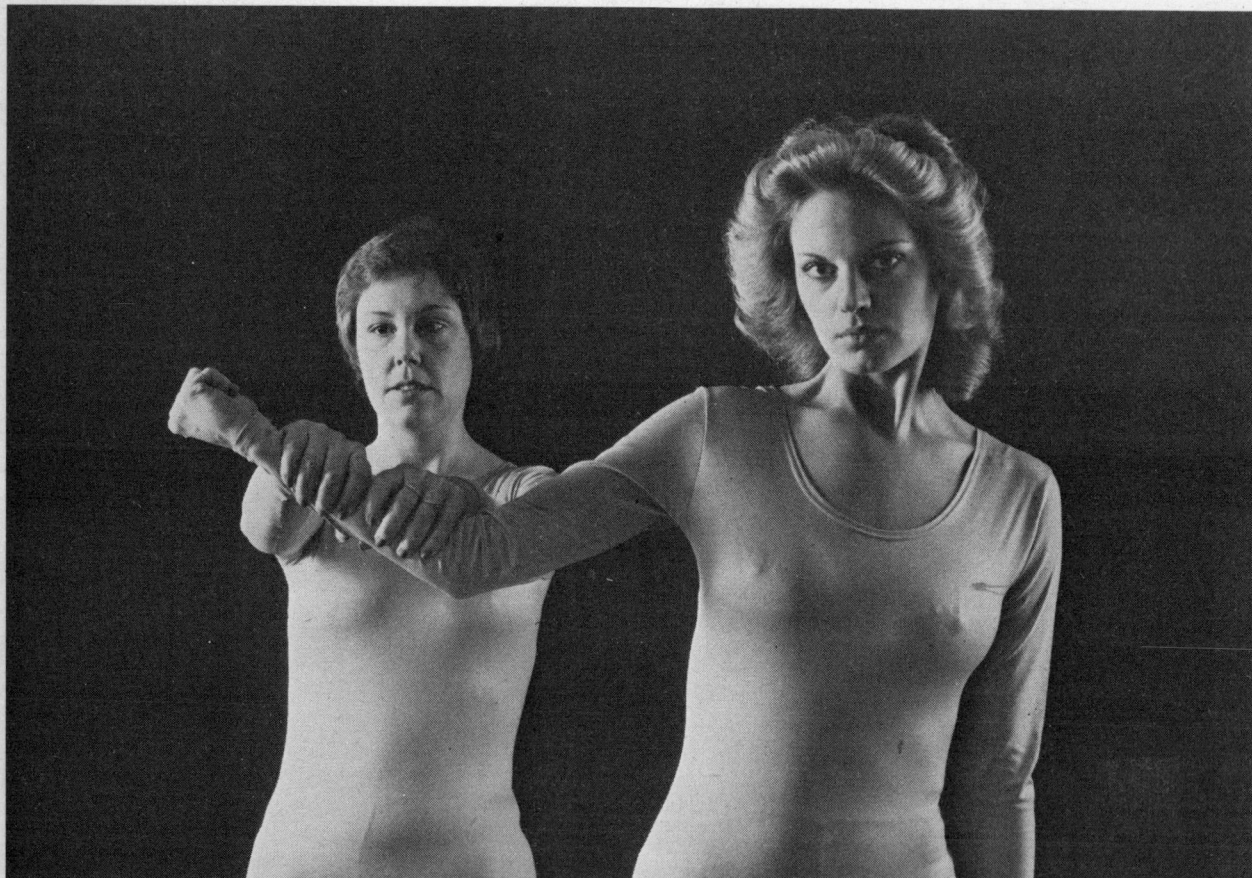

Whiplash (rear neck muscles)

1. Stand erect, back to wall or other support, feet spread comfortably apart, hands on hips, head bent forward, chin resting on chest.
2. Partner clasps hands behind your head and provides resistance while you pull your head backward as far as possible.

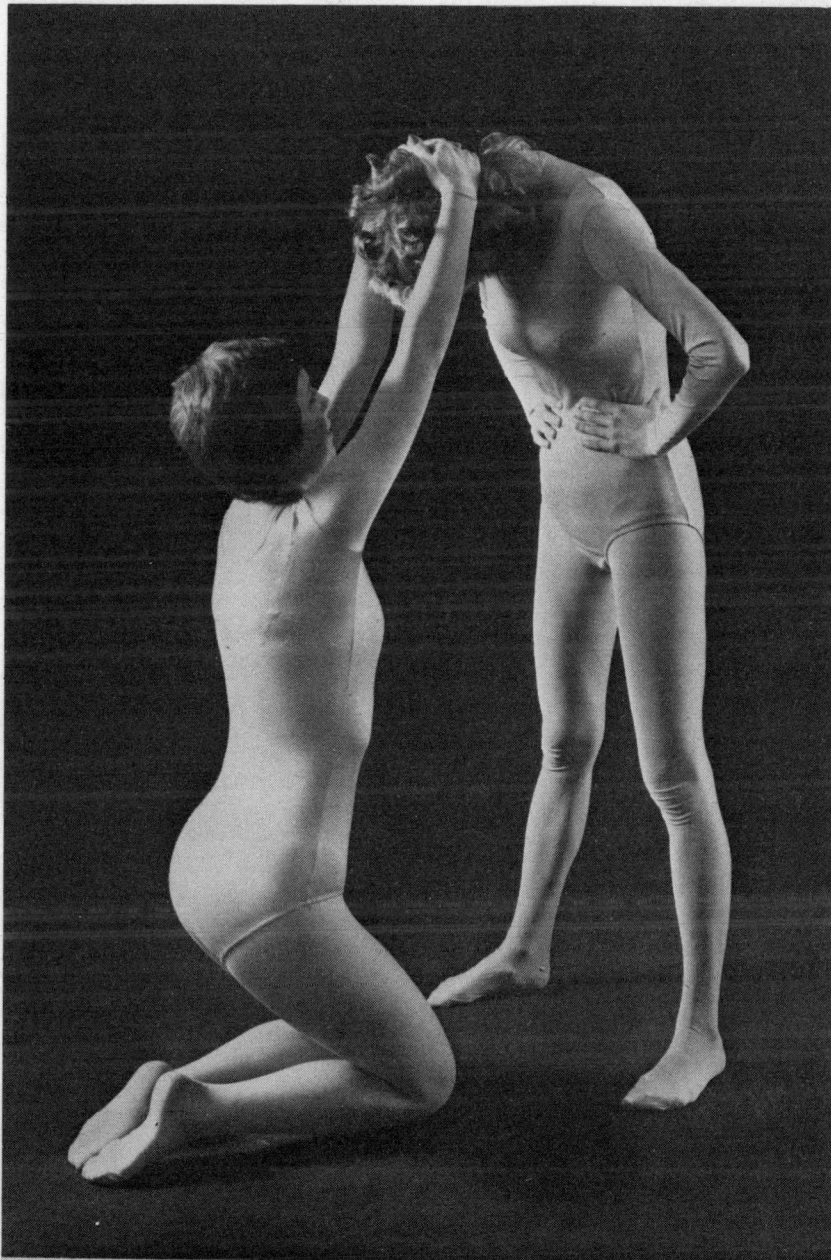

Neck Pull (front neck muscles)

1. Stand erect, feet spread comfortably apart, hands on hips, head bent backward, as far as possible.
2. Partner clasps hands around your forehead and applies resistance while you pull your head forward until chin rests on chest.

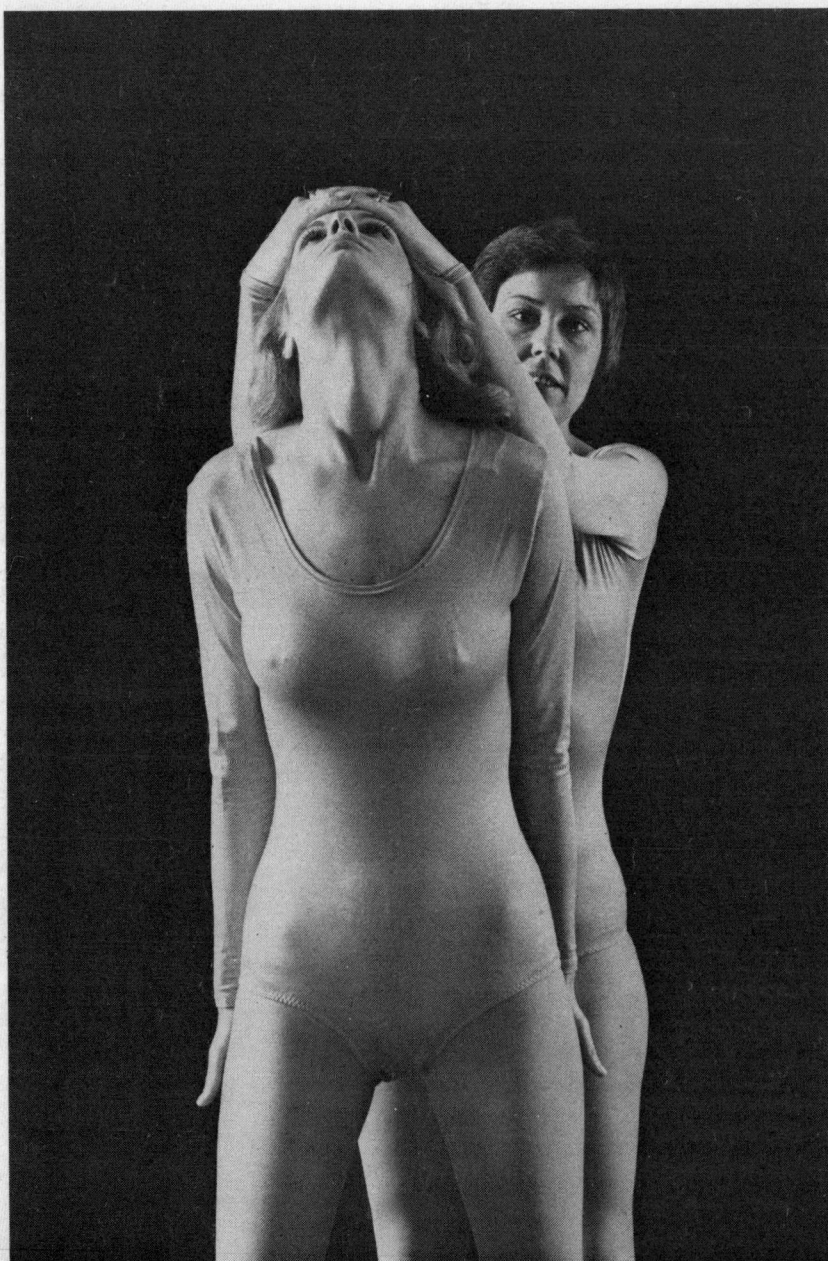

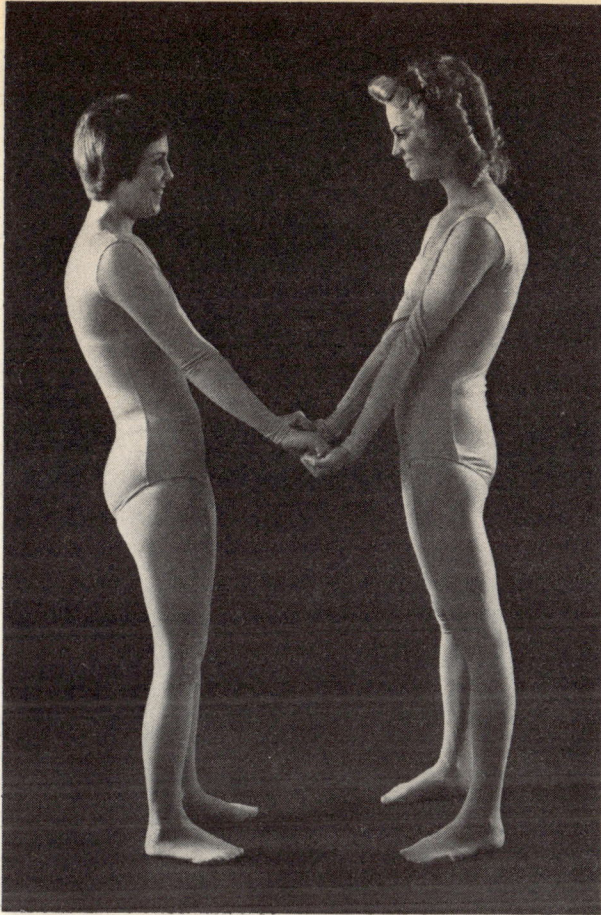

1

Arm Curl (biceps and forearm muscles)

1. Stand erect, feet comfortably apart, elbows bent slightly.
2. Partner stands facing you and interlocks his hands with yours—your hands palms up, his palms down.
3. While partner provides resistance, raise your arms to chest by bending elbows.

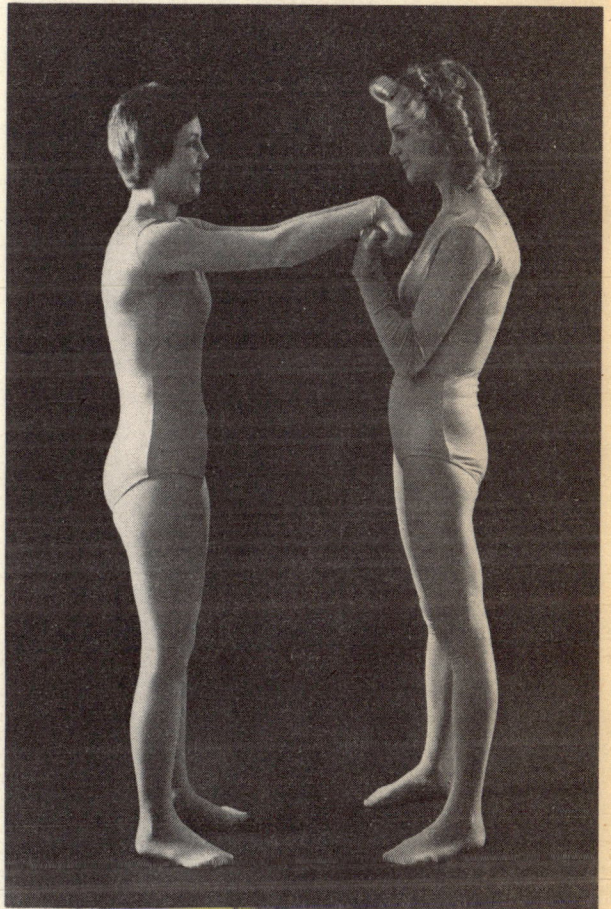

2

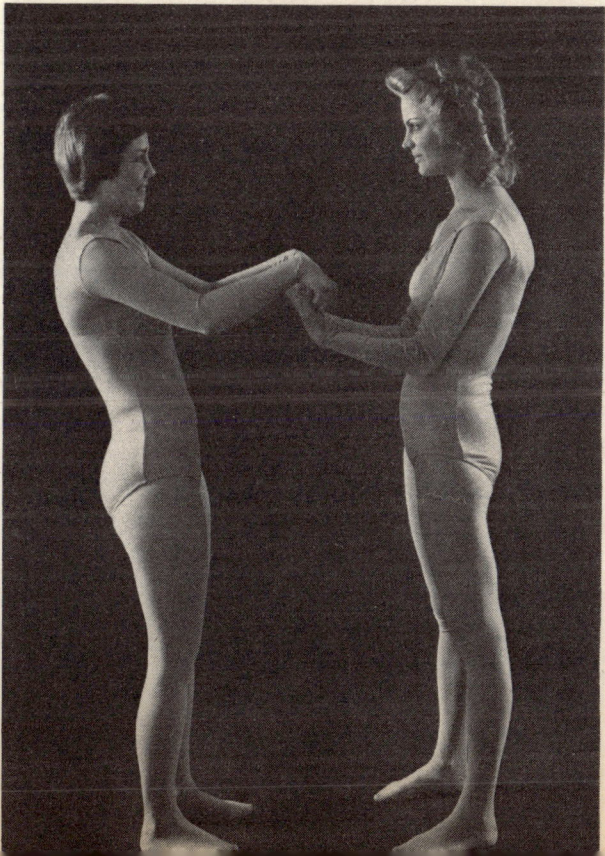

3

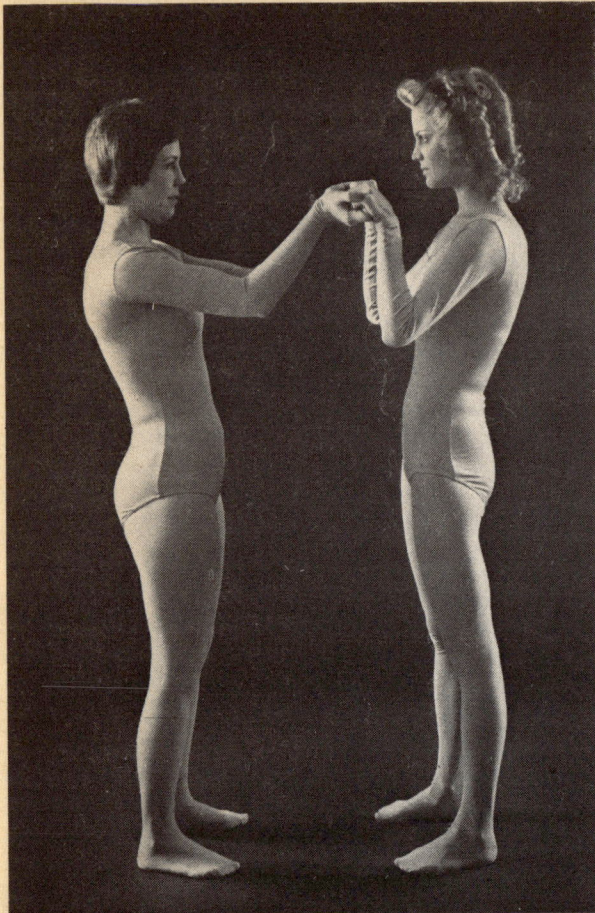

1

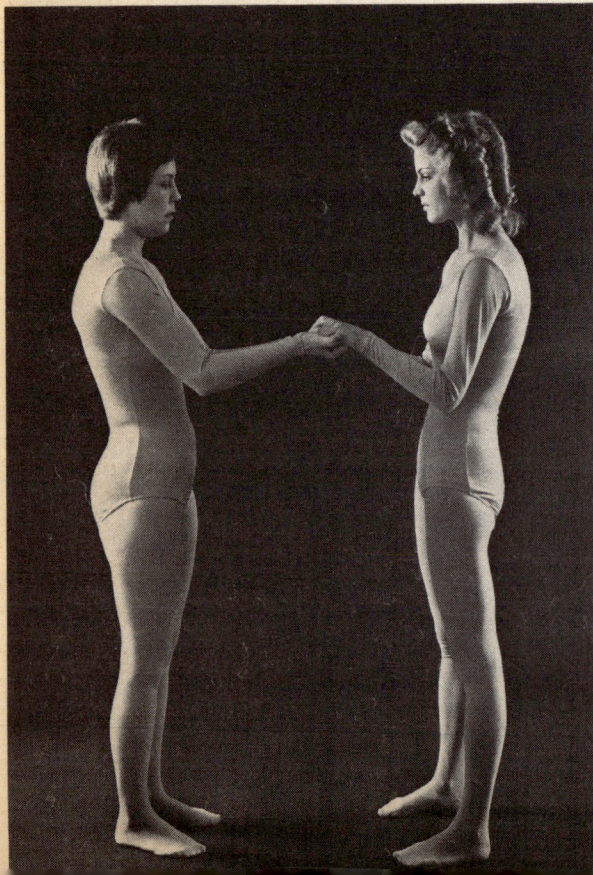

2

Arm Extension (rear forearm muscles)

1. Stand erect, feet comfortably apart, arms bent at elbows, fists chest high.
2. Partner stands facing you and interlocks his hands with yours—your hands palms down, his palms up.
3. While partner provides resistance, lower arms to sides by bending elbows.

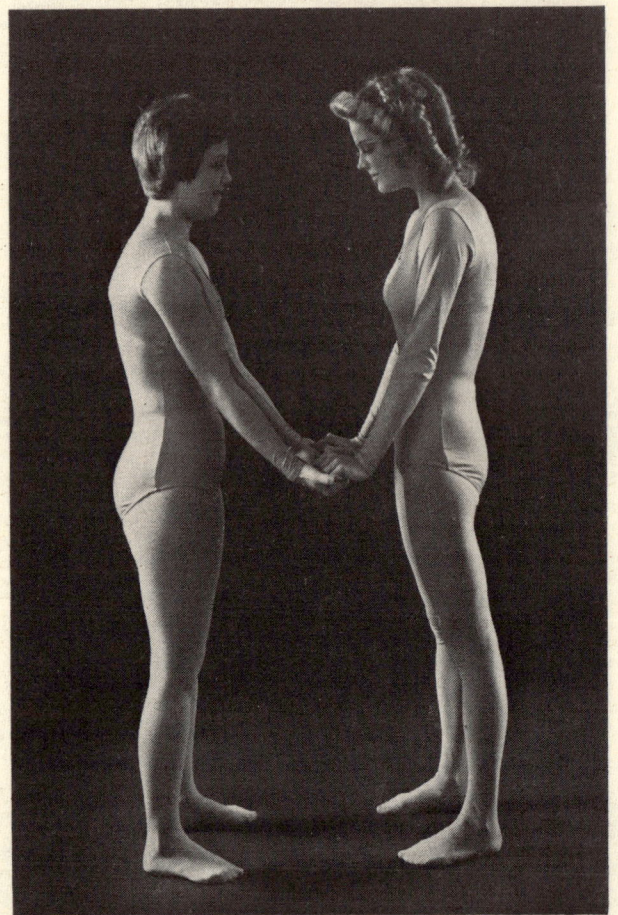

3

Leg Extension (leg muscles)

1. Sit on table or bench (high enough so feet are off the floor), hands gripping sides of table.
2. Partner stands facing you with hands gripping right leg.
3. As partner provides resistance, raise leg parallel to floor.
4. Repeat exercise with left leg.

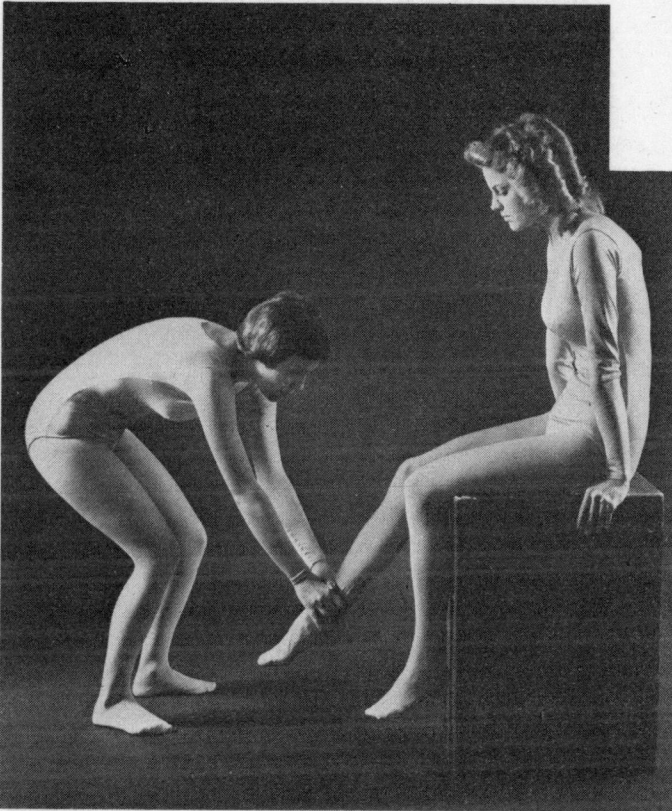

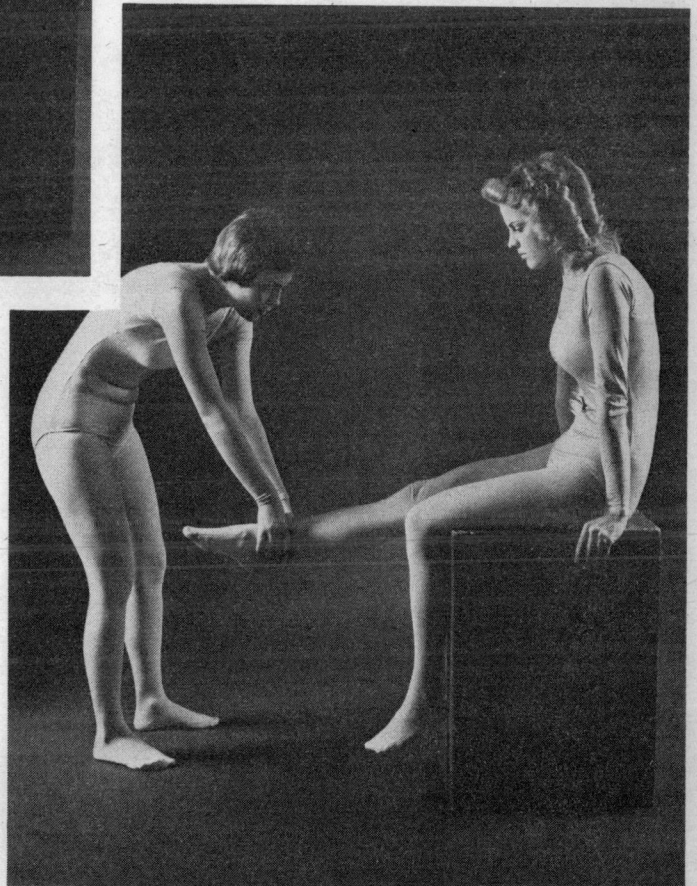

Leg Flexion (leg muscles)

1. Sit on table or bench (high enough so feet are off the floor), hands gripping sides of table and right leg extended parallel to floor.
2. Partner stands facing you with hands gripping right leg.
3. As partner provides resistance, lower leg to side of table.
4. Repeat exercise with left leg.

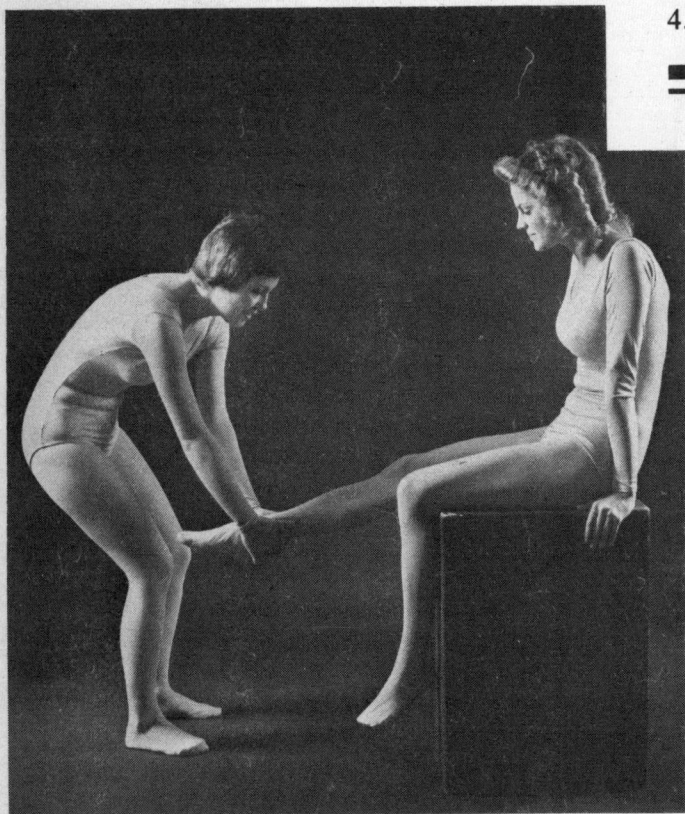

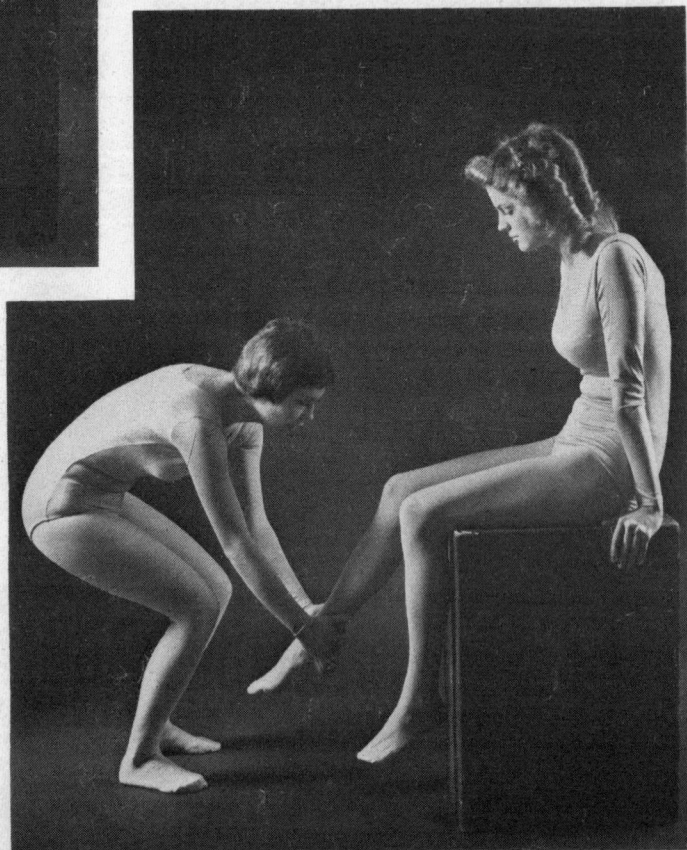

Pushup (arm and shoulder muscles)

1. Lie face down on floor, palms on floor under shoulders, feet straight out behind you with toes on floor.
2. Partner stands facing you with hands on shoulders.
3. While partner provides resistance, extend arms, pushing body off floor, keeping back straight, supporting weight on arms and toes.

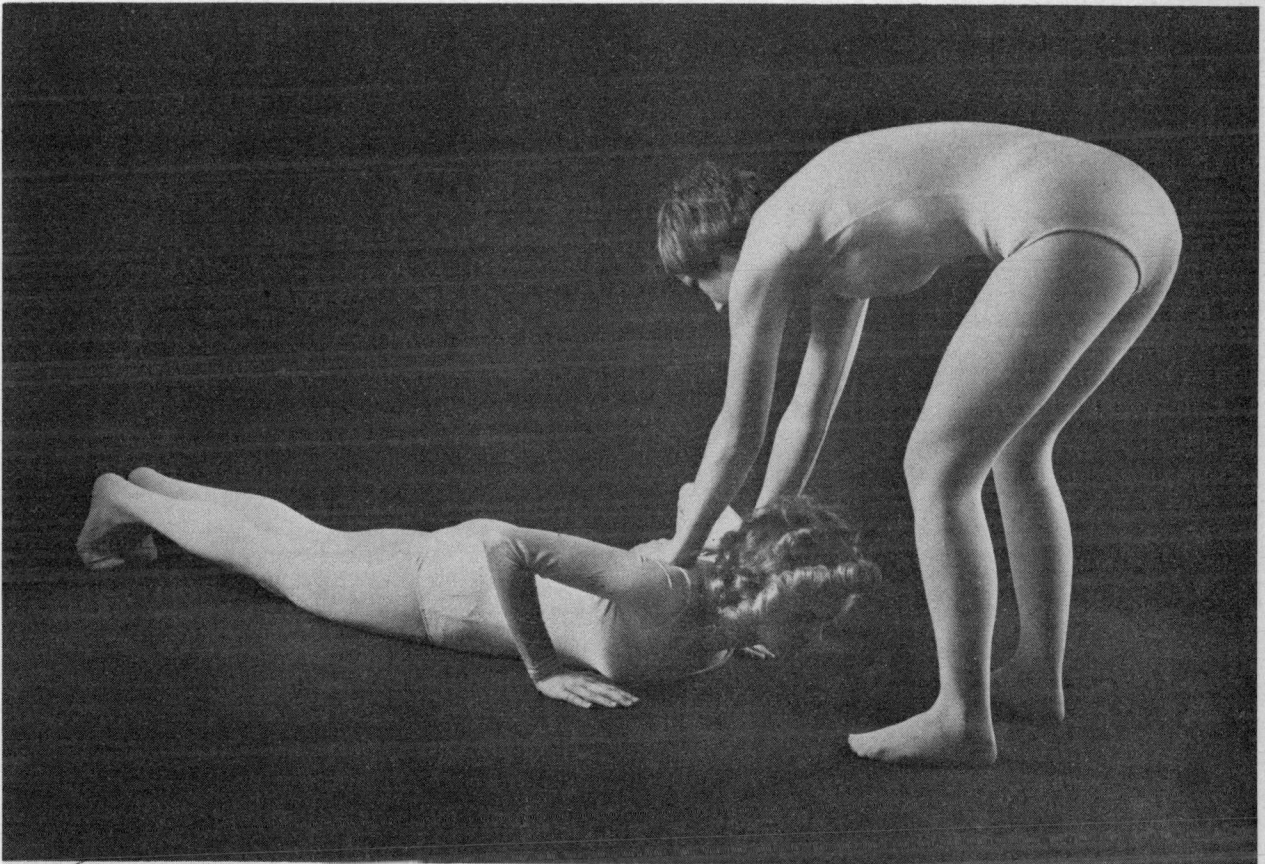

Isokinetics (Exercise Machines and Gadgets)

Much exercise machinery that has been marketed in the past has been of little or no actual value, but it has always had a market of sorts.

The new, ultra-sophisticated, very expensive exercise equipment is quite a different story. Because of its cost, the manufacturers had no idea it would sell as well as it has.

Of course, it's much too expensive for most people to have in their homes, but the gyms that have invested heavy cash in it have gotten a good return on their money and have built up a substantial clientele.

If you consider barbells and dumbells as machinery, which I don't, there's no question about the good they do in developing strength. In addition to what they do for muscular strength, they can also be used to develop endurance. Some of the machines that use a system of ropes and pulleys, together with weights, are excellent and are in a medium price class. They have applications for strength building for all parts of the body.

I don't happen to know any exercise authorities who are highly enthusiastic about rowing machines. Those that are sold for home use for the most part use rubber resistance, which wears out, with the rubber cables losing their tension. A common objection to them is that they exercise a limited number of body areas. They work specifically on the legs, arms, back and to a lesser degree the hips.

The stationary exercise bicycle is one of the best machines within the price range of the home user. It is excellent for building cardiovascular pulmonary endurance—for the lungs and the heart—and also has some effect on toning the muscles of the legs and hips.

So-called chest expanders are better than rowing machines to exercise the arms and shoulders, and are much less expensive. They're also portable. Some of my friends have built their own, at modest cost, and they're quite efficient. Aside from what they do for the arms and shoulders, their effectiveness is limited.

Vibrator belts, sold as an easy short-cut for spot reduction, are, in the opinion of the experts I've consulted, almost worthless. These people tell me that a vibrator belt has no effect whatsoever in removing fat, that it doesn't increase strength or endurance, and that it can be danger-

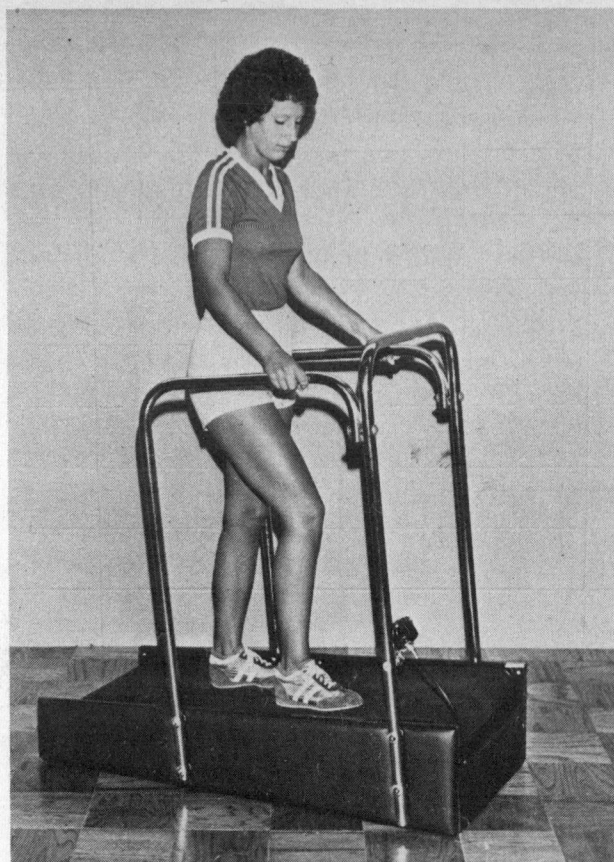

Pro-Gym's Pace-Setter Treadmill is for those days it is too cold, rainy or snowy to jog or walk. A speedometer helps you pace your exercise.

ous if used for too long a time on a specific area of the body, because it can damage blood cells.

Exercise wheels, which are inexpensive, will strengthen the stomach muscles if used regularly, and to a minor degree, the chest and back muscles.

Our conclusion is that for home use, within a reasonable price range, the two exercise machines worth consideration are the stationary bicycle and weights.

If you're working out in a gym, exercise machines that help only one area of the body are quite all right to use as a part of your routine. You're paying a fee, and you might as well avail yourself of everything.

There's a type of person for whom mechanical gimmicks have great appeal. If these people find what looks like a clever piece of equipment, they'll use it, instead of doing a simple physical exercise to accomplish the same purpose.

Aside from weight equipment and cycles, most exercise machines' widest appeal is to those who want to get results without any great physical effort. The success manufacturers have enjoyed is proof that many such people exist.

Some equipment, mostly sold by mail order, is possessed of some merit but fantastically overpriced. For example, one advertiser has sold a piece of equipment for strengthening the arms and shoulders, promoting flexibility there, and developing the chest. The price is $9.95 plus postage. What the buyer receives is a piece of tire inner tube and a little 16-page booklet.

Another advertiser sells a piece of equipment for strengthening the legs and arms, and building cardiovascular pulmonary endurance. It sells for an even $10. And it turns out when it arrives to be a jump rope with handle grips at both ends. The slim booklet that accompanies it contains the same rope skipping exercises that are to be found in most exercise books.

Any exercise machine of some kind may help you, but it will almost never accomplish any more than you could do without it by doing simple types of exercise intended to accomplish the same things.

If you're interested in a piece of equipment, the practical thing to do is to get complete information on it, including manufacturer's specifications, instead of relying on what is nearly always extravagant advertising.

One other piece of equipment may be designated as exercising machinery, and that's a slant board. The slant board has some value, particularly in advanced exercise. Here again, however, an old solid wooden door or a piece of heavy plywood can serve the purpose, if propped at one end against something of the right height.

I don't classify a whirlpool bath unit as a piece of exercise equipment because it doesn't really exercise you. It will do what it claims to do, however.

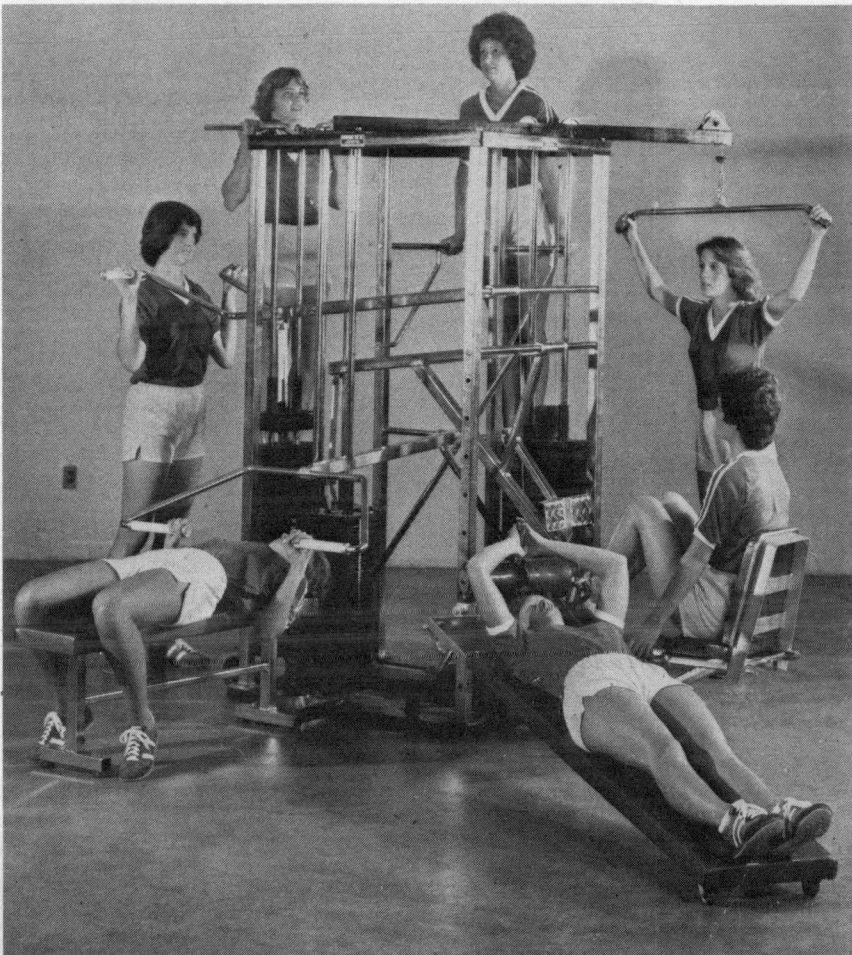

Pro-Gym's Blue Chip model weight training machine offers from 6 to 13 exercise stations with the basic model including a leg press, chest press, shoulder press, high lat, quad low pulley and chinning.

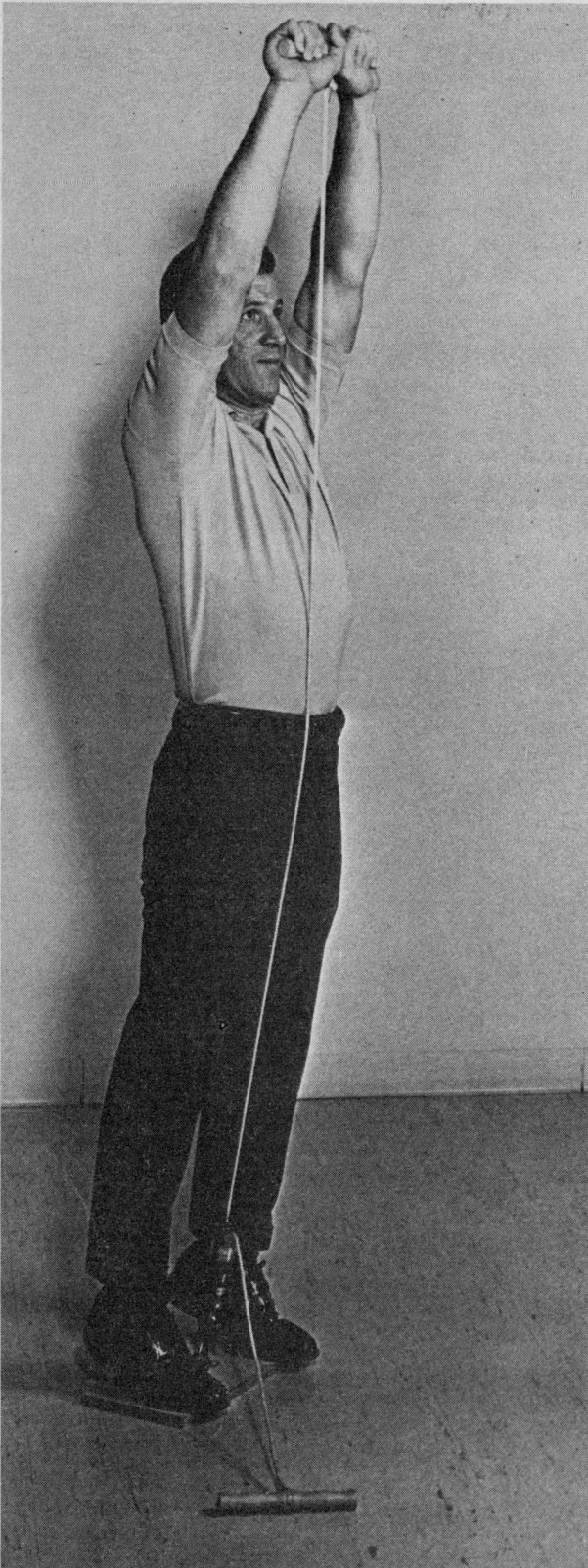

The Exer-Genie weighing only 2 pounds offers a wide variety of controlled resistance exercises which can be done at home, in the office, or at the gym. Copyright © 1970 Exer-Genie, Inc. USA.

Vibrator massage units are favored by some people, but being massaged is not an exercise. I've found that the massage I get with a Water-Pik shower unit after vigorous exercise is both soothing, and stimulating, as well as a temporary reliever of tense muscles. I don't happen to know anybody who has such a unit who would want to be without it.

Earlier in this discussion of exercise machines, I mentioned an ultra-sophisticated piece of equipment that's much too expensive for most people to have in their homes. It's the Nautilus, produced by Nautilus Sports Medical Industries of DeLand, Florida. It's an amazing piece of equipment that can give the exerciser full-range resistance, direct resistance, balanced resistance, omnidirectional resistance, rotary-form resistance and negative work potential. It operates with a cam system, an automatic pulley, spiral-shaped, that automatically changes the resistance the instant any movement occurs. Consequently, it works on *all* of a muscle. The selected weight can be as much or as little as required. The rotary-form resistance offered by the Nautilus gives the exerciser an advantage over barbell exercise in that the exercise can always match the functions of the muscular structures.

The Exer-Genie, produced by Exer-Genie, Inc., of Fullerton, California, provides resistance by the friction from a specially braided nylon line winding around a shaft. The degree of resistance is shown on a calibration chart, and can be varied by an uncomplicated pin arrangement. It requires very little space and provides a considerable variety of isotonic and isometric exercises for special muscle groups.

The Super Mini-Gym Exerciser, produced by Mini-Gym, Inc., of Independence, Missouri, employs isokinetics, which offers a maximum load on a muscle at every point in its full range of motion.

The Gladiator Gym Machine, produced by Universal Athletic Sales Co., Inc., of Fresno, California, requires a 12- x 18-foot working space and has 15 different exercise stations that can be used simultaneously, so that 15 people can be working on one machine at the same time.

The various stations offer a leg press up to 160 pounds, a chest press to 230 pounds, a shoulder press to 230 pounds, a high lateral pull to 210

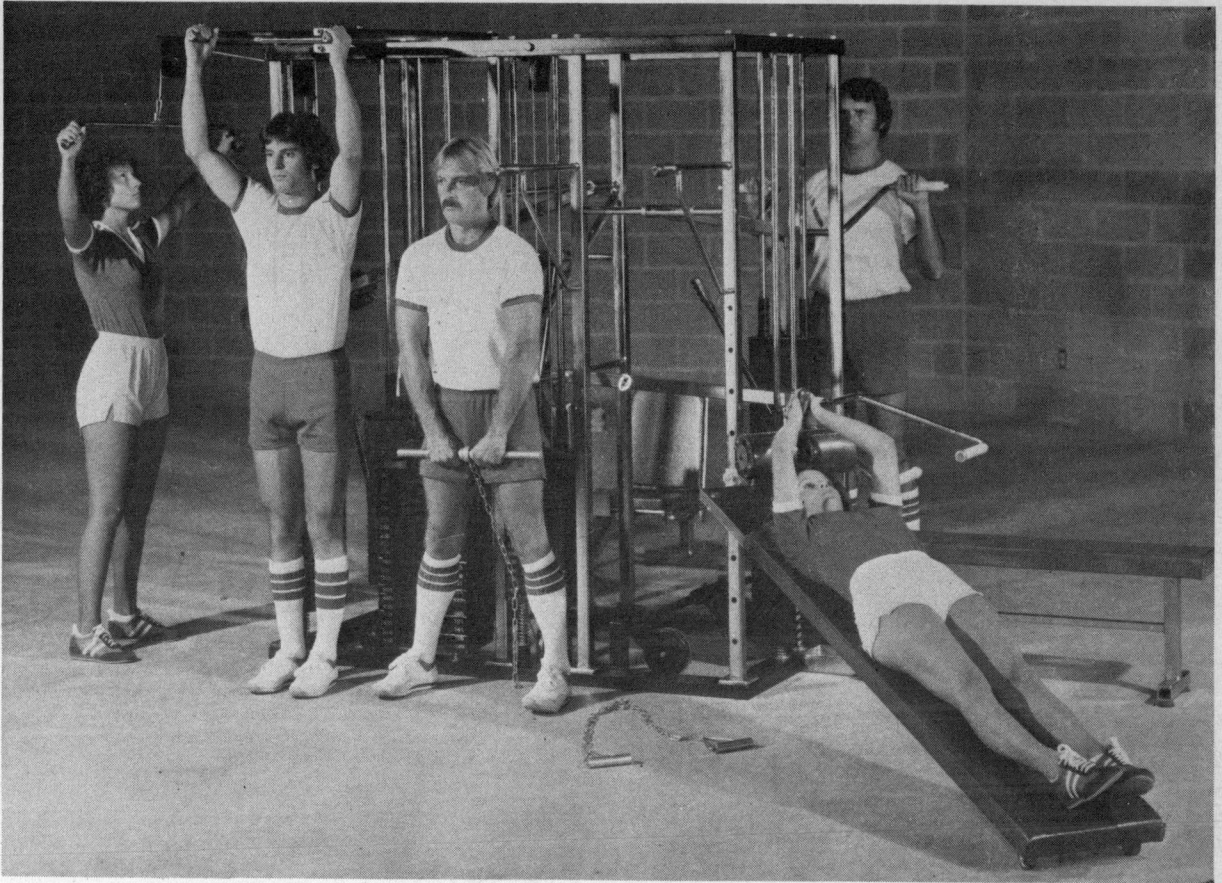

Pro-Gym's Pro Model weight training
machine with 12 basic training stations.

pounds, a quadriceps and dead lift to 160 pounds, chinning, dipping, hip flexor, incline board abdominal conditioner, thigh and knee pull to 160 pounds, back hyperextension and swimming kick, rowing wrist and forearm pull to 160 pounds, wrist conditioner over 150 pounds, neck conditioner to 70 pounds and hand gripper to over 150 pounds.

A gym that has any of these more sophisticated machines will be well equipped in other areas.

Once you've developed a reasonable amount of strength, you're ready to proceed to the fitness element that is, in our opinion, the most important of all—cardiovascular pulmonary endurance. If you don't move ahead into it and are content to go no further than the development of strength, you're cheating yourself. With all the pressures of today's world, endurance is the most important physical attribute you can develop.

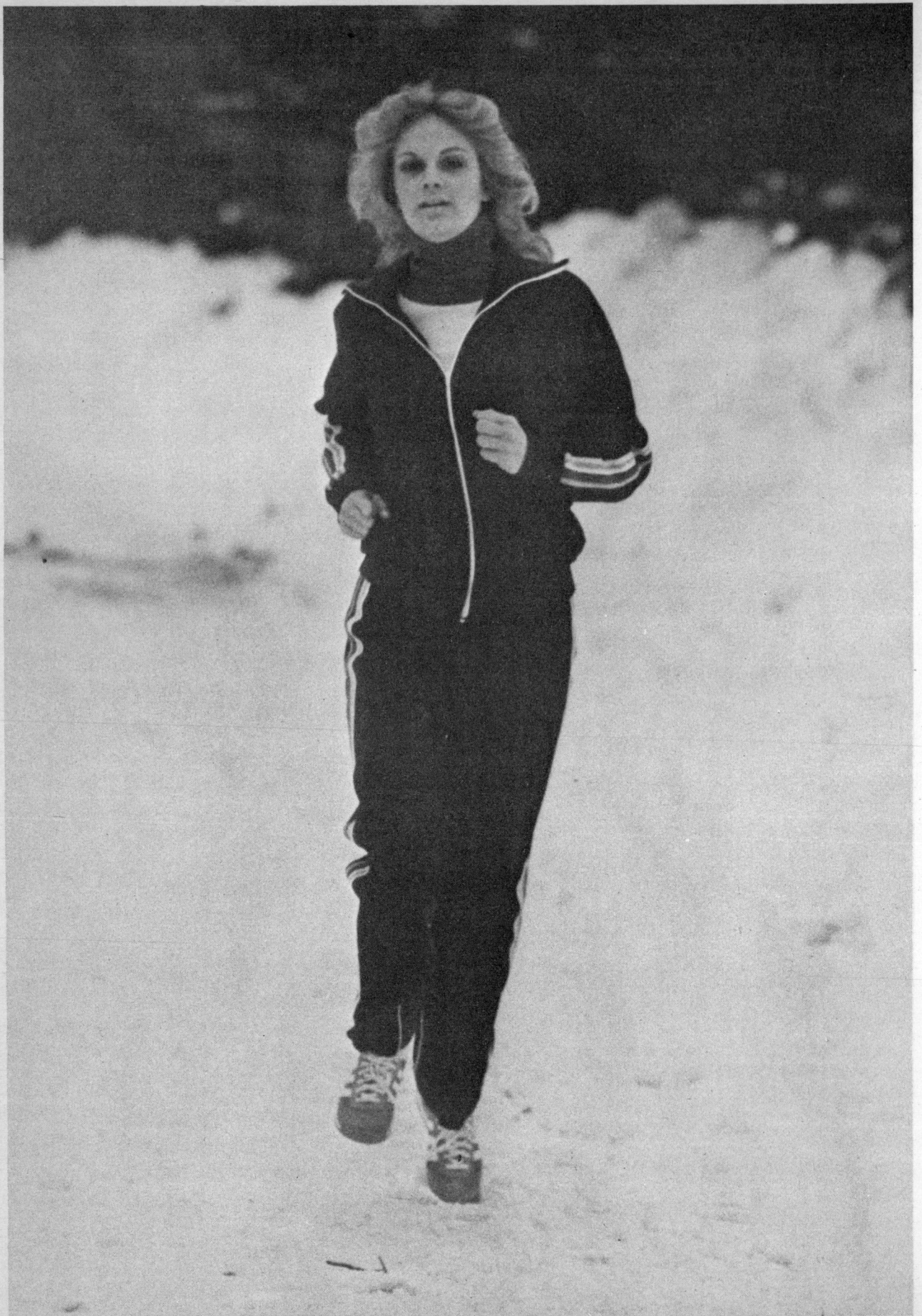

Endurance

ENDURANCE, to put it simply, is the capacity to sustain intense activity for a period of time without excessive fatigue. Endurance is measured by the length of time a muscle or muscle group can sustain a type of activity—for example, how many times a person can repeat an exercise such as situps or pushups, or how long or how far a person can run, swim, or bicycle. Two types of muscle systems are involved in endurance training—skeletal and cardiovascular. Your skeletal muscles are those needed for movement—neck, arm, trunk and leg muscles. The cardiovascular muscle system includes your heart, lungs and circulatory system. The two muscle systems are interrelated—exercises to improve endurance of one system put demands on the other. However, the exercise methods most effective in building the endurance fitness of the two systems are quite different in nature. To build endurance of the skeletal muscles, exercises such as situps, pushups (calisthenics) or bicep curls and bench presses (weight training) are implemented. Dynamic exercises—running, jogging, bicycling, walking or rope jumping (aerobics)—are the only exercises which effectively improve cardiovascular endurance. It is important to realize that to perform a dynamic exercise, such as jogging, you must develop a certain endurance fitness level in your leg, back and abdominal muscles or jogging for long distances becomes impossible. The same holds true for exercises to improve endurance of the skeletal

muscles. A certain level of cardiovascular fitness is necessary to do a prolonged series of situps or pushups because of the demands placed upon your heart and circulatory system.

Why do you need to develop endurance? Endurance improves your efficiency and therefore productivity. As your endurance fitness level improves, the energy required to perform a given amount of work decreases. You can perform a task longer with less fatigue. Raking leaves, gardening, painting your house, playing touch football with the kids, tennis, racquetball, even your chosen occupation all demand a certain amount of endurance. A typist, for example, must have enough arm, shoulder and back muscle endurance to type 8 hours a day. A construction worker needs a high degree of endurance to sustain his vigorous work level for 8 hours a day. Even the top executive needs to maintain a certain level endurance.

How do you know whether or not you need to improve your muscular and/or cardiovascular endurance? Ask yourself these questions:

1. Do I tire during the work day?
2. Am I tired at the end of the work day?
3. Do I have enough energy left over after work for hobbies or other leisure-time pursuits?
4. Do I have the energy for weekend chores and some left over for fun or sports activities?

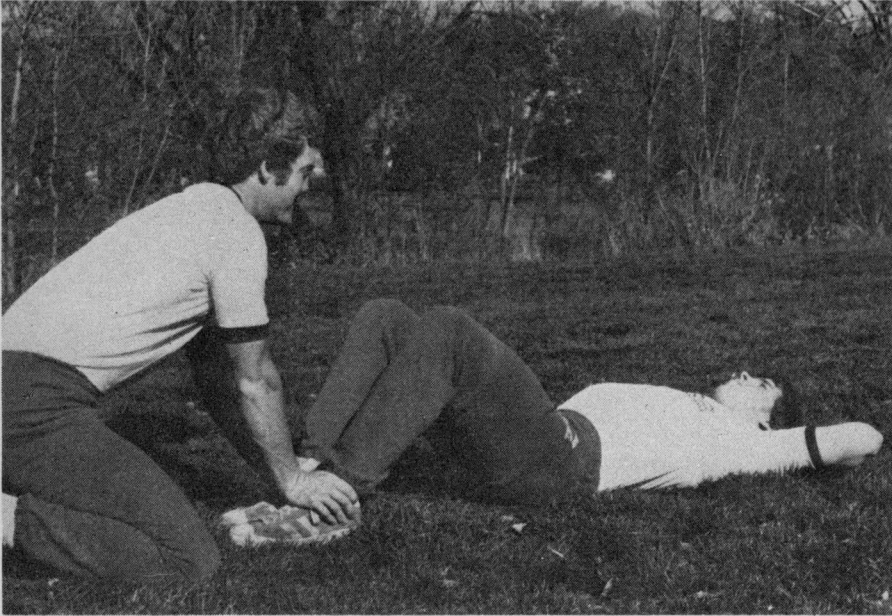

Skeletal muscle endurance involves those muscles needed for movement—neck, arm, trunk and leg muscles. How many situps (left) and/or how many pushups (below) you can do in one exercise period is an indicator of the amount of endurance you possess in your abdominal muscles and arm and shoulder muscles.

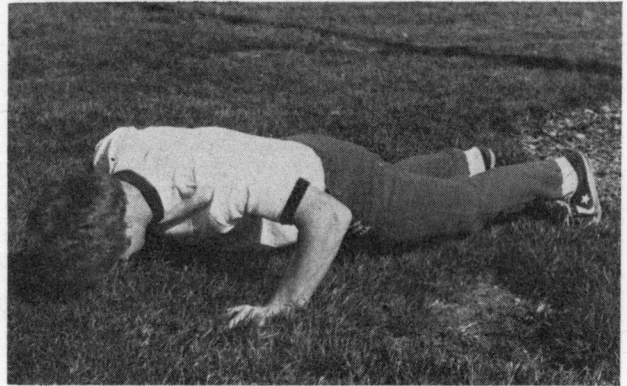

If you seem to tire easily without good reason, if you seem to need lots of naps, if you lack the energy to join the kids or friends in an active game, you need to improve your endurance.

SKELETAL MUSCLE ENDURANCE

Before you attempt to improve the endurance of a specific muscle or muscle group, you must possess adequate strength. Review your scores on the Strength Test in Chapter 1. If you failed any part of the test, you should do exercises to build your muscle strength in that area. Muscle strength is a prerequisite for endurance exercises.

The calisthenic, weight training and isokinetic strength building exercises described in Chapter 3 are also used to build muscular endurance. The main difference between exercising for strength and for endurance is in the number of repetitions. Muscle endurance is developed when a muscle or muscle group works against a light resistance with many repetitions. Strength exercises involve heavy resistance with few repetitions. Endurance exercises should be done at about a rate of 30 per minute. If you are exhausted prior to the 1-minute goal, the resistance or work load is too heavy and you're building strength instead of endurance. If, on the other hand, you are not exhausted at the end of 1 minute and could exercise longer, the resistance is too light and should be increased.

Using the weight training exercises to build endurance, you decrease the amount of resistance and increase the number of repetitions. For example, if you can do 6-10 situps holding a 20-pound weight, reduce the weight to 5 pounds and attempt to do 30 situps in 1 minute. If you are not exhausted at the end of the minute, increase the amount of weight and/or the number of repetitions and the allotted time. By doing this, you are employing the overload principle—as the endurance capacity of a muscle or muscle group increases, the intensity of the exercise is also increased. If you prefer to use calisthenics or isokinetic exercises to increase endurance, do the maximum number of repetitions possible, still using the 30 per minute rate, rest and then repeat. Always strive to increase the number of repetitions.

Unlike strength exercising, where a 50 per-

Fitness and Health

Activities that lead to improved aerobic fitness such as jogging and swimming also:

- Reduce the risk of heart disease.
- Improve circulation and respiration.
- Reduce the problems of overweight.
- Strengthen bones, ligaments and tendons.
- Reduce tension and psychological stress.
- Minimize fatigue.
- Enhance self-concept and body image.

cent gain in strength is difficult to attain, muscle endurance gains are many times dramatic. After a few weeks, it is possible to triple or quadruple the number of repetitions of a particular exercise.

CARDIOVASCULAR ENDURANCE

Cardiovascular pulmonary endurance is the *most important* aspect of any total physical fitness program. Exercise helps your heart, lungs and circulatory system to perform more efficiently—more work with less effort. With the proper exercise, your heart, which is muscle tissue, increases in strength and can pump more blood through your system in fewer beats per minute, whether you are at rest or engaged in physical activity. For example, the heart of an unconditioned person may pump only 70 percent of the blood in each heart chamber, whereas the heart of a physically fit person may pump 80-90 percent. The heart of the conditioned person doesn't have to work as hard (beats less often) to supply the body with blood. This increase in efficiency enables your heart to respond more effectively and safely to a sudden demand.

In addition to strengthening your heart and improving its efficiency, exercise also improves your ability to take in, transport and utilize oxygen. This is known as aerobic capacity. Your respiratory system becomes more efficient—taking in more air with each breath, thus getting

more oxygen into the blood. The increased efficiency of your circulatory system—arteries, capillaries, blood vessels—better distributes blood throughout the body. Increased heart output plus improved distribution leads to an improved supply of oxygen to the muscles. The muscles, which need oxygen to sustain intense activity, can then better respond to long periods of exercise without excessive fatigue.

There is only one exercise method which will effectively build your cardiovascular pulmonary endurance—aerobics. Aerobic exercise includes running and/or jogging, bicycling, swimming, walking, running in place or jumping rope. They are all dynamic, rhythmical activities which will cause a *sustained* increase in heart rate, respiration and muscle metabolism. A sustained exercise will increase the strength and endurance of your heart, lungs and circulatory system and can also reduce body weight by burning a large number of calories in a short period of time.

To benefit from any of the aerobic exercises,

Aerobics and the Heart

The heart is a muscle. Exercise strengthens it, making it a more efficient pump. This allows the heart to get more rest between beats. Exercise reduces the total work done by the heart.

Unconditioned: heart rate = 70 beats a minute × 60 minutes an hour × 24 hours = *100,800* beats a day.

Conditioned: heart rate = 50 beats a minute × 60 minutes an hour × 24 hours = *72,000* beats a day.

As physical activity increases, the risk of heart disease declines. Proper diet, weight control, no smoking or smoky rooms, and reduced tension and stress also are factors in preventing heart disease. So your life-style may be as important as physical activity.

the *intensity*, *duration* and *frequency* of the exercise must be sustained and maintained. The proper *intensity* is best indicated by the heart beat rate you sustain throughout the exercise period. The intensity of your exercise should be based upon your training heart rate. (See Chapter 1 to determine your proper training heart rate.) You must increase your heart beat rate to its training rate and then sustain that rate for at least 15 minutes before you can benefit from any aerobic exercise.

To determine if your heart rate has reached the training rate, do 5 minutes of aerobic exercise and then immediately take your pulse for 15 seconds. Multiply that number by four. If your heart rate is below that suggested, you should pick up the pace of your exercise—i.e., if bicycling, pedal at a faster pace. If your heart rate is higher than suggested, slow down your exercise pace. If your heart beat rate is 30 beats *over* the suggested training rate, you have reached your *maximum* heart beat rate. *Slow* down your exercise pace. Take another count after another 5 minutes of exercise to see if you are within your training heart beat range. You should not overstress your heart.

The *duration* of exercise can be expressed in time, distance or the number of calories burned. We've already stated that an aerobic exercise should be sustained for a minimum of 15 minutes in order to build cardiovascular strength and endurance. In terms of calories, it is recommended

Aerobic Fitness Prescription Chart

Fitness Category		Intensity (in beats/min)	Duration (in calories)		Frequency
			Men	Women*	
Excellent			Over 400†	Over 300†	6 days weekly
	Age 20	164-178			
	25	162-176			
	30	160-174			
	35	157-171	— Exercise duration and frequency		
	40	154-168	remain the same regardless of age —		
	45	151-164			
	50	148-161			
	55	145-158			
	60	143-155			
Average			200-400	150-300	6 days weekly
	Age 20	153-164			
	25	151-162			
	30	148-159			
	35	145-157			
	40	142-154	— Exercise duration and frequency		
	45	139-151	remain the same regardless of age —		
	50	136-149			
	55	133-146			
	60	130-143			
Poor			100-200	75-150	Every other day
	Age 20	140-154			
	25	137-151			
	30	134-148			
	35	130-144			
	40	126-140	— Exercise duration and frequency		
	45	122-136	remain the same regardless of age —		
	50	118-132			
	55	114-128			
	60	110-124			

*Caloric expenditure is less for women, because they are smaller than men and burn fewer calories in a given activity.

†For long duration workouts (over 400 calories), training intensity may be reduced to a comfortable level.

	Calories per minute*	Time taken to burn approx. 200 calories (in minutes)
Calisthenics	5.0	40
Walking (3½ mph)	5.6	36
Cycling (10 mph)	8.5	24
Swimming (crawl)	9.0	22
Skipping Rope (120/min)	10.0	20
Jogging (5 mph)	10.0	20
Running (7.5 mph)	15.0	14

*Exact calories burned depends on efficiency and body size.

that if you rated poor on the Step Test in Chapter 1, your aerobic exercise should last long enough to burn 100 to 200 calories; if average, 200 to 400 calories; and if you rated excellent, you should burn more than 400. To see how many minutes of aerobic exercise it takes to burn 200 calories, see chart at left.

How frequently should you engage in an aerobic exercise period? For beginners, two or three times a week is enough. As you progress, you can begin to exercise more; the more frequently you exercise, the more progress you make toward fitness. As you can see from the Aerobic Fitness Prescription Chart below, those who rate average or excellent should exercise 6 days a week.

Aerobic Activities

Run		Jog		Bicycle		Swim		Walk	
Distance (miles)	Time (min)	Distance (miles)	Time (min)	Distance (miles)	Time (min)	Distance (yd)	Time (min)	Distance (miles)	Time (min)
3.4+	27+	3.4+	40+	7.8+	47+	1,600+	45+	4.2+	72+

— Distance and time remain the same regardless of age —

| 1.7-3.4 | 14-27 | 1.7-3.4 | 20-40 | 3.9-7.8 | 24-47 | 800-1,600 | 22-45 | 2.1-4.2 | 36-72 |

— Distance and time remain the same regardless of age —

| 0.8-1.7 | 7-14 | 0.8-1.7 | 10-20 | 1.9-3.9 | 12-24 | 400-800 | 11-22 | 1.0-2.1 | 18-36 |

— Distance and time remain the same regardless of age —

SAMPLE AEROBIC TRAINING SESSION

Warm-up, aerobic exercise, cooldown—those are the elements of your training session. Let's look closer at a typical session, say for a 35-year-old man in the average fitness category and see how these sessions lead to fitness.

His fitness prescription would be: *intensity,* 145 to 157 beats a minute; *duration,* 200 to 400 calories; *frequency,* every other day at the beginning, then 5 or 6 days a week with 1 day off for good behavior (refer Aerobic Fitness Prescription Chart). He has picked jogging as his aerobic exercise. After his warm-up he will jog at a 12-minute-per mile pace for 20 minutes (1.67 miles) to burn 200 calories (20 minutes at 10 calories a minute). He can vary his sessions by jogging in different locales, working at the upper edge of his training zone for shorter duration, or at the lower edge for longer. After his run, he will cool down with easy jogging, walking and stretching. It won't take too many sessions like this before he begins to experience a *training effect.*

Heart and lungs improve as the body adjusts to regular exercise, and he will soon be able to complete his session at a lower heart rate. As this happens, it's necessary to do something to insure a continued training effect. In the case of our 35-year-old jogger, he could: (1) jog the same distance at a faster pace (but calories burned remain the same); (2) cover a greater distance at the same pace (calories burned increase but intensity falls *below* training zone); (3) slowly increase both pace and distance, thereby keeping heart rate in training zone while increasing calories burned.

In practice, #3 usually occurs naturally. You increase pace without knowing it. You find yourself running faster without a greater sense of effort or fatigue. As fitness improves, it becomes easy to extend the duration of a workout. When you find this happening, you're ready to increase the intensity, duration, and frequency of your training sessions; or periodically retake the Step Test or run the 1½ miles for time to pinpoint your fitness level.

aerobic training session

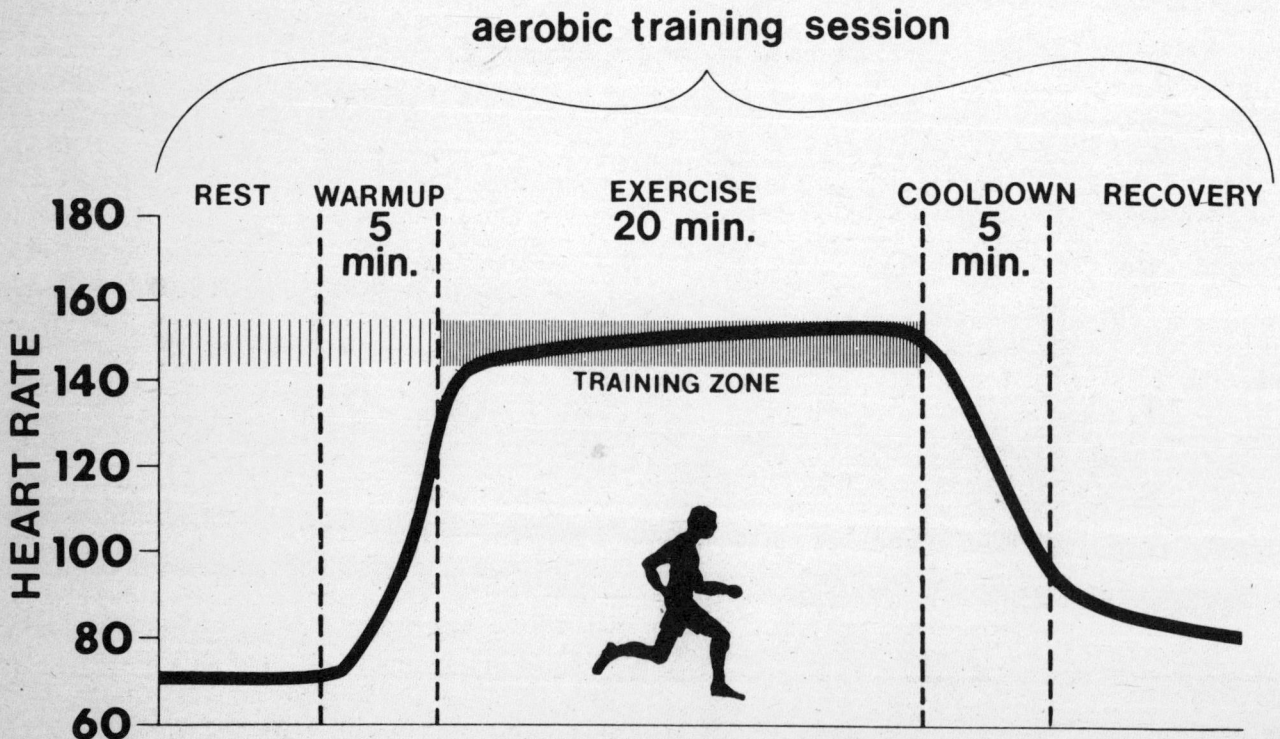

WHICH AEROBIC EXERCISE?

Now that you know how aerobic exercise will benefit your cardiovascular system and how long and how frequently you must participate in aerobic activity, your next decision is which aerobic exercise you will engage in to achieve cardiovascular fitness. First of all, consider your body type, which was discussed in Chapter 1. For each type of body, exercises were given which best suited each body type. This may influence your decision on which type of aerobic exercise you choose. But more importantly, you should choose an exercise that you enjoy. If you select an exercise you don't particularly have fun doing, you're not going to stay on a physical fitness program for long.

We'll try to help in your decision by looking at each of the aerobic exercises—when, where and how to do each and what equipment you need in order to participate in each.

As physical activity increases, the risk of heart disease declines. Make daily physical activity a part of your life-style.

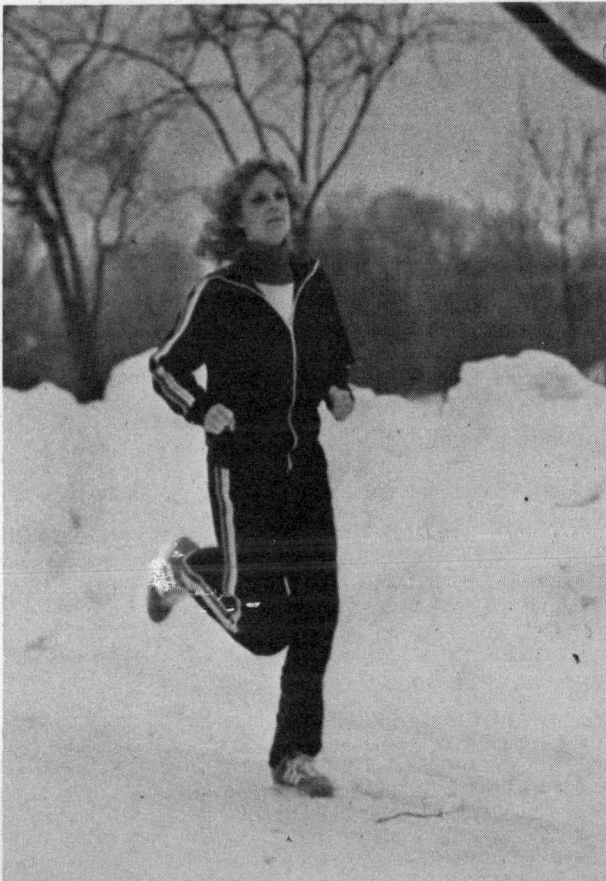

Aerobics and the Lungs

Respiratory muscles become more efficient. Fit individuals take in more air per breath, breathe deeper, and ventilate a greater proportion of their lungs, getting more oxygen into the blood. Oxygen transport in the blood is improved by an increase in hemoglobin and total blood volume.

The body learns to better distribute the blood to working muscles. This redistribution, accompanied by increased heart output, leads to an improved supply of oxygen to the working muscles. Aerobic exercise may increase the number of capillaries serving individual muscle fibers.

RUNNING AND JOGGING

Running is the most instinctive form of cardiovascular pulmonary endurance exercise known to man. Primitive man didn't even know what cardiovascular pulmonary endurance was. He ran not for that reason but to flee from danger. Even the early American Indians did a lot of running, as couriers and in chasing wild game. Here again, their continued welfare and sometimes their lives depended on the ability to run. They didn't think about it—they just did it.

Savage tribes in Africa often saved their lives by running away from an enemy that had them outnumbered. Running from danger was the natural thing to do.

And all of these early people had tremendous cardiovascular pulmonary endurance. When they died, it was rarely from a heart attack but usually from lack of medication for diseases, from an imbalance in diet or from battle wounds. Today in our automated society, few Americans walk, let alone run, to get from one place to the next. And in America today, coronary heart disease is the number one killer. Coincidence?

147

GOT THE BLUES? EXERCISE THEM AWAY, EXPERTS SUGGEST*

Has a blue funk gotcha? Exercise it away.

Two groups of investigators recently published documentation to underpin previous personal testimonials on the value of exercise in relieving depression, a disorder that is almost an epidemic in our society.

"When we run, blue moods lift, anxiety and anger melt away and creative thinking often occurs," said Dr. John Greist of the University of Wisconsin.

Swimming, cycling and dancing, all of which involve the rhythmic movement of large muscle masses, probably will produce the same mood effect, he said, but his studies have been limited to running.

Depressed men and women, ages 18 to 30, were divided into three groups. One group received 10 sessions of standard psychotherapy, the second group received an unlimited amount of psychotherapy, and the third group got a running treatment from a therapist who was not a psychiatrist.

"During runs, discussions ranged over the usual subjects that runners talk about, such as weather, running gear, different running routes, pace, distance, terrain," Greist said, adding that depression was never discussed.

Six of the eight patients who ran were essentially cured within 3 weeks. A seventh patient recovered during the 16th week of study. The eighth patient, while running conscientiously according to prescription, showed neither improvement nor deterioration in depression, although she did increase her level of fitness.

"These results compare favorably with those patients in psychotherapy and have persisted for at least a year in follow-up."

In the December issue of the *Physician and Sportsmedicine,* Dr. Robert S. Brown of the University of Virginia gave students a battery of psychological tests, including depression and personality exams, before and after a 10-week period of running three times a week, 30-minutes a day, or engaging in some other form of exercise.

"Depression scores decreased with wrestling, mixed exercise, jogging and probably with tennis," Brown said. "However, there was no change in depressions in the softball team members or the group that had no exercise routine."

The most significant reductions in depression scores occurred in the group that jogged for 5 days a week for a 10-week period.

*Reprinted with permission from the *Chicago Sun-Times.* Article by Arthur J. Snider.

Hardly. Lack of exercise, vigorous exercise, is directly related to the rise of heart disease. Running and jogging are not a panacea for heart disease but they can reduce your risks of having a heart attack by strengthening the heart muscle, lowering your body weight, reducing the amount of fat in the blood, and possibly reducing stress and strain.

Before you begin a running or jogging program, you must know what condition your heart and circulatory system is in. The first order of business should be a visit to your physician. With his OK, take the Step Test in Chapter 1 to give you a rough indication of your cardiovascular condition. Another self-testing method is Dr. Kenneth Cooper's 12-minute Run/Walk Test. You simply see how much distance you can cover by running and walking in a 12-minute period. If you cover less than a mile, you are in very poor condition. If you traverse 1¾ miles and up in the 12-minute period, you are in excellent condition.

If you are overweight, have diabetes, lower back pain, liver or kidney problems but still want to run, see your doctor before trying the Step Test or Cooper Walk/Run Test. Very likely your doctor can prescribe a walking and/or running program which will best fit your needs.

You may also want to know what the difference is between running and jogging. Not much really. When you run, you move at a pace of roughly 7.5 mph. Jogging is a slightly slower pace—5 mph. If you are a beginner or if your physical fitness rating is poor, you should begin by jogging—after all, the purpose of cardiovas-

Before You Run/Jog

Running (or jogging), the most instinctive and primitive exercise known to man, is simple. All the advice and instruction you need is extremely brief. Let's review it:

1. *Before you start, get the approval of a qualified physician, probably following a complete physical examination.*
2. *Get your feet in condition. Get rid of corns, bunions and painful callouses. Strengthen the feet by exercise if necessary.*
3. *Strengthen the muscles most used in running by a simple exercise program. Aim especially at strengthening the legs, abdomen and upper chest.*
4. *Limber up by doing the simple flexibility exercises described in this book. What this amounts to is stretching any muscles that seem to be taut. Passive stretching, with a prolonged pull on them without motion, is better than active stretching.*
5. *Always do a warm-up before running or jogging and a cooling-off at its conclusion.*
6. *Don't try too much too soon.*
7. *Don't use a sprinter's style. Come down on your heels rather than your toes.*
8. *Of the little special equipment and apparel needed, see that it's of good quality, properly constructed, and that it fits you correctly.*
9. *Set your own pace. Don't try to compete against runners who are in better condition, have more natural ability or are younger than you are.*
10. *For maximum effectiveness, run or jog from 15 to 30 minutes three times a week.*
11. *If you get hurt, lay off for a few days until the damage is corrected.*
12. *Since running is a natural, instinctive exercise, rely on your instincts to guide you.*
13. *Make it fun. Jog outdoors rather than inside whenever possible. Run or jog on grass or dirt in preference to cinders or pavement, particularly when you're getting started.*
14. *Make running or jogging a habit, a regular part of your life rather than something you're going to do long enough to better your physical condition.*
15. *Last, while it's not a specific point, run or jog for about 3 weeks before you make up your mind to get your cardiovascular pulmonary endurance exercise from such activity. Then if you decide it's not for you and that swimming or bicycling or long, brisk walks would be more fun, by all means follow the dictates of your instinct.*

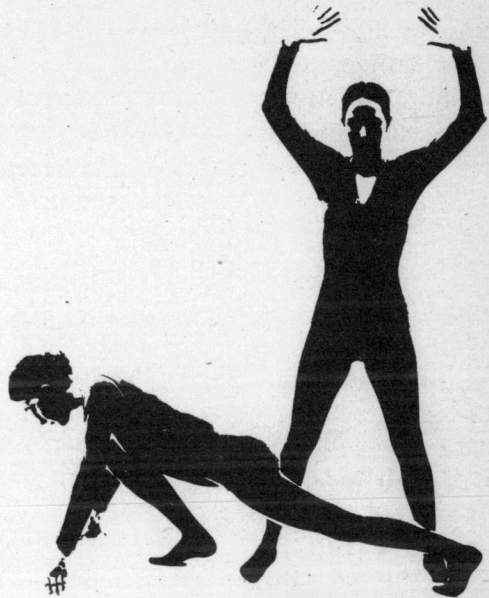

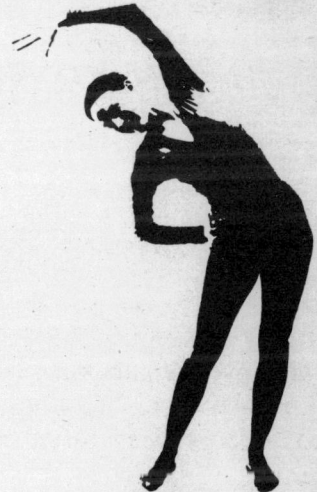

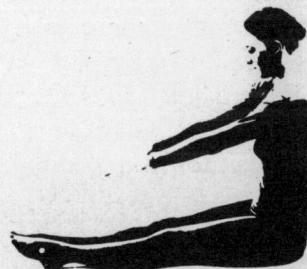

cular exercise is rhythmic and sustained activity. If you began by running, you probably could not sustain that fast pace for very long.

With your doctor's OK and an evaluation of your physical fitness condition, you are ready to begin running or jogging.

Before You Jog or Run—The Warm-up

The warm-up, which should last about 5 minutes, gradually prepares the body for the exercise to come. Begin with easy stretching exercises and then, as body temperature, circulation, and respiration adjust to the increased activity, move to more vigorous calisthenics (see Chapter 2 for suggested warm-up exercises). Pay particular attention during the warm-up to:

- Stretching the lower back to reduce back problems.
- Stretching hamstring and calf muscles to prevent soreness and reduce the risk of injury.
- Increasing tempo of exercise gradually to adjust body to higher levels of intensity.

Where to Jog or Run

If possible, avoid hard surfaces such as concrete and asphalt for the first few weeks. Running tracks (located at most high schools), grass playing fields, parks and golf courses are recommended. In inclement weather, jog in church, school or YMCA gymnasiums; in protected areas around shopping centers; or in your garage or basement. Varying locations and routes will add interest to your program.

When to Jog or Run

Run whenever it suits your fancy. Some like to get up early and do several miles before breakfast. Others elect to run during the lunch hour, then eat a sandwich at their desk. Many prefer to wait until after work, when running can help cleanse the mind of the day's problems. A few are night owls who brave the dark in their quest for fitness; they are quick to point out that the run and shower help them to sleep like a baby. We would only caution you to avoid vigorous activity 1 or 2 hours after a meal, when the digestive organs require an adequate blood supply, and when any fat in the circulation hastens the risk of clotting.

What to Wear

The most important piece of running "equipment" is the running shoe. Because it is so important, we're covering running shoes separately. Here, we'll talk about the type of clothing you should wear when jogging or running.

Jogging doesn't require fancy clothing. One of running's attractions is the fact that you don't need to spend much money. Nylon or cotton gym shorts and a T-shirt are adequate in summer. For winter running, a sweat suit or jogging suit serves until temperatures fall below 20 degrees Fahrenheit. Some runners prefer cotton

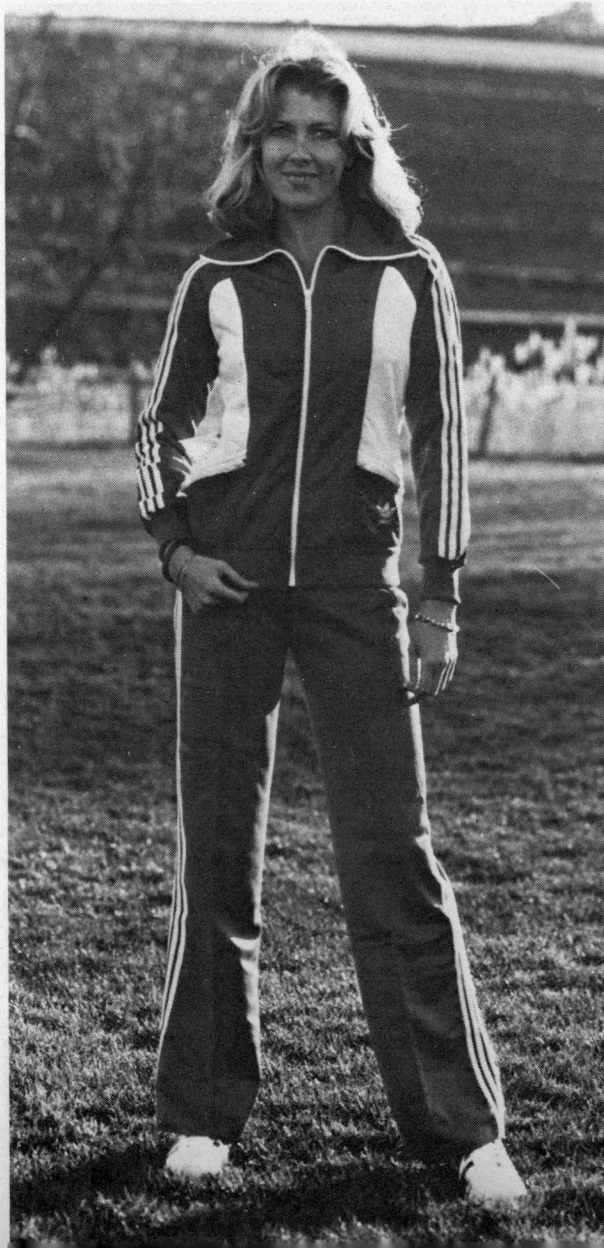

For winter running, a warm-up suit will keep you warm until the thermometer dips below 20 degrees Fahrenheit. (Photo courtesy of Adidas.)

Aerobics for Overall Fitness

Aerobic exercise influences other organs and systems: the nervous system learns to use muscles efficiently; the endocrine system learns to support your efforts with the appropriate hormones. Bones, ligaments, and tendons get tougher.

The physique and body composition can be altered. Body fat diminishes, muscles tone up, and appearance improves. Along with improved appearance and the feeling of well being go some subtle psychological changes: improved self-concept and body image, reduced anxiety, improved vitality, increased self-confidence, and joy of living.

There is evidence that some of the effects of aging may be temporarily offset with a vigorous aerobic fitness program, so the increased capacity and adaptability associated with aerobic fitness can add life to your years, not just years to your life.

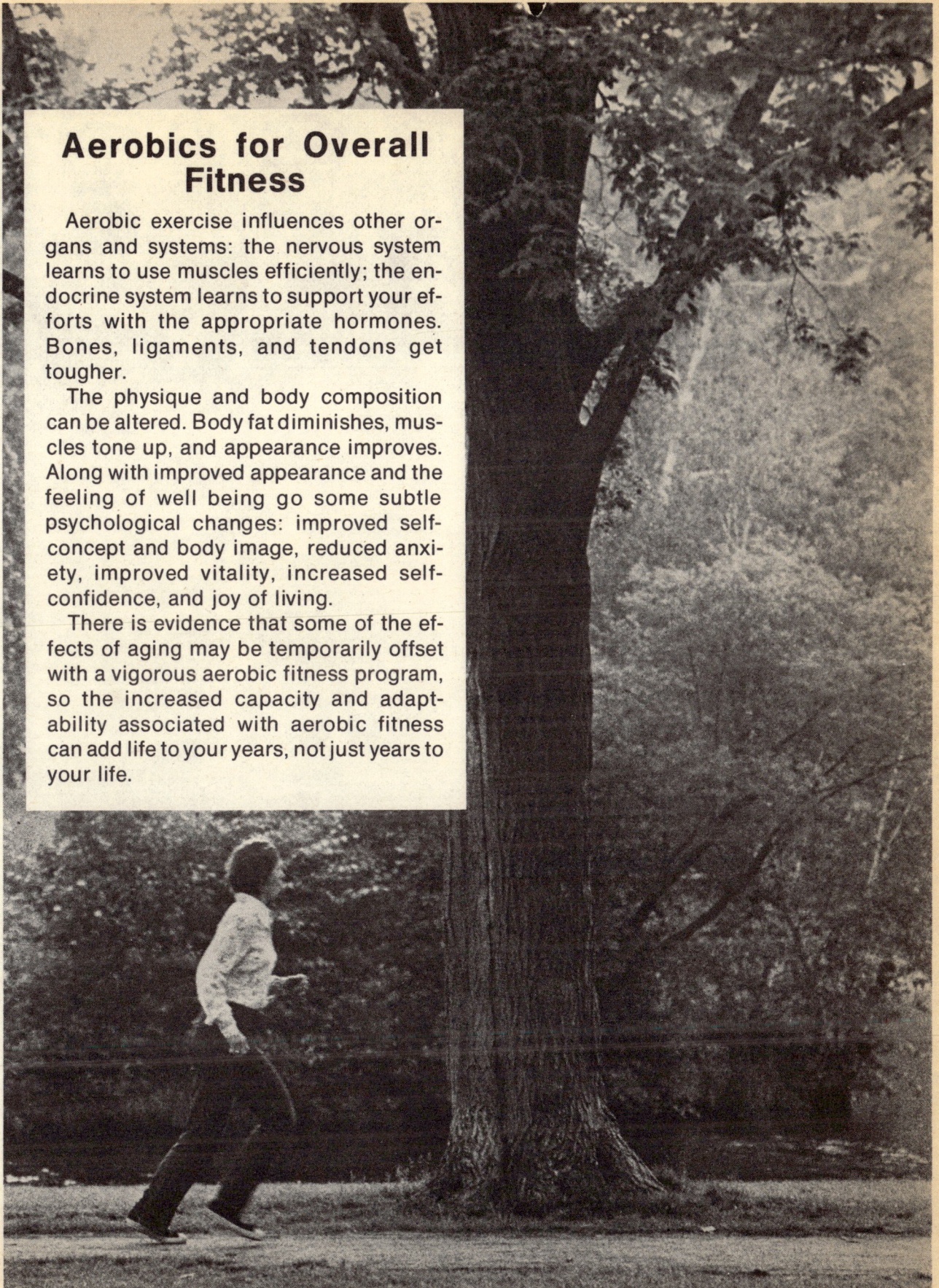

thermal knit long underwear under their running shorts. Several layers of lighter apparel are preferable to a single heavy garment. Add gloves and a knit cap in colder temperatures. When the wind blows, a thin nylon windbreaker helps to reduce heat loss. A cap is particularly important in cold weather, since a great deal of body heat is lost through the head.

When temperatures fall below 20 degrees Fahrenheit, you may choose to wear both the underwear and the sweat suit. Many continue to run despite subzero temperatures. There is no danger in doing so provided you are properly clothed, warmed-up, and sensitive to signs of wind chill and frostbite.

Never wear a rubberized sweat suit in any weather. The water lost through perspiration

The Running Bra by Formfit is designed to minimize bounce, skin irritation and collagen tissue breakdown which results in sagging.

doesn't contribute to long term weight loss, and your body's most effective mode of heat loss is blocked.

Special Clothing Considerations for Women

An American Medical Association study of female athletes and the need for special bras showed that every step a runner took caused the breasts to rise and then fall against the chest. Such a movement, the study concluded, always caused soreness. Women athletes have commented that on the occasions when the bouncing isn't pronounced enough to be painful, it's always psychologically uncomfortable.

Since the best custom fit bras for running cost from $20 to $25, some women are reluctant to spend the money. But a well-fitted bra should be considered a necessary part of the woman's running equipment. Since right and left breasts are never identical, a custom fit bra for the serious runner should be considered.

In addition to being individually fitted, the best bras shouldn't have underwires or anything that puts weight on the shoulders. It should limit both up and down and lateral motion and be made of firm, elastic material that's nonabrasive and nonallergenic, with either velcro fastening or a placket to protect the skin from fasteners.

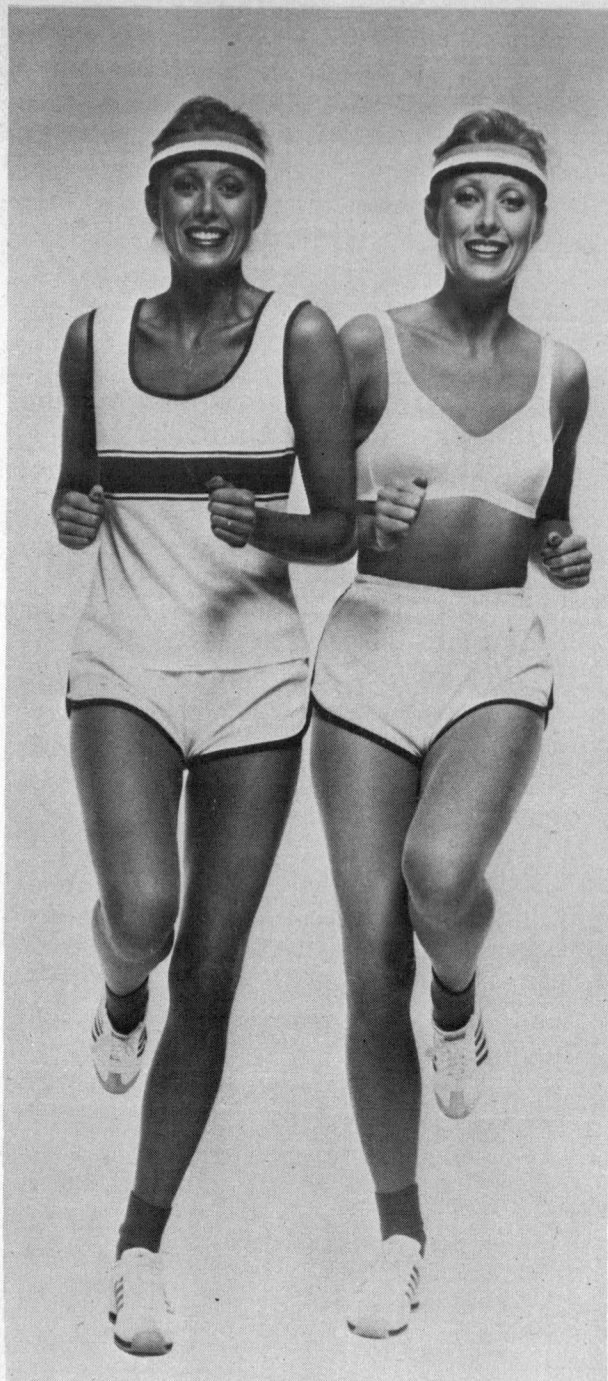

There are less expensive substitutes. For those who aren't allergic to synthetics, there's a Warner's bra of firm elastic with adjustable straps. Sears, Roebuck & Co. sells their Step-In Sports Bra with an all-around stretch nylon bottom band that holds the bra in place—no fastener is needed. Also on the market is Form-Fit's Running Bra for around $10.

Running Shoes

Everyone agrees that the most important piece of equipment for a runner is the right pair of shoes. There are many good, durable, well-made running shoes on the market. Probably your best bet for finding the right pair for you is a sporting goods store or shoe store, unless you trade at a well-stocked department store. However, few stores carry *all* the well-accepted brands of running shoes. The beginning runner can expect to do a considerable amount of shopping around, particularly in a nonmetropolitan area, in order to find the brand or type of shoe that fits best.

Some runners buy their shoes by mail-order and find their purchases most satisfactory. You don't just send your shoe size and width but also a pencil outline of each foot, since the right and left feet are seldom identical. If the shoes aren't right for you when they arrive, send them back immediately. You will find a list of the top running shoe manufacturers at the end of this section.

If you're trying on running shoes in a store, wear your running socks. If you wear both an inner and outer pair of socks when running, as some runners do, wear both when you're getting fitted. Again, it's a good idea to take with you a pencil outline of each foot. Comparing the bottom of a shoe with your tracing can often show you a great deal about the shoe's conformity to your foot.

When you try a shoe on, pay special attention to the toe area. Cramped toes can cause trouble. When standing, there should be at least ¾-inch between the tips of your toes and the end of the shoe.

One "must" is foot comfort, so you should walk around the store to ascertain how comfortable—or uncomfortable the shoe is.

Everyone agrees that good foot support is vitally important since your feet will be hitting the ground hard many times during the running session. Nearly all running shoes have some support, but the amount is by no means standard. While it's possible to *add* support after you've bought shoes, it's certainly preferable to have what you want already in the shoe as it comes from the manufacturer.

Training flats, the shoes worn from day to day in running sessions, are considerably heavier than racing flats, which are built light to give a racer greater speed. The racing flats aren't recommended for the less experienced or noncompetitive runner.

But even in the training flats, there can be a vast difference in weight. Extra weight can

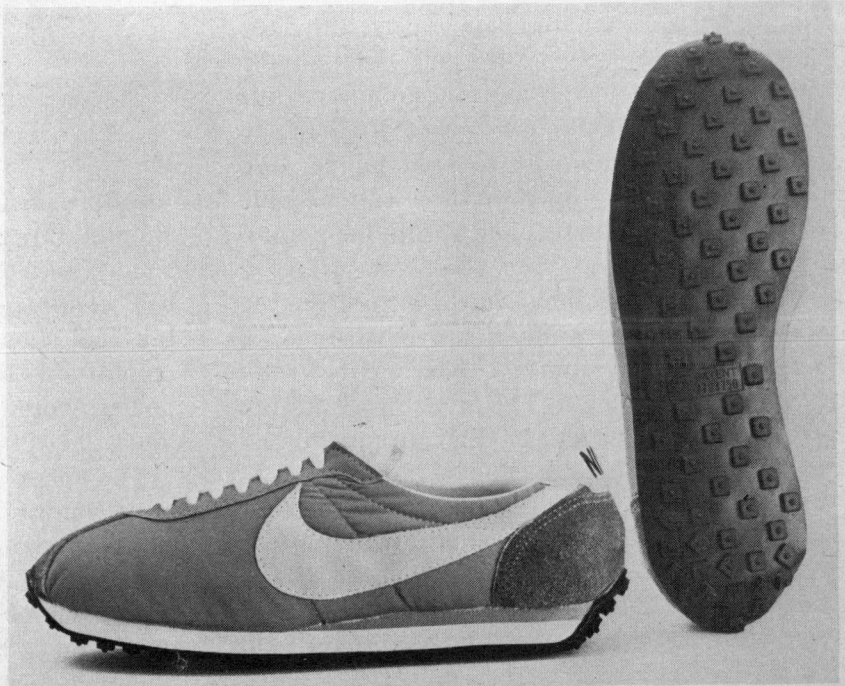

Nike's Waffle Trainer is particularly good for traversing rough terrain. The Waffle Trainer is lighter than most other training flats.

The racing flat, such as the Nike Elite (right), is designed for speed and is really not needed by anyone other than the serious competitive runner. A racing flat is lighter weight than the training flat and it will usually have a thinner sole.

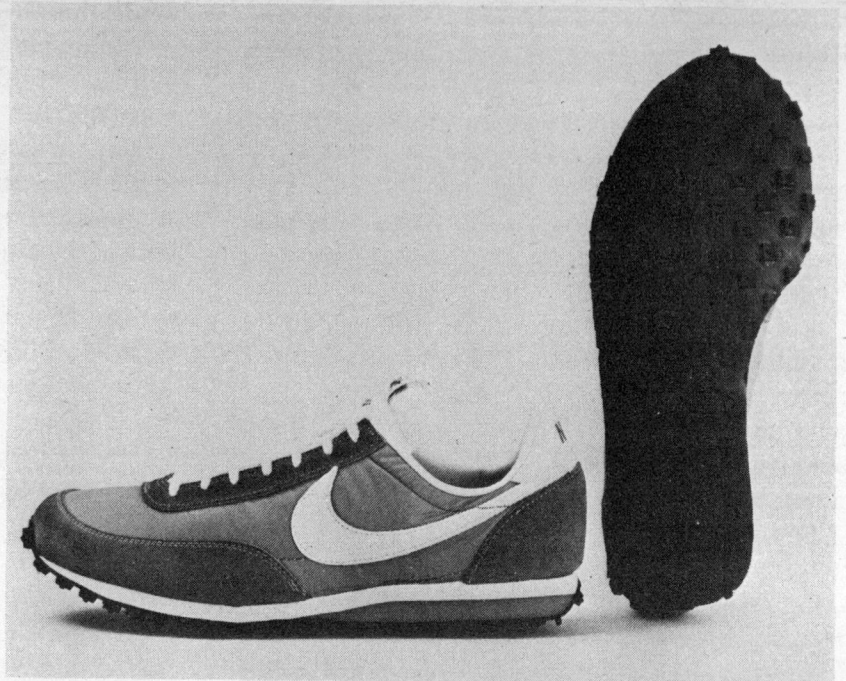

Adidas' Formula I training flat (below right) is highly recommended because of its high heel lift which helps relieve strain on the Achilles tendon — a common problem area for most joggers and runners.

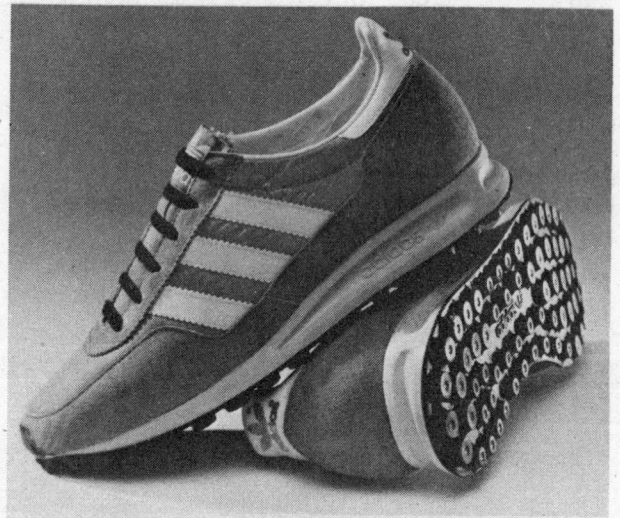

exhaust you on a long run. The lightest weight training flats that fill the bill in other respects will be your best choice.

All-over fit is one of the requirements—and nobody except the wearer can be absolutely sure that a shoe fits him perfectly for running and jogging. A shoe that doesn't come in a variety of widths as well as lengths is one to be wary of.

A shoe must have flexibility, especially in the sole. If the sole doesn't bend easily, the shoe can create great problems for you. Soles should provide both protection and cushioning, while staying flexible. Some shoes have more than one sole—a tough outer sole to fight impact and wear, and one, two, or even three softer inside layers to cushion the foot and absorb the pounding.

Treads on shoe soles vary. Currently, the most popular is the waffle tread, consisting of a series of raised grippers. The waffle tread provides good traction. The grippers absorb the first part of the impact and can consequently be considered part of the cushioning process.

Spikes are recommended only for experienced competitive racers and are definitely much more jarring than rubber treads.

While you might think that a narrow heel would be preferable, it's now been established that wider heels give more stability. The heel should, however, hold the heel of your foot snugly, to avoid blisters. A somewhat elevated heel is now considered preferable. The back of the heel should hit the back of your foot at a comfortable level. If it is too low, the shoe will not provide the support you need. If too high, you will be plagued by blisters.

The upper of the shoe is often the selling feature, simply by eye-appeal, but the upper must be functionally correct, too. It must be firm enough to hold the foot in position but soft enough to be comfortable. Thick seams in an upper can be uncomfortable and irritating.

Uppers come in nylon, leather or a combination of the two. Most runners prefer nylon because ot its light weight and the fact that it permits air to circulate more freely. It's also more water-resistant than leather and easier to clean.

Prices for training flats vary from the mid-twenties up to $40.

No one shoe has everything. One of the best, with high-quality workmanship, has a three-layered sole, a waffle tread, the wider heel with an outside groove to further reduce shock, a nylon mesh upper, and great strength and durability. However, it is available in just one width. The price is around $40.

A shoe that won first place in the *Runner's World* magazine's evaluation comes in narrow, medium and wide widths, has two layers of sole under the forefoot and three under the heel, a

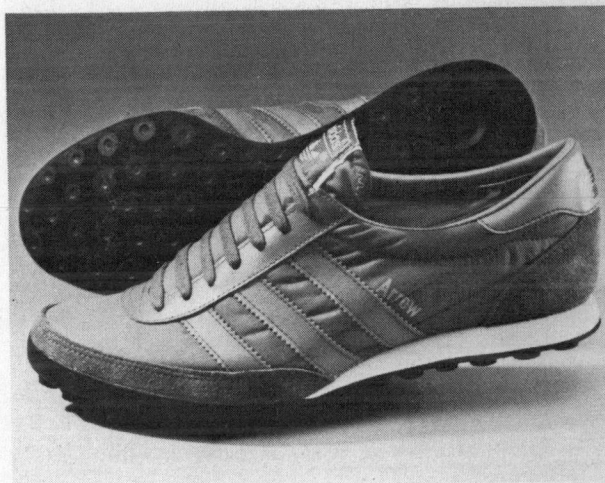

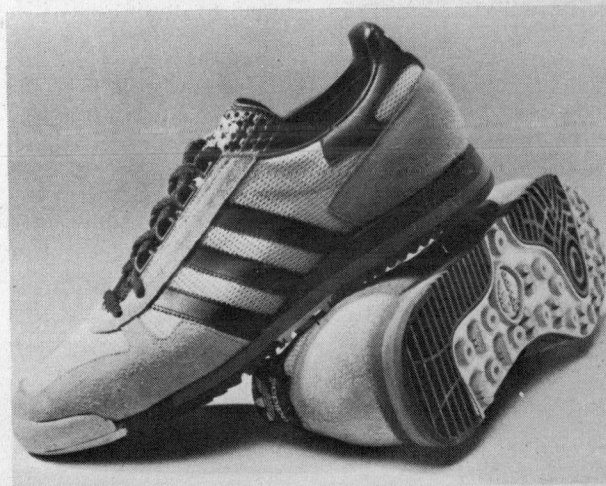

The Adidas Arrow (above) is a spikeless racing flat with nylon uppers and velour reinforcement. For women there is the Adidas Lady Runner (below).

Running Shoe Manufacturers

Adidas USA Inc.
2382 Townsgate Road
Westlake Village, CA 91361
(805) 497-9575

Brooks Shoe Mfg. Co.
Factory and Terrace Streets
Hanover, PA 17331
(717) 632-1755

Converse Rubber Co.
55 Fordham Rd.
Wilmington, MA 01887
(617) 657-5735

E.B. Sport International
Lydiard Enterprise
Box 180
Basking Ridge, NJ 07920
(201) 324-9011

Etonic
Eaton Co.
147 Centre St.
Brockton, MA 02403
(617) 583-9100

New Balance Athletic Shoes
38-42 Everett St.
Boston, MA 02134
(617) 783-4000

Nike
8285 S.W. Nimbus Ave.
Beaverton, OR 97005
(503) 641-6453

Pony Sports & Leisure Inc.
251 Park Ave. South
New York, NY 10010

Puma
Beconta Inc.
50 Executive Blvd.
Elmsford, NY 10523
(914) 592-4444

Saucony Shoe Mfg. Co.
14 Peach St.
Kutztown, PA 19530
(215) 683-8711

Tiger
2052 Alton Ave.
Irvine, CA 92714
(714) 754-0451

special innersole that molds itself to the runner's foot, and nylon mesh uppers. However, the sole is less durable than one would expect on such a high quality product. The price is around $35.

Probably one of the best buys on the market has an excellent built-in arch support. The heel is well-cushioned, but the forefoot cushioning isn't as good. The waffle tread rates high on durability, along with the nylon and suede upper. Available sizes are 6 to 13, in narrow, medium and wide widths, the price running around $30.

Although the sole durability and flat tread are disadvantages, another shoe has the advantage of coming in all the standard widths of ordinary shoes, from AA to EEEE. It also has good shock absorption, a one-piece polyester and suede upper with a padded tongue for comfort and a padded heel for excellent support. The price on this one, too, is moderate, running around $30.

The manufacturer who introduced the waffle tread has another shoe that's particularly good for running over rough surfaces. The upper is nylon and suede. The shock absorption in the heel is below average, but the weight is about 10 percent lower than that of most of the good running shoes. Again, the price is around $30.

One of the best buys in a recommended shoe is strong and durable but short on cushioning, although it has a four-layer heel. The upper is very strong, and the price is only around $28.

Another of the lower-priced training shoes has a good waffle tread and flared heel, with fairly good forefoot cushioning and excellent heel cushioning. The nylon mesh upper gets a high rating on durability and comfort, and the price is only around $25, but it comes in medium width only.

Another which rates well in everything except sole durability comes in narrow, medium and wide widths and is only around $23.

Training flats for women are for the most part in the $25 to $30 price range. One developed by a dedicated woman runner is both lightweight and rugged. It has a star waffle pattern, good traction and a wide heel for stability. The upper of nylon mesh trimmed with suede is both durable and comfortable. The shoe has a contoured arch support, comes in narrow, medium and wide widths and is priced at around $28.

Heel-and-Toe

A doctor who jogs regularly says he didn't like that form of exercise at first, much as he wanted to. He studied the foot movements of those who enjoyed jogging. "When I began to imitate their jogging style," he says, "it made all the difference in the world. For the first time, I began to enjoy the exercise. The right heel-and-toe motion is, I think, the most important phase of jogging."

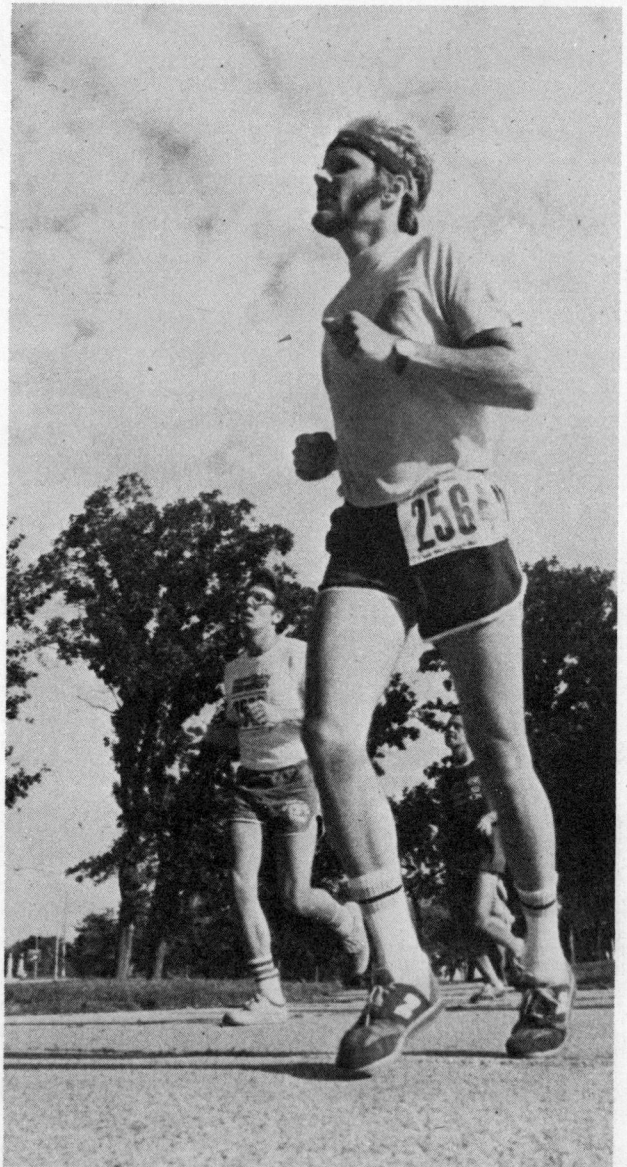

A marathon is probably the most gruelling and brutally demanding event a runner can enter into. Twenty-six miles 385 yards, non-stop.

THE JOY OF RUNNING

In spite of the criticism against running as an exercise by some orthopedic surgeons and a few internists, the number of serious runners seems to go upward every day. Such popularity must be deserved.

The basic theme of runners seems to be Joy! They all talk enthusiastically about how happy running has made them. Some of them go so far as to lyricize how running has taught them to enjoy pain. People all over the United States are quick to tell what running has done for them — and the testimonials are not from any one segment of society. They all say that the psychological benefits at least equal the physical ones. Running, they say, has given them more self-respect. It has increased their confidence in themselves, it has made them friendlier, it has made them think more clearly, and it has improved their dispositions, while relieving their tensions.

There is so much ardent testimony from runners that anyone who investigates its effects is forced to the conclusion that the exercise must have considerable merit.

And the stamp of approval for running isn't given solely by young, vigorous athletes. People in their 70's and even their 80's are running devotees. Constantly increasing numbers of both the young and the old are participating, and running marathons all over the country get so many entrants that the courses are jammed — at least at the outset.

One of the leading recruiters for runners would have to be James E. Fixx, author of that publishing phenomenon, *The Complete Book of Running,* which enjoyed weeks of the enviable number one position on the Best Seller lists. Mr. Fixx is a zealous missionary for the sport, seeking — and getting — many converts.

Joe Henderson is another leader. As editor of *Runner's World,* he determines the editorial make-up of a magazine that is sometimes called the runner's bible. Nobody in the publishing field would have given a plugged nickel for its chances when it began, because its potential subscription list seemed much too limited. Even successful as it is today, magazine publishers would still give it a low rating on the basis of editorial make-up, writing and layout. But runners swear by it and keep their dog-eared back issues.

One of Henderson's best promotions has been what he calls Fun Runs, held in somewhere from 70 to 80 cities throughout the United States and in a few foreign cities. There's no registration fee, no qualifying and none of the red tape that often ties up such an event. Naturally, *Runner's World* is prominent at every Fun Run. To get information on how to get a Fun Run going in your community, simply send a query to Bob Anderson, *Runner's World,* Box 366, Mountain View, California 94042. Incidentally, the subscription price to *Runner's World* is $9 a year.

If cross-country running is your dish, there's *The Harrier,* Box 188, Eltingville Station, Staten Island, New York 10312, at $8 a year.

The Jogger, a newsletter published by the National Jogging Association, 1910 K Street NW, Washington, D.C. 20006, is given to paid-up members of the association.

Running, a quarterly published in Salem, Oregon, Box 350, 97308, is $5 a year.

Running Times, 12808 Occoquan Road, Woodbridge, Virginia 22192, is a monthly at $10 a year aimed particularly at runners in the East.

Yankee Runner, Box 237, Merrimac, Massachusetts 01860, is designed to cover running in the New England area.

As you can see, when you become a runner, you're not alone. If you have the feeling that running will make you something unique, forget it. You're joining a big fraternity.

A few runners get discouraged and quit early in the game, almost always because they got off to a bad start, without proper advice or supervision. There's really little excuse for that because competent guidance is now available everywhere.

Every experienced adviser will tell you that you don't get instant results. The first few days of running are difficult for the beginner, who is almost never in good physical condition, but improvement after the start is rapid.

Another that comes in sizes from 3½ to 10½ and widths from AAAA to EEEE gives excellent shock absorption and excellent heel cushioning. The price is around $28.

There are also a great many racing flats for men and women, in roughly the same price range as the training shoes, but of lighter weight. By the time a runner is ready for racing flats, he or she will have seen enough variety in these shoes to have a general idea of what is wanted.

Running/Jogging Technique

An upright posture while running conserves energy. Run with your back comfortably straight, your head up, and shoulders relaxed. Bend your arms with hands held in a comfortable position; keep arm swing to a minimum during jogging and slow running. Pumping action increases with speed. Legs swing freely from the hips with no attempt to overstride. Many successful distance runners employ a relatively short stride.

No aspect of running technique is violated more often by neophytes than the footstrike. Many newcomers say they can't or don't like to jog. Observation of their footstrike often reveals the reason: they run on the ball of the foot. While appropriate for sprints and short distances, this footstrike is inappropriate for distance runs and will probably result in soreness. The *heel-to-toe* footstrike is recommended for most runners. Upon landing on the heel, the foot rocks forward to push off on the ball of the foot. This technique is the least tiring of all, and a large percentage of successful distance runners use it. The flat-footed technique is a compromise where the runner lands on the entire foot and rocks onto the ball for push-off. Check your shoes after several weeks of running; if you're using the correct footstrike, the outer border of the heel will be wearing down.

Hot Weather Running

At moderate temperatures the body heat generated by exercise or work is easily dissipated. As temperatures increase, the temperature-regulating mechanisms increase perspiration rate to keep the body temperature from climbing above tolerable limits (about 102.5 degrees Fahrenheit). (As perspiration evaporates it cools the body.) When humidity is high, it doesn't evaporate, and no heat is lost. At that point, excessive sweating only contributes to the problem. Perspiration comes from the blood and reduces blood volume. Also, salt and potassium needed by the cells are lost in perspiration.

During work in the heat, it's common to lose more than a quart of sweat an hour. During vigorous exercise in a hot, humid environment, sweat rates can approach 3 quarts an hour for short periods. A good estimate of fluid loss is the body weight difference after work in the heat. Athletes often lose 6-8 pounds in a single workout. Adequate replacement of water, salt and potassium is vital to maintain exercise or work capacity and to avoid heat cramps, heat exhaustion or heat stroke.

To replace salt loss, drink lightly salted water (¼-teaspoon of salt per quart of water), and use the saltshaker at mealtime. Avoid salt tablets. Potassium must be replaced with citrus fruits or juices. Some commercially available drinks supply fluid and electrolyte (inorganic chemicals for cellular reactions) needs. Another approach is to lightly salt lemonade or to drink tomato juice and water (or tomato juice, then water) in volumes comparable to the fluid loss.

The body adjusts or acclimates to work in the heat. Gradual exposure to exercise in a hot environment leads to changes in blood flow, reduced salt loss, and increased perspiration. After 5 to 7 days your heart rate for the same amount of exercise may decline from 180 to 150 beats per minute. Physically fit individuals acclimate more readily to work in the heat, their well-trained circulatory systems make them better suited to its demands. Acclimated individuals should be able to replace salt loss with the saltshaker at meals.

Altitude and Running

As you ascend to higher elevations to run or jog, be aware of limitations imposed on work capacity by reduced oxygen supply.

During the first few weeks of exposure to altitude, your ability to perform is impaired. It can be improved over a period of several weeks by training at that altitude. Altitude acclimatization leads to improved lung function, increased red blood cells and hemoglobin, and increased numbers of capillaries in the working muscles. These changes reduce but never eliminate the effect of altitude on aerobic capacity.

Air Pollution and Running

Avoid exercise in a polluted atmosphere. Carbon monoxide takes the place of oxygen in the red blood cells, which reduces aerobic ca-

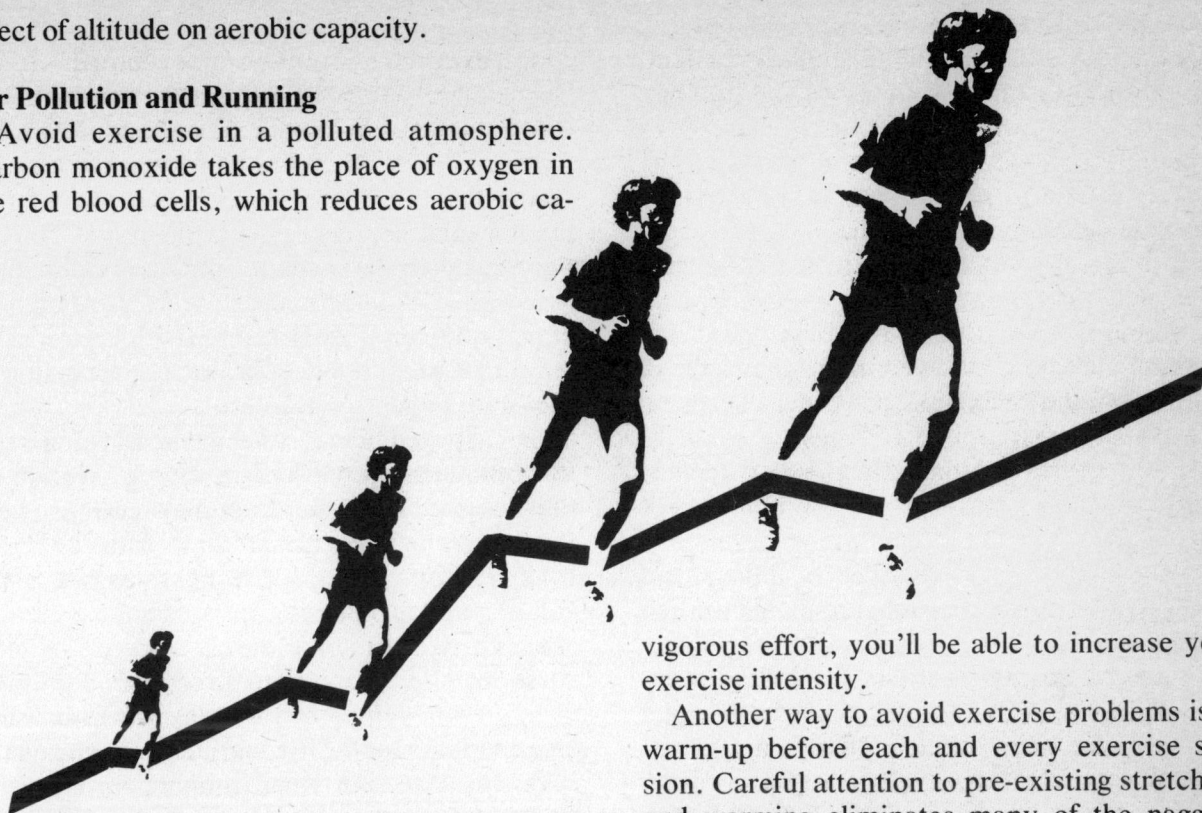

pacity. Air pollution can:

- Irritate airways (bronchitis).
- Break down air sacs in lungs (emphysema).
- Reduce oxygen transport.
- Cause cancer.

One source of pollution can do all these things—the cigarette. It's probably the worst single source of air pollution.

The U.S. Surgeon General has stated that the effects of smoking also may be harmful to the nonsmoker who is exposed to the smoke of cigarettes, cigars, and pipes. Pipe and cigar smoke is particularly unhealthy because it hasn't been inhaled into the smoker's lungs, which helps to filter out some of the harmful ingredients in the smoke.

Running and Jogging Problems

Previously inactive adults often encounter problems when they begin exercising. You'll avoid such problems if you vow to make haste slowly. It may have taken you 10 years to get in the shape you're in, and you won't be able to change it overnight. Plan now to make gradual progress. At the start, too little may be better than too much. After several weeks, when your body has begun to adjust to the demands of

vigorous effort, you'll be able to increase your exercise intensity.

Another way to avoid exercise problems is to warm-up before each and every exercise session. Careful attention to pre-existing stretching and warming eliminates many of the nagging complications that plague less patient individuals. Never forget to cool down after each workout. In short, prevention is the most effective way to deal with exercise problems.

Blisters can be prevented by wearing good, properly fitted shoes. At the first hint of discomfort, cover the area with some moleskin or a large bandage. If you do get a blister, puncture the edge with a sterilized needle to drain the accumulated fluid, treat with an antiseptic, cover with gauze, circle with foam rubber, and go back to work. It's wise to keep the items needed for blister prevention at hand.

Muscle soreness, usually due to exercise after long inactivity, may be caused by microscopic tears in the muscle or connective tissue, or to contractions of muscle fibers. It's almost impossible to avoid soreness when you first begin exercising. Minimize it by exercising modestly, at least at first, and by doing mild stretching exercises when soreness does occur. Stretching can be used to relieve soreness and to warm-up for exercise on the following day. Massage and warm muscle temperatures also seem to minimize the discomfort of soreness.

Side stitch is commonly experienced by the beginner or unconditioned runner. A sharp pain felt just beneath the rib cage, it is thought to be a muscle cramp in the abdominal area, perhaps the diaphragm muscle. If you can stand the pain, keep on running; there is nothing to worry about and it will eventually go away.

Muscle cramps are powerful involuntary muscle contractions. Immediate relief comes when the cramped muscle is stretched and massaged. However, that does not remove the underlying cause of the contraction. Salt and potassium are both involved in the chemistry of contraction and relaxation. Cold muscles seem to cramp more readily. It's always wise to warm-up before vigorous effort and to replace salt and potassium lost through sweating in hot weather.

Bone bruises are experienced by hikers and joggers usually on the bottoms of the feet. Such bruises can be avoided by careful foot placement and by quality footwear. Cushioned inner soles also help. A bad bruise can linger, delaying your exercise many weeks. There's no instant cure once a bruise has developed, so prevention seems the best advice. Ice may help to lessen discomfort and hasten healing. Padding may allow exercise in spite of the bruise.

Ankle problems especially in the case of a sprained ankle should be iced immediately. A bucket of ice water in the first few minutes may allow you to work the next day. A serious sprain should be examined by a physician. High-topped gym shoes reduce the risk of ankle sprains in games such as basketball, tennis, handball; low-cuts with thick soles invite sprains. Ankle wraps and tape allow exercise after a sprain, but again, prevention is a more prudent course.

Achilles tendon injuries have become quite common. Some high-backed running shoes have been implicated in the rash of *bursa* injuries among runners. The bursa is located beneath the tendon and serves to lubricate its movements. When rubbed long enough, it becomes inflamed. Once inflamed, it may take weeks or months to return to normal. Ice helps, but continued activity is often impossible for several weeks. Rupture of the achilles tendon seems to be more frequent in recent years. Partial rupture occurs when some of the fibers of the tendon are torn. Complete rupture results when the tendon, which connects the calf muscles to the heel, is

completely detached. Prevention is the only approach to these problems since surgery is the only cure. An inflammation of the tendon could lead to partial or complete rupture if left untreated or abused. Also, individuals with high serum uric acid levels seem prone to achilles tendon injuries. Those with high levels should have ample warm-up before exercising and should avoid sudden starts, stops, and changes of direction during their exercise.

Shin splints are pains on the lower portion of the shin bone. They're caused by a lowered arch, irritated membranes, tearing of muscle from bone, a muscle spasm due to swelling of that muscle, a hairline fracture of the bones of the lower leg, muscle strength imbalance, or other factors. Rest is the best cure for shin splints, although taping or a sponge heel pad seem to help in some cases. Preventive measures include exercises to strengthen shin muscles, gradual adjustments to the rigors of exercise, running on softer surfaces, occasionally reversing direction when running on a curved track, and using the heel-to-toe footstrike.

Knee problems are chronic sources of irritation for many athletes. A knee injury suffered early in life can affect the ability to exercise. For example, a knee injured playing high school football may lead to signs of arthritis in the late 20s or early 30s. Such degenerative changes often restrict the ability to run, ski or engage in other vigorous activities. Those of you with knee problems should consult your physician for ways to relieve the limitations they impose. Some have found that aspirin effectively suppresses the inflammation and pain often associated with exercise. Ice helps to reduce the inflammation and speed your return to activity. Knee problems also can result from improper footstrike, worn shoes, or improper foot support. If knee problems, persist, see a doctor.

Low back pain that besets millions of Americans is caused by lack of physical activity, poor posture, inadequate flexibility, and weak abdominal or back muscles. Specific exercises can strengthen one muscle group or stretch another to remove the muscular imbalance and improve the posture. By improving abdominal strength and stretching back muscles the forward tilt of the pelvis can be reduced.

Stressful exercise is anything stressful that is

Good Shoes Help Prevent Foot and Leg Injuries

A doctor who is a recognized authority on sports medicine says emphatically that jogging is the one sport likely to inflict the most injuries, because of all the foot, ankle, leg and knee difficulties – shin splints, jogger's heel, etc. Most of the injuries, he states, happen to beginners who don't know how to get started. A bad pair of tennis shoes used on pavement may lead quickly to an inflammation of the supporting structures of the arches. Shin splints, he says, are most often developed by people with flat feet.

More serious is what he calls a "compartment syndrome," which can kill a muscle in the leg, when increased pressure inside the muscle compartment shuts off the blood supply to the tissue. The injury symptom in the first stage is pain in the leg, numbness, and a tense feeling of the muscle. If the situation isn't corrected quickly, it may call for corrective surgery.

He says joggers should have a built-up section in the heel of their shoes to protect the achilles tendon, as well as good arch support and a firm sole that is flexible.

Even with that precaution, he says joggers should condition themselves on grass or dirt.

A further precaution he issues is that substantially overweight people should take off weight before they try to jog. He further advocates flexibility exercise before starting to run, as well as a cooling-off routine at the completion of a run.

You can jog or run practically anywhere —country roads, parks, in the city or on inside tracks. However, if possible, avoid hard surfaces such as concrete and asphalt for the first few weeks.

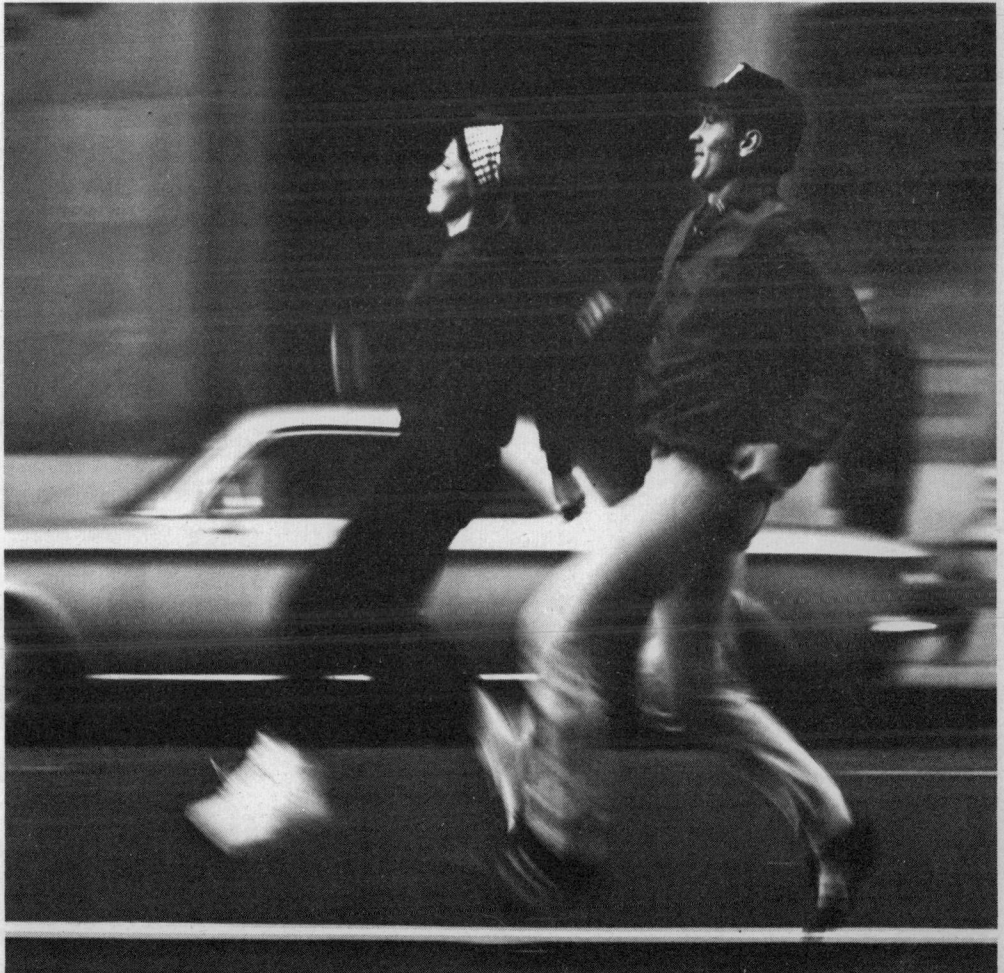

MARATHON RUNNING

A marathon is the most gruelling and brutally demanding event a runner can enter. Twenty-six miles, 385 yards, non-stop covered by the best runners in just over 2 hours. The distance is always the same – the courses, however, vary considerably.

It's been said that if four or five runners start a discussion on training methods for, say, a marathon, no two of them will be in complete agreement. Marathon running, they all agree, is vastly different from a 4- or 5-mile jog.

Some marathon runners train by alternating fast sprints with long-distance runs. Some follow strict schedules, with specific mileage goals, while others run at their convenience.

Some run 3 days a week while others run every day of the week. Some try for the best possible time every outing, while others grind out the mileage without worrying about time until the actual race.

Some fast for days before a marathon. Others load up on carbohydrates about 2 hours before the start of the race. Some eat a light breakfast several hours before a race that starts in the morning and then have a light snack an hour before the race starts. One runner has a formula of fasting for 1 day, 7 days before a race, then eating nothing but pure protein for the next 3 days, followed by a couple of days of carbohydrates, fruit, with lots of fruit and vegetable juice in the morning before the race.

They all agree that a marathon runner should drink lots of liquid before the start of a race, quite the opposite of what was considered good training 10 years ago. Some drink fruit juices, some plain water, some drink Gator-Ade, while others load up on beer.

One school of thought says sprints are necessary to develop any speed, while another group insists that the speed will come if you run enough training miles. Both groups can point to runners who seem to prove their side.

Running in marathons has become so popular that one travel agency is now offering

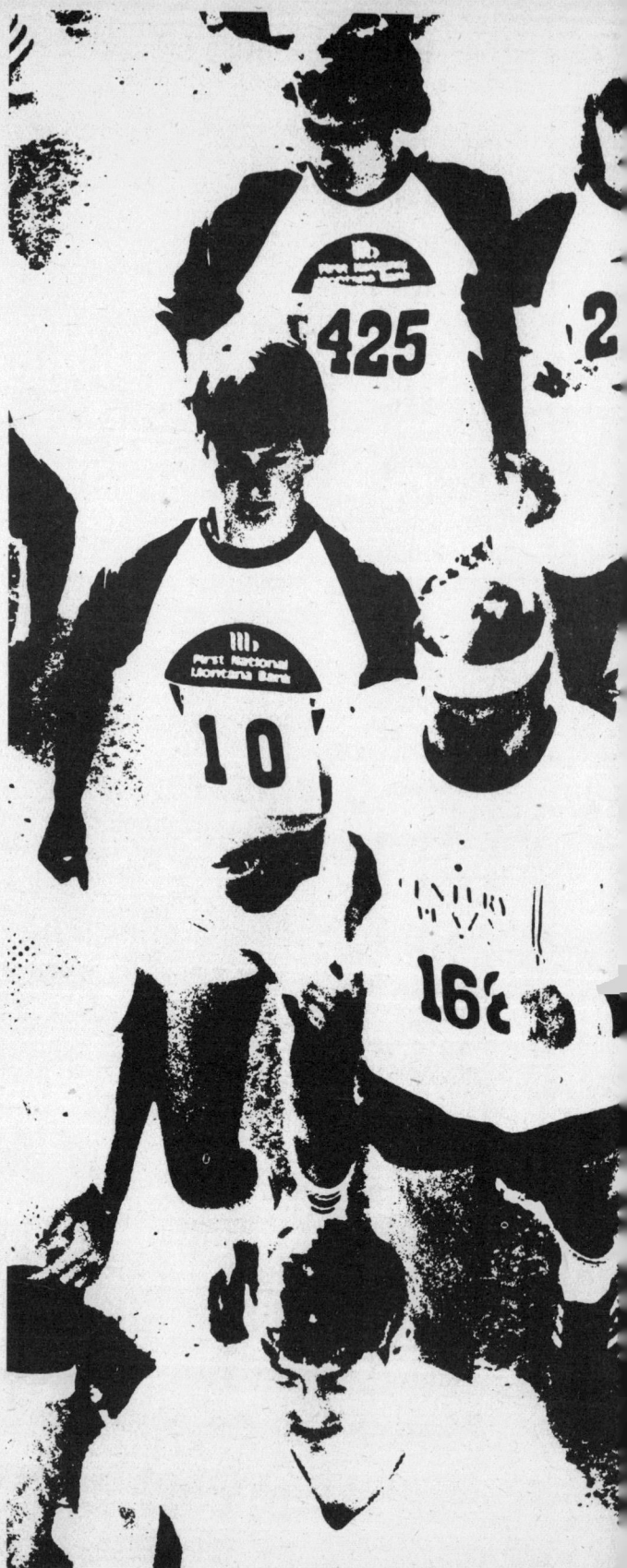

overseas package tours that put the tour buyers in marathon races that are world-famous.

One popular tour takes the runners to Greece for the Athens Marathon, from the plains of Marathon to Athens. Another to New Zealand winds up with participation in the Eclipse Marathon at Hamilton, after several days of running with a running club, the Auckland Harriers.

Tours now being offered range from under $1,000 a person to more than $2,000 and the response has been good.

With the tremendous popularity of running, a good pair of shoes is about the only major expense that's necessary, but astute merchandisers have found that giving runners other ways to spend some money can be highly profitable.

One manufacturer of expensive clothing for runners says, "It's no different from what's happened in amateur photography. You can take pictures, some of them excellent, with a cheap box camera — but middle class and even poor camera nuts today put thousands of dollars into camera equipment."

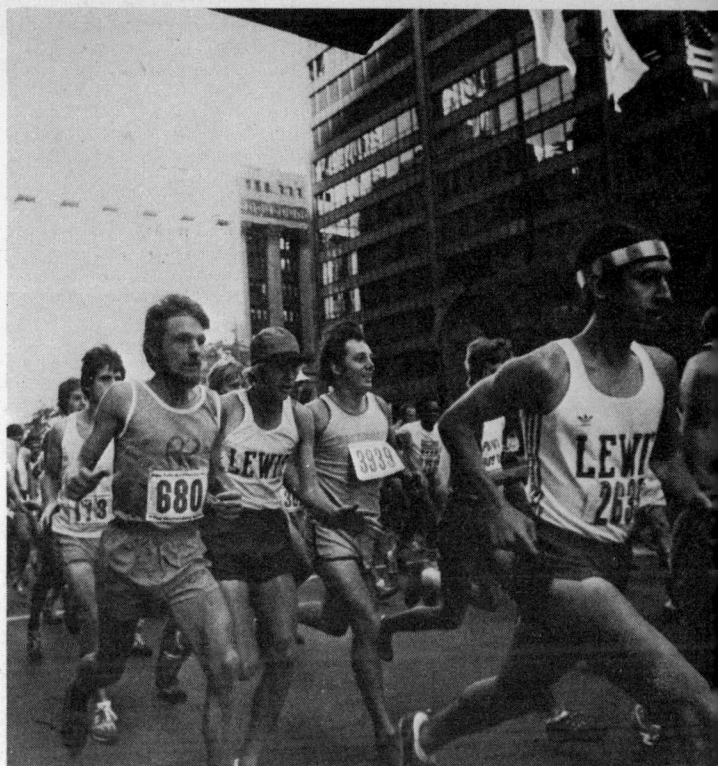

They're off—in Chicago's Mayor Daley Marathon!

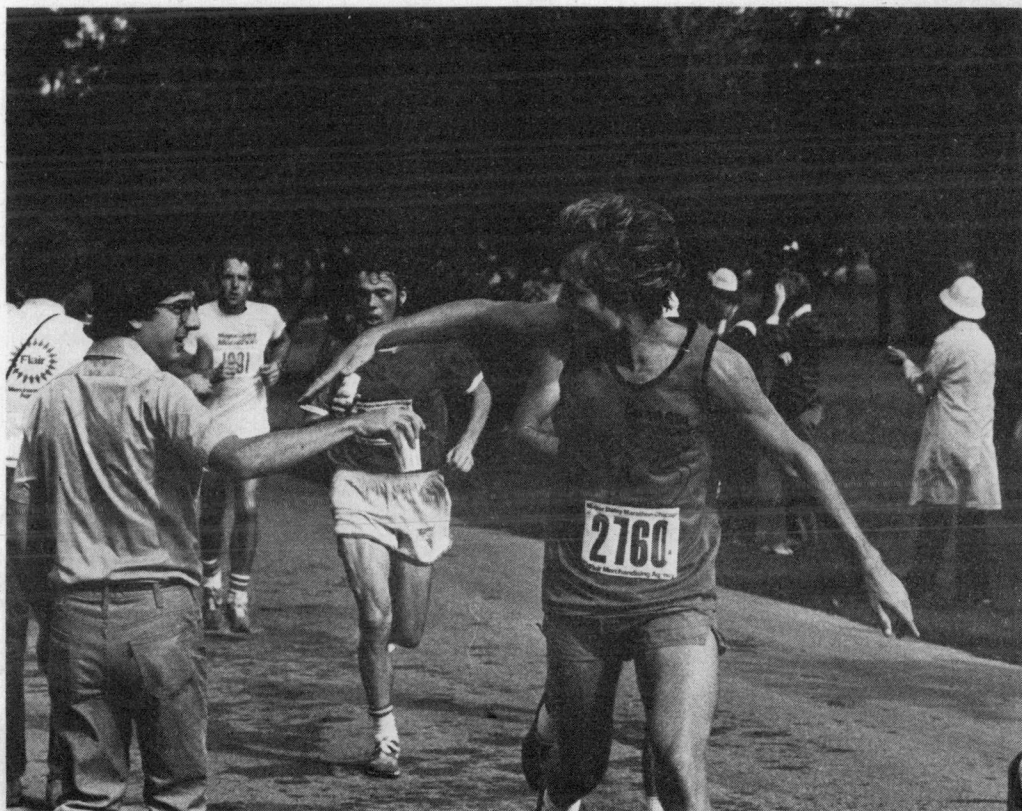

During a marathon run it's possible to lose more than a quart of sweat an hour. In addition to losing water your body is also being depleted of salt and potassium. It is important that this lost fluid be replaced throughout the run in volumes comparable to the fluid loss.

"perceived" as a threat. One of the body's responses to stressful situations is the secretion of several "stress" hormones. Associated with this response is an acceleration of the clotting time of the blood. Exercise may be stressful when it's unfamiliar, exhaustive, or highly competitive. Older individuals should begin participating in unfamiliar activities gradually, avoid exhaustion, and postpone competition until fitness and familiarity provide the proper background.

Sudden vigorous exercise is any sudden vigorous exercise, such as shoveling snow, which creates special kind of stress. Failure to warm-up properly leads to cardiac abnormalities caused by an inadequate oxygen supply to the heart. A 5-minute warm-up eliminates the problem.

Running and the Respiratory System

In the human body, unlike in simple organisms, a unique and different respiratory system is needed to supply the oxygen to meet metabolic needs. This gas transport and distribution comes from the lungs to the tissues by way of the blood. This gas transport is the responsibility of the cardiovascular system.

First, let's consider external respiration where the air goes through the nose into the nasal cavity where it's warmed and agitated. Air is conducted past the glottis into the trachea, and the trachea is divided into two sections, one going to the left lung and the other to the right. So the lungs perform two vital functions, conduction of air and respiration. Within the lung, two extremely thin endothelial layers separate the air from the blood in the capillaries.

During exercise, when metabolic requirements are greater, the depth and rate of breathing are increased sufficiently by the accessory breathing muscles. The recoil of the ordinary breathing muscles is greatly helped by contractions of the abdominal muscles. They aid by raising the inter-abdominal pressure to produce strong expiration. They also draw the lower ribs downward.

Movement of the human body plays a major part in bringing about the increased ventilation that takes place during heavy exercise.

As body temperature goes up, so does the ventilation rate. While resting, the rate of breath-

They're Married, They Both Jog – But Don't Jog Together

The author's daughter and son-in-law are both ardent joggers, regardless of the weather. When they jog, they both wear jogging suits, which as far as I can see, are glorified versions of sweat shirts and sweat pants. I suppose one important difference is that they're colorful, easily seen by motorists, and give the wearer a psychological lift. Since the suits are used only for jogging, keeping them clean and fresh isn't much of a problem.

They both agree that a good warm-up with some flexibility exercises before getting under way is important to them.

For their warm-up, they do a little stationary jogging (or running) until they begin to perspire. Then they do flexibility exercises of the same kind as those done by runners.

Since they're getting plenty of other exercise, they usually jog only 3 or 4 miles a day and think that's enough for them to get big benefits from jogging. They insist that a day when they don't jog is a poorer day all around than those days when they follow their usual routine.

They do *not* jog together, however. They've tried that and say they keep wondering if they're going fast or slow enough for each other. Jogging alone, they set their own pace, one that they like.

Polly has interested a number of her feminine friends in jogging, but says most of them go much too slow for her.

Jim, on the other hand, enjoys jogging with a group of his male friends. "There's no competition," he says, "and nobody tries to keep up or beat anyone else. There's a definite companionship about it."

Editor's Note: The lung and heart capacities of a woman are lower than those of a man. Because of this, women do not have to jog or run as hard as a man does to attain the same fitness level. Unlike men, women reach their heart training rate much more quickly. So when a man and woman run together, the man may be running comfortably within his training heart rate, but the woman is exceeding hers due to the fast pace of the run. This can lead to the woman overexerting herself. If they were to slow down so the woman is comfortable, the man may not be able to reach his target training rate.

Jogging — Two Approaches

Of all the endurance exercises, jogging and running are probably the least expensive. They require no real coaching or supervision once a physical examination has been passed satisfactorily, and the program can be very flexible.

One experienced jogger has a stock answer when somebody asks him how to go about beginning to jog. He takes the person to a nice, attractive bicycle trail fairly close to his home. Then he says, ''Now, put one foot in front of the other one in a running motion. Keep going, straight ahead. Stay on the path.''

They usually turn and stare at him, trying to think of another question. He never lets them ask it. He quickly says, ''What I've just told you is that the way to start a jogging routine is to start jogging. That's all there is to it.''

And it is, despite what one methodical young man in my community did. First he read the Fixx book and then went to the library and asked for any more material they had on jogging. He read it all. Then he bought special apparel, based on what he thought would be best from what he'd read. Then he visited six different sporting goods and shoe stores and asked to see their jogging footwear. He examined it all, asking dozens of questions, most of which the clerks couldn't answer. After all that, he bought a pair of shoes.

Then he did flexibility exercises for 20 minutes a day for 3 weeks. Following that, he tried three different ways of warming-up for 2 weeks, until he decided one method suited him best.

Finally, he started jogging – but even there, he did research. He jogged on grass, on boards, on pavement and even a cinder track before he settled on a bicycle path.

And now he jogs happily, certain that his approach to the exercise has been much better and more scientific than that of other joggers.

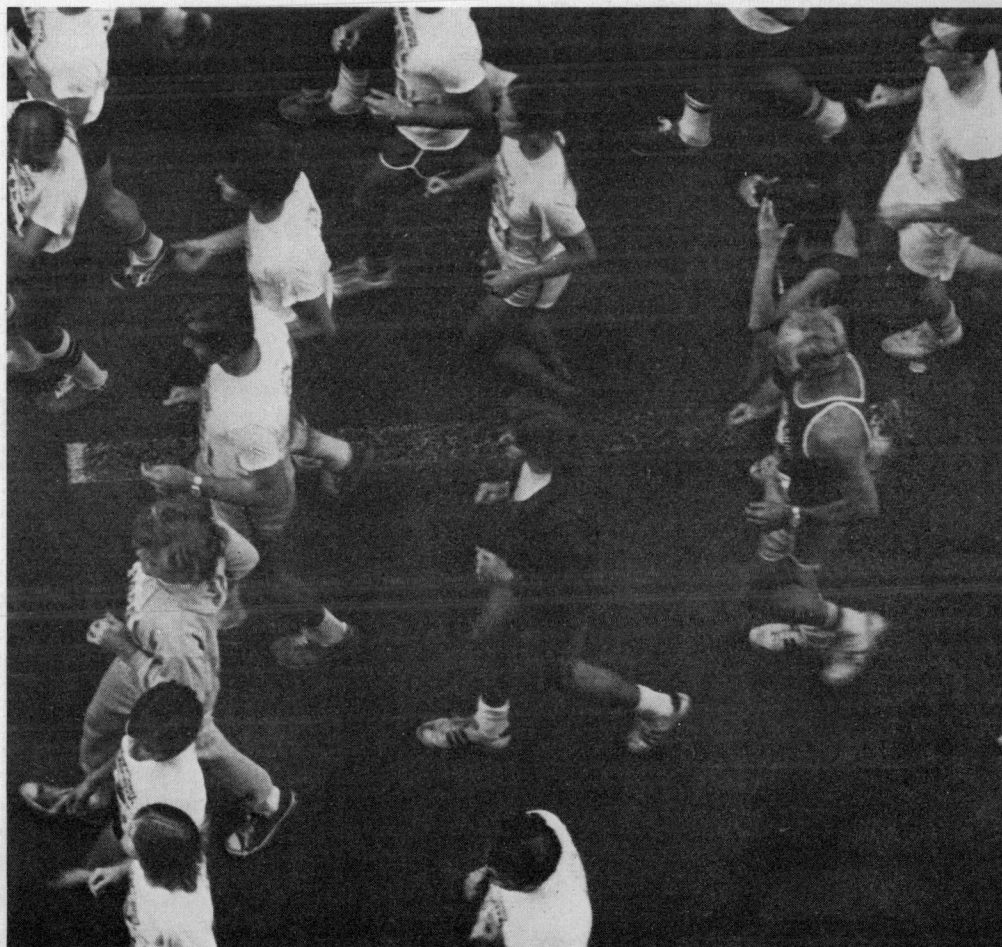

Training for a marathon involves long, slow distance training. You combine the features of underdistance running (a short run at a fast pace) with overdistance running (a long run at a slow pace).

Distance Runs — "Just Proud to Finish"

While it's alarming that so many people are plunging into jogging without any pre-conditioning, it's also encouraging that they've become sold enough on the exercise to do so. In a local shopping news this morning, I read an ad addressed to the general public: "FUN JOG, 5 miles, every Tuesday at 6 PM. Meet at northwest corner of county road F. Everyone welcome."

Many local celebrities around the country have received widespread publicity on entering 20- or 25-mile distance runs. While they haven't won, they've finished, and I haven't read about their suffering any ill effects.

One of these men said to me after completing a 20-mile run, "I didn't think I was going to be able to finish. I guess personal pride was the determining factor. I felt proud of myself that I made it. As to endangering my health, there's an element of risk in almost everything we do. Walking across a busy street can be dangerous. But you can't curl up and live in a cocoon."

ing is usually from 12 to 20 breaths per minute. With exercise, it rises as much as up to 50 or 60 per minute. The total lung ventilation goes up from 7 liters per minute to as much as 150 liters per minute in heavy exercise. While resting, the muscular work of breathing is almost minute. But as exercise becomes more strenuous, the body must work harder. Athletic trainers, particularly running coaches, try to develop maximum breathing efficiency. Great breathing efficiency is believed to have been an important contributor to the long sought after 4-minute mile run.

Your "Second Wind"

All experienced runners talk about getting their second wind. Physiologists say that while there's no satisfactory scientific explanation for it, it probably comes with metabolic adjustment to the increased work load of the exercise. It may also be due to a change in the muscular efficiency as the body heats up. The faster relaxation of the muscles while working against each other in the reciprocating motion required of them may be the cause of second wind.

Running/Jogging and Obesity

Since running demands the physical effort of carrying the body around and necessarily pounds the skeletal muscles and bones when the runner comes down on each heel, weight reduction is a wise preliminary for anyone who's 10 percent or more overweight.

If the obese person wants to get into running before his weight is down to normal, the best way to start is probably a jog-walk combination. This routine has an advantage over diet alone in that it causes a loss of much greater amounts of fatty tissue and the beginning of more solid tissue.

The ideal combination is probably exercise plus diet. For those runners who feel a need to take off weight, Chapter 5 on nutrition and weight control gives practical guidelines.

It should be emphasized that for an overweight person, running should be done only with a gradual increase from lower to higher levels of energy consumption—but always vigorous enough to produce sweating.

Running/Jogging, Heart Attacks and High Blood Pressure

People who don't run have been heard to say that they'd be afraid a vigorous running program might bring on a heart attack. Results of tests would indicate quite the contrary. The Laboratory of Physiological Hygiene at the University of Minnesota conducted a study of American railway employees. The results showed that in 191,609 man-years of risk and 1,978 deaths, the age-adjusted deaths for arteriosclerotic heart disease were respectively 5.7, 3.9, and 2.8 for clerks, switchmen and section men. The clerks' jobs were sedentary, the switchmen's mildly active and the section men's extremely active.

In another test, it was learned that 6 months in a San Diego State fitness program brought high blood pressure decreases of systolic pressure of almost 12mmHg and 13mmHg in diastolic values.

Runners/Joggers and Pain

Runners generally experience two different kinds of pain as the result of exercise—pain during and immediately following a running session, and another localized kind of soreness that doesn't show up until 1 or 2 days later. The first type of pain is of short duration, quickly relieved.

The second is much more annoying. It is quite often caused by a localized motor spasm when the muscle after hard exercise stays in its contracted condition. A session of stretching the muscles in which the spasms have occurred will often bring quick relief. However, don't try to stretch them by immediate running. A *bouncing* stretch can be even more painful. A slow, steady pull is much more effective. Always, of

Never rush from a vigorous workout into a hot shower! The flow of blood to recently exercised muscles combined with the flow to the skin to dissipate heat may result in inadequate flow to the brain or heart. Always cool down after a workout.

Jogging Helped Him Cut Down His Smoking

One man I know who used to smoke at least two packs of cigarettes a day has cut down to about half a pack since he started to jog, without any prompting or urging from anyone. I said, "Ed, it doesn't seem to me that you smoke as much as you used to. What's happened? Did the doctor scare you into cutting down?"

"Not at all," he replied. "I've been doing well with my jogging, and trying to do better. And I found that cutting down on cigarettes improved my wind. I may quit smoking altogether before long. I don't know. I still enjoy a cigarette."

This is a man who hates detail and regimentation, although he regiments the people who work under him and insists on their attention to detail.

"From what I read and heard, I decided that jogging would be good for me. I knew I was in lousy physical condition. I needed something like jogging. But if somebody'd told me, 'To make a jogging program effective, you should get out on the road every Monday, Wednesday and Saturday morning at 7:15 AM and jog until 7:45, covering a specific number of miles in that time,' I'd have told 'em to go fly a kite. But nobody did that. Friends I asked about a routine all said, 'It's up to you. How far you jog, when you do it, the number of minutes you spend jogging, even where you jog are all up to you.' And when I asked about how quickly and how much I should increase my jogging schedule, everybody said, 'That's strictly up to you. Follow your own instincts.' "

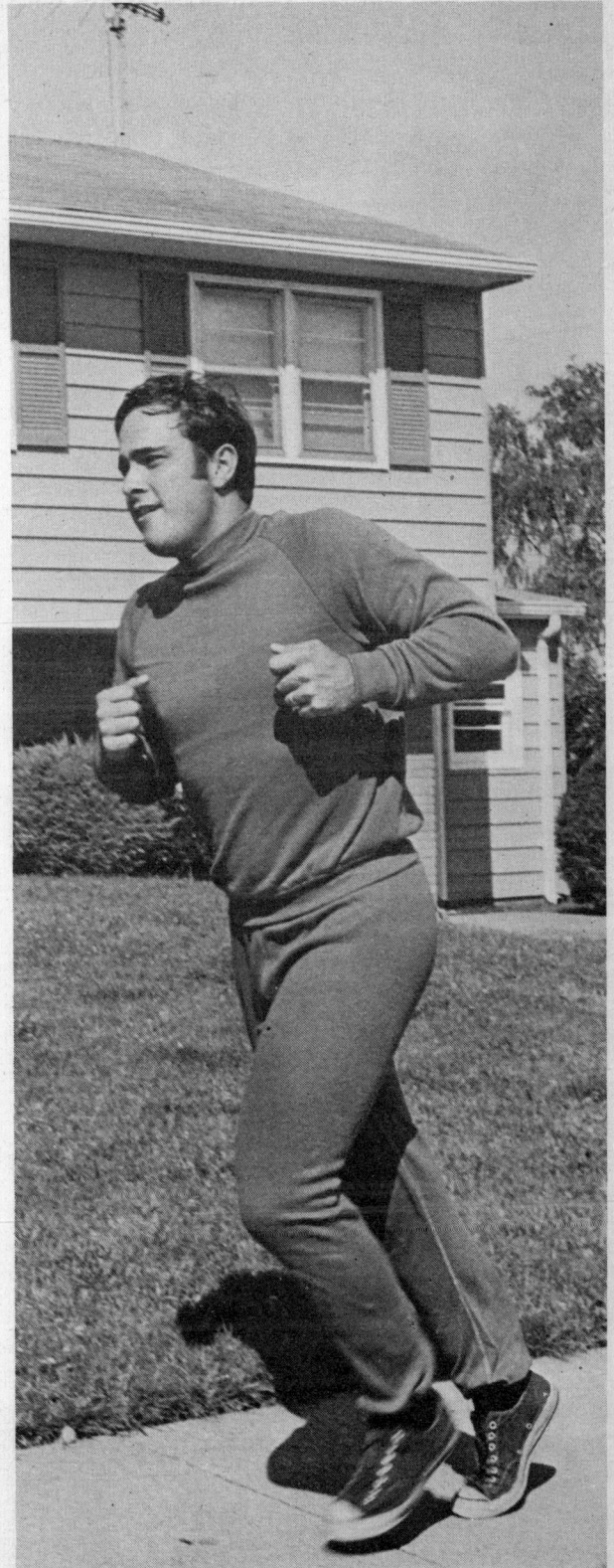

course, a good warm-up before running minimizes any muscle soreness.

Running/Jogging for People 65 and Over

As far as the effect of age on the cardiovascular system is concerned, runners point with pride to Clarence De Mar, a famous marathon runner who ran 12 miles a day throughout his adult lifetime. He competed in 25-mile distance runs when he was 65 and he ran a 15-kilometer race at 68, 2 years before his death from cancer. The autopsy showed that the running had developed a superb myocardium, that the valves were normal and the coronary arteries much larger than normal size.

As with the obese, a gradual upward trend in exercise is indicated for those 65 and over. Using the overload principle, senior citizens can

---

Jogging as Arthritis Preventive

An elderly friend of mine who has arthritic tendencies says he's kept his arthritis from getting worse by jogging 3 miles a day, every other day. Some doctors tell their arthritis patients that regular physical activity is the best preventive measure against arthritis that presently exists.

---

build up to a point they wouldn't have dreamed possible at the outset.

One expert on geriatric exercise and the author of an excellent book, *The Physiology of Exercise,* is Herbert A. de Vries of the University of California. He has devised an exercise regimen for the elderly with a warm-up done by calisthenics and static stretching to improve joint mobility and to avoid muscle problems. The program is to be done three times a week. Here's the run-walk schedule by progression.

Series 1: 50 steps running, 50 steps walking (1 set).
  a. Five sets the first day (250 steps running, 250 steps walking).
  b. Each day for 5 days, increase the number of sets by one until 10 sets have been com-

pleted so that at the end of 6 days you will complete 500 steps running, 500 steps walking.
  c. At the end of the first 6 days, begin Series 2 (50 steps running, 40 steps walking), doing 5 sets the first day and increasing the number of sets by one until 10 sets have been completed. Follow the same procedure for each new running-walking series.
Series 2: 50 steps running, 40 steps walking (1 set).
Series 3: 50 steps running 30 steps walking (1 set).
Series 4: 50 steps running, 20 steps walking (1 set).
Series 5: 50 steps running, 10 steps walking (1 set).
Series 6: 75 steps running, 10 steps walking (1 set).
Series 7: 100 steps running, 10 steps walking (1 set).
Series 8: 125 steps running, 10 steps walking (1 set).
Series 9: 150 steps running, 10 steps walking (1 set).
Series 10: 175 steps running, 10 steps walking (1 set)
Series 11: 200 steps running, 10 steps walking (1 set).

While this program is intended for those who are 65 years and over, it could be a safe start for anyone 35 or over who is in poor physical condition.

Once-a-Week Jogging May Do More Harm Than Good

The benefits of jogging do not continue indefinitely after a jogging program is stopped. Once good physical condition is reached, it may be reduced, if the aim is simply to maintain a certain condition without improving it, but benefits won't last without continuation.

One athletic coach observes, "I've seen businessmen who jog every Saturday, with no exercise throughout the rest of the week. I don't think they're accomplishing anything. My secret belief is that such exercise may do more harm than good."

BICYCLING

Bicycling can be an excellent fitness activity to build cardiovascular endurance. Unlike jogging or running, it is a safe exercise for the obese, overweight or unfit and, like running or jogging, can provide the strenuous type of workout needed to condition the carviocascular system. You noticed we used the word "can." If you wish to use bicycling as your cardiovascular endurance exercise, you *must* cycle over 8 miles per hour for any benefit to take place. How fast you pedal depends on your physical condition and how much work it takes to get your heart beating at your training rate. If you pedal at 10 mph and at the end of 5 minutes haven't reached your training rate, you'll have to pedal faster. Trial and error and pulse checks will tell you when you are working hard enough to effect beneficial results. Like calisthenics, the only resistance you are working against is the weight of your body. To increase that resistance, ride up hills or put your cycle in a gear that offers more resistance.

One other *must* if you have chosen bicycling—flexibility exercises for the hamstring and leg muscles. This can't be overemphasized. When you pedal, you don't get the maximum extension of the ankle and foot, which can result in a shortened hamstring and a loss of leg flexibility. So prior to cycling and after cycling, flexibility exercises for the hamstring and lower leg should be done. See Chapter 2 for exercises specific to these areas.

In addition to being such an excellent cardiovascular pulmonary exercise, outdoor bicycling is *fun*. While you can do it alone, it's also great family exercise.

My son, his wife and two young sons have four 10-speed bikes as well as a tandem bike. In addition to the exercise, those bikes have contributed much to family togetherness. There are now good bicycle trails practically everywhere.

My daughter, her husband and their 10-year-old son all have 10-speed bicycles and their 5-year-old daughter has a beginner's bicycle with which she's remarkably efficient. The husband and wife do a lot of mountain road cycling which is strenuous, dangerous and not recommended for novices.

As this is being written, the two families are planning a 60-mile trails trip in northern Wisconsin on a bicycle trail built on an old railroad bed. The tour takes the riders through three long tunnels where they must get off their bicycles and walk and it is said to be magnificently beautiful. You can get information on all kinds of bicycle tours from vacation and recreational information bureaus in every state that is making an effort to attract tourists.

One word of caution is necessary. Get a bicycle that is the right size for the person who's going to use it. Otherwise, the rider is going to be so uncomfortable that the bike won't get much use. Also, there are several different types of bicycle seats. Some are heavily padded and some aren't. Some are wide and some are narrow. If the seat that comes on a bicycle you like isn't comfortable, it's simple to buy a seat you like and replace the offending one with it.

In addition to being such an excellent cardiovascular pulmonary exercise, bicycling is also a great family exercise.

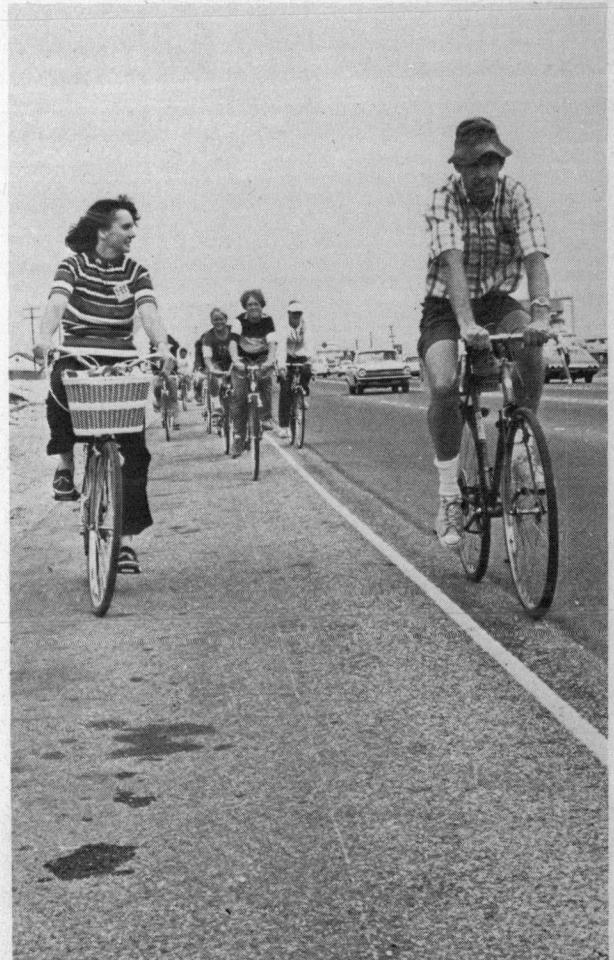

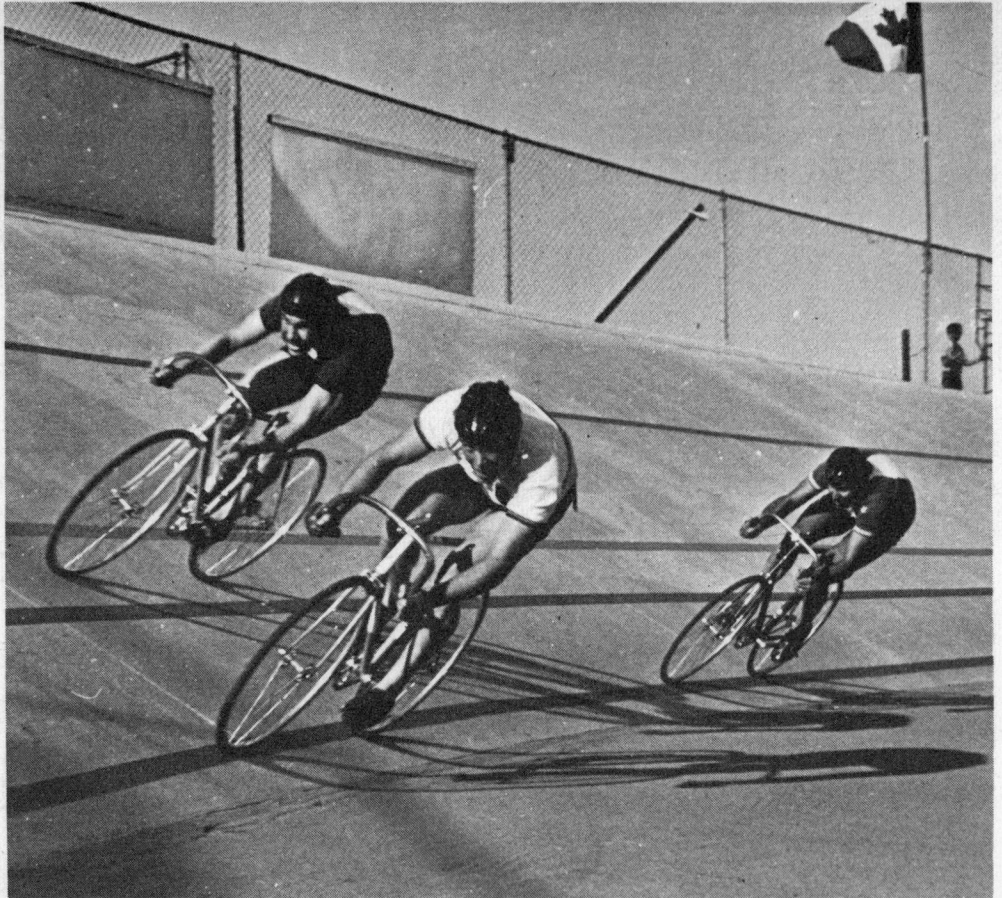

Professional bicycle racing requires a high degree of cardiovascular pulmonary endurance as well as excellent leg muscle strength and flexibility.

Do *not*—I REPEAT, DO *NOT*—buy a bicycle because it's the lowest priced one you can find. Today's multi-speed bicycles are complicated mechanisms with a number of things that can go wrong. We have tested all kinds of bicycles and have reached the conclusion that in multi-speed bikes, the lowest-priced models don't compare with better ones. Only in the standard old one-speed bicycle does a low-priced model give customer satisfaction, and even here, the more expensive models often have better tires and better features that make them well worth the extra cost.

Starting with poor equipment is a costly mistake.

On the other hand, it's entirely possible to go overboard by buying a better bicycle than you need, particularly in what are referred to as racing bicycles. Professional racers spend small fortunes on their equipment and have reached a point where they pay a great deal more money for a slightly better piece of equipment. It's unlikely that you're going to be a professional racer, and unless you are, investing in a professional racing bike would be a waste of money. Even if you plan to do some racing against friends, their equipment will seldom fall into the professional category.

Now we come to a problem that every rider must solve for himself—a choice between a three- or four-speed touring bike and a 10-speed racing bike.

It's been my experience that most women greatly prefer the touring bike. The rider's position on a racing-type bicycle is completely foreign to anyone who learned to ride on the old standard one-speed bicycle.

Actually, you're most comfortable on a 10-speed bike when you're pedaling all-out, in racing position, However, when traveling at a leisurely pace, you may be extremely uncomfortable.

A friend of mine decided he and his wife would take up cycling and he bought two good 10-speed bicycles, one for his wife and one for himself. After five or six brief trials, his wife refused to use hers. She said riding it hurt her back. My friend finally sold his wife's bicycle and bought her a 3-speed touring bike. Now she's happy and rides even more than he does.

If you're in your 30's or older, haven't done any bicycle riding in recent years and decide to take it up again, my advice would be to start with a touring bicycle. It will give you all the exercise you want, and you won't feel awkward or uncomfortable with it.

Actually, from an exercise standpoint, there's certainly nothing wrong with the old standard one-speed bicycle. All in all, you'll exert just as much energy—maybe more—than you would with one of the more modern bicycles.

For really rugged exercise over rough terrain, there's the moto-cross bicycle. There are now many moto-cross competitions around the country. But be careful what you buy if you're going to engage in moto-cross competition. Be sure it's an approved moto-cross bicycle and not a "moto-cross style" bicycle.

Moto-cross cycles have become especially popular with young boys who aren't allowed to drive motorcycles because of their age. The closest they can come to achieving their desire is to operate a moto-cross bike.

Most children don't have to be encouraged to get exercise with their bicycles.

Adults who aren't in top physical condition should start their bicycle exercise by riding a mile a day—approximately 12 city blocks. They should quickly cut the amount of time it takes to cover the mile and then increase the number of miles covered. This is one exercise that most people can do every day without inconvenience.

The one problem is weather. And that brings up the subject of the stationary exercise bicycle.

A couple of years ago, when my wife had started to recover from a coronary, the doctor encouraged her to walk briskly for 10 minutes a day at first and then build up slowly to ¼-hour every day.

There was no question but that this routine brought quick and marked improvement in her physical condition. The big problem was the weather in the Chicago area.

Our winters are rugged, with low tempera-

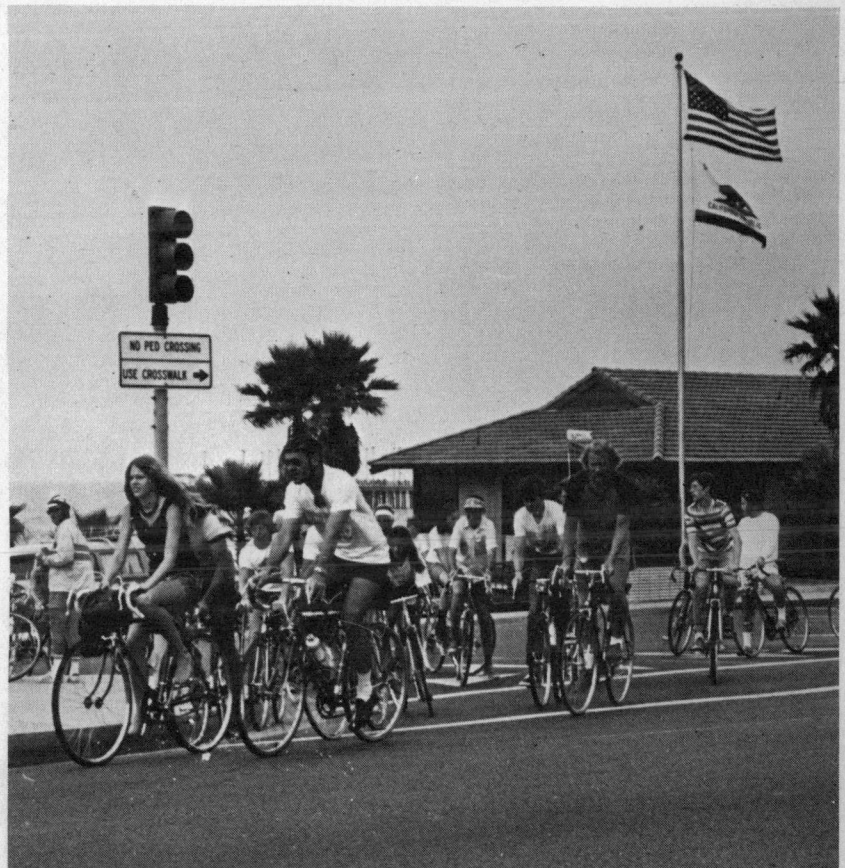

Undoubtedly the reason some people prefer bicycling to running or jogging is that they get more enjoyment out of it. It doesn't seem to them to be exercise as much as it is recreation.

tures which aren't good for people recovering from heart attacks. They shouldn't be braving the elements, but neither should they be without exercise.

Our doctor had my wife buy a stationary exercise bicycle to use during the winter and during inclement weather at any other time of the year. We kept it in a convenient corner of the breakfast room. Both she and I began to ride it regularly.

So sold was the doctor on this form of exercise that he later had her buy a second exercise bike to keep at our summer home in Wisconsin, to use on rainy days and whenever she hadn't been able to get enough brisk walking during the day.

The first bike was a Schwinn, in the $150-$170 price range, a beautifully made piece of precision equipment with adjustable pedal tension, a speedometer and a mileage counter as well as a timing device you could set for whatever length of time you chose. A bell rang at the end of the period. You knew how fast you'd been going, and how far you'd gone during the elapsed time.

The second bike was in the $80 price range. To nobody's surprise, it wasn't as nice a product as the first one, but it filled its purpose adequately. I found the ideal pace for me was 5 miles at 15 to 20 miles per hour.

Guests in our home who wanted to try the bike started out at high speed and got carried away. It was so easy, they told us. Nothing to it! And the next day, they were invariably tired and sore.

Athletic coaches I've talked to all pick bicycle riding as superior to either bench stepping or treadmill running or walking for the promotion of cardiovascular pulmonary endurance.

Undoubtedly, the reason some people prefer it to running or jogging is that they get more enjoyment out of it. It doesn't seem to them to be exercise as much as it is recreation.

People of advanced age who aren't suffering from arthritis or bone deterioration at the joints tend to like both running and cycling.

Regardless of age, a cycle tour vacation offers a maximum of health-producing and maintaining exercise, at the opposite pole from a summer or winter resort vacation where food, sun-bathing, bridge, night-club entertainment and inactivity form a rather common routine.

In order to improve your cardiovascular system when bicycling you must cycle over 8 miles per hour for any benefit to take place. Remember to warm-up with flexibility exercises for the hamstrings and calves.

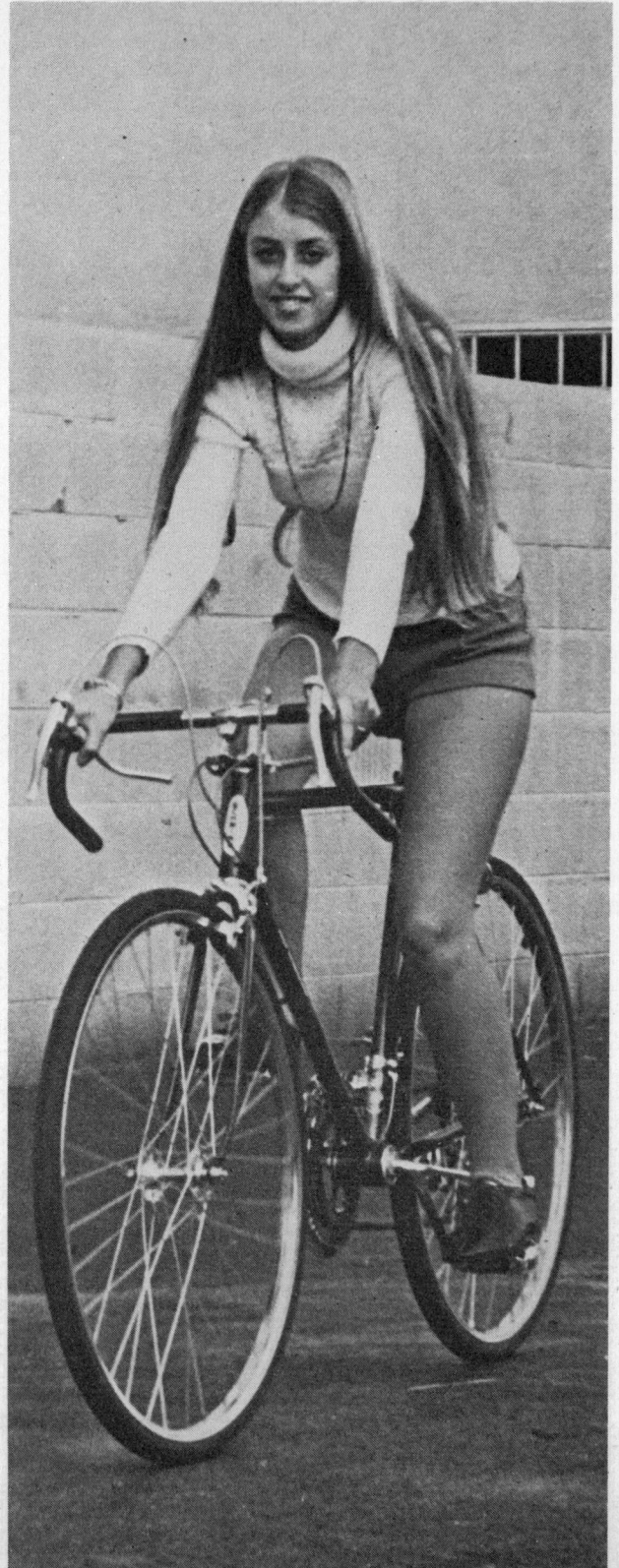

BICYCLING AND HEALTH*
by
Paul Dudley White

The late Dr. Paul Dudley White was recognized as one of the world's most respected cardiologists, especially in the area of diseases of the heart. Dr. White attended Harvard University, graduating with an A.B. degree in 1908 and M.D. degree in 1911. He had served as chairman of a National Red Cross committee on cardiovascular disease; executive director of the National Advisory Heart Council; was a member of the American Academy of Arts and Sciences, American Medical Association; past president of the American Heart Association. He was a member of the Royal Society of Medicine (England), Royal College of Physicians (London, Ireland), was founder and past president of the International Society of Cardiology. He had authored several books, including *Heart Disease, Heart Disease in General Practice, Electrocardiography in Practice, Coronary Heart Disease in Young Adults, Clues in the Diagnosis and Treatment of Heart Disease, Fitness of the Whole Family, Hearts: Their Long Follow-Up,* and *My Life and Medicine.*

I have welcomed the invitation to prepare a chapter for this book on the subject of the effect of bicycling on the health of the cyclist. I must begin, however, with the warning that everyone should insist that the bicycling must be safe and preferably done on special paths and trails. A decade or more ago a few of us in metropolitan Boston incorporated a Committee for Safe Bicycling and during the years that have passed have helped to establish safe paths, usually for both cyclist and pedestrian together since as a rule they can use the same path if it is wide enough, not only in' Massachusetts but in many other parts of the USA.

Accidents, which usually involve motor car and cyclist, have often not been the fault of the motor car driver. In many cases they have been due to the carelessness and illegal action of the cyclist him-or-herself. I have seen much reckless cycling by individuals of all ages riding against the traffic, or too fast, ignoring the traffic signals, failing to signal on turns, and not being equipped with adequate lights or horns or bells. I believe that the great majority of the bicyclists

*Reprinted from *Bicycle Digest.*

of today do obey the rules, but the minority—and they are too many—are the offenders and they bring discredit on the others. I hope that this book will have a very wide circulation so that it will be read by the careless as well as by the careful.

And now to turn to the more pleasant and interesting effect of cycling on the health, both general and special. First, the physiology of the process: I find that relatively few individuals have ever been told about the wonderful pumping mechanisms with which nature has endowed us, to aid the heart in maintaining a proper circulation of blood to our brain, our lungs, our heart itself, and to the muscles. Over 400 years ago in Italy anatomists and physiologists discovered that the veins of the arms and legs have been supplied by nature with valves which prevent the blood from accumulating by gravity in the lower part of the body. William Harvey of England, who had studied in Padua, Italy, from 1599 to 1603, had been shown these valves and after his return to London used their function to complete one of the greatest discoveries of all time, namely the circulation of the blood, which he presented in a small book in 1628.

When the leg muscles of the thighs and of the calves contract as in simple walking, running, bicycling, swimming, tennis, golf or other sports, they squeeze the deep veins within them and, because of the presence of valves in the veins, the blood is pumped up towards the heart and thence to the brain by the heart. Thus the heart is not the only pump in the body. It has been estimated that this muscular action of the legs relieves the heart of about one-third of its work by the simple exercise of walking, and the same should be true of bicycling.

A third pumping mechanism in the body is dependent on the muscle of the diaphragm in making the cavity of the thorax into a suction pump by causing a negative pressure therein during deep inspiration. This suction action not only brings air into our lungs but also helps to bring blood up from below. This vital action of the diaphragm should not be impeded by obesity in the abdomen, emphysema or other diseases of the lungs, or by generally poor physical fitness. Moreover, the pollution of the inspired air with tobacco smoke results in the contamination of the oxygen by carbon monoxide gas which, as it enters the blood, drives out the oxygen from the hemoglobin in the red blood corpuscles. This lowered oxygen content in the blood can have catastrophic results if the coronary or other cardiac reserve happens to be low. Thus the physiology of the circulation of blood enters into the physical exercise of bicycling in a major way and needs clear understanding.

Having discussed the physical benefit of cycling, I would like now strongly to emphasize the mental or psychological benefits. The best antidote for emotional stress or fatigue is the physical exercise of the legs in walking or running or cycling a few miles. If it cannot be done safely outdoors, one may use an exercise bicycle or a treadmill indoors. It is better than a tranquilizer drug in most cases unless the mental fatigue is profound. One psychological advantage that the cyclist has over the pedestrian is

the exhilaration of going further in a short time and in exploring more of the countryside. But of course it is possible to go too far and to become physically exhausted. Much common sense is needed in this recommendation.

Another beneficial effect of bicycling on the psyche is the satisfaction of using the legs in transportation, thereby saving money, not polluting the air, and simultaneously aiding one's health. It is not necessary to be a champion racer or to have a ten-geared bicycle—it is possible to maintain one's health by riding an old-fashioned single or three-speed bicycle and one can get plenty of benefit in riding slowly as one can in walking slowly. Still another nice custom of camaraderie associated with group riding as in bicycle tours in this country or abroad has been established by the Youth Hostels and other organizations with which I have been associated. This adds also to international friendship, a goal of world peace we all seek.

Group riding as in bicycle tours has even reached to overseas riding tours established by the Youth Hostels and other organizations.

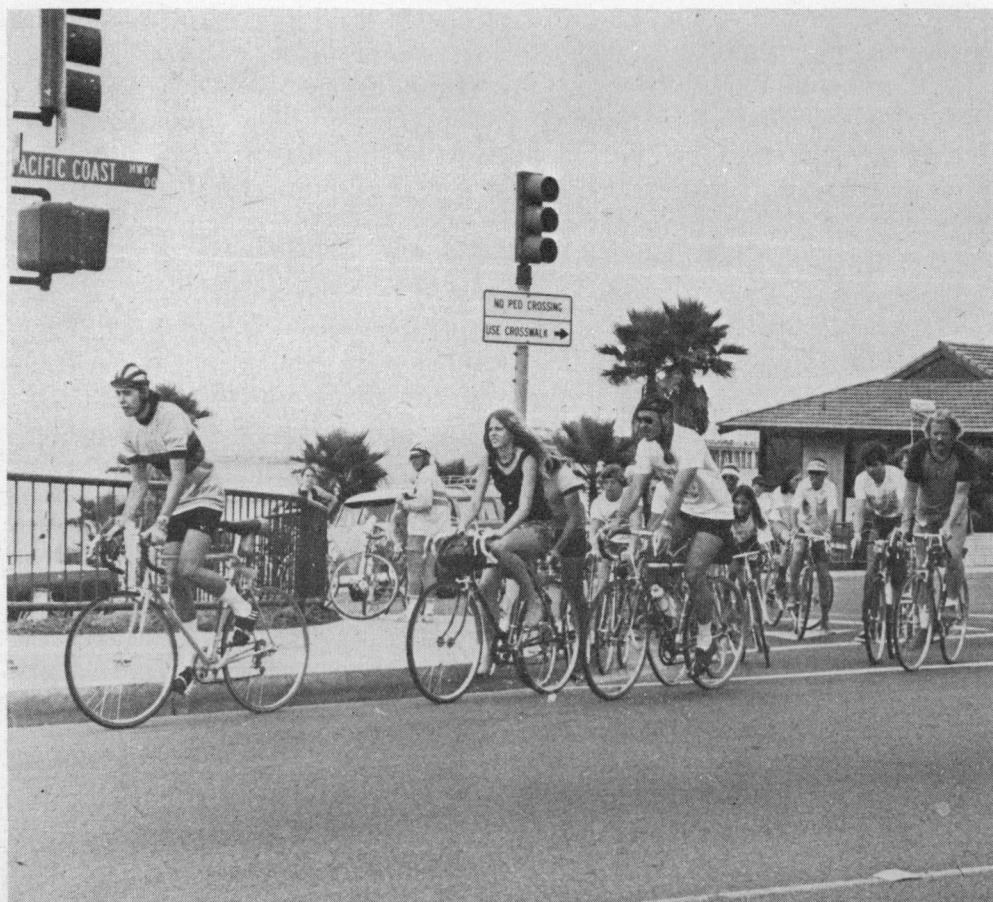

SWIMMING

Swimming is recognized as America's most popular active sport. It is one of the best physical activities for people of all ages and for many persons who are handicapped. Vigorous water activities can make a major contribution to the *flexibility, strength,* and *circulatory endurance* of individuals. With the body submerged in water, blood circulation automatically increases to some extent; pressure of water on the body also helps promote deeper ventilation of the lungs; and with well-planned activity, both circulation and ventilation increase still more.

In order to improve cardiovascular endurance via swimming, you must use one of the five recommended strokes—the crawl, the breaststroke, backstroke, butterfly or sidestroke. The swimming strokes should be performed rhythmically and continuously with the swimmer covering about 30 yards a minute. Just as is true for all aerobic exercises you must swim at your training heart rate for a minimum of 15 minutes for any fitness improvement to take place.

Since each of these swimming strokes utilizes all the major muscles in the body, warm-up exercises for flexibility and strength are extremely important. They will help you avoid being stricken with muscle cramps and soreness during and after your swimming session. You can either pick exercises from Chapters 2 and 3 for flexibility and strength or you can pick from the pool activities which follow. However, whether you choose activities from previous chapters or from those exercises which follow, you should concentrate on back stretching and strengthening exercises. Most swimming strokes cause the back to be in a hyper-extended position. Thus static stretching exercises for the back are highly recommended. One excellent deckside back stretching exercise is to stand with legs apart, extending the hands high over head and reaching as far as possible, holding

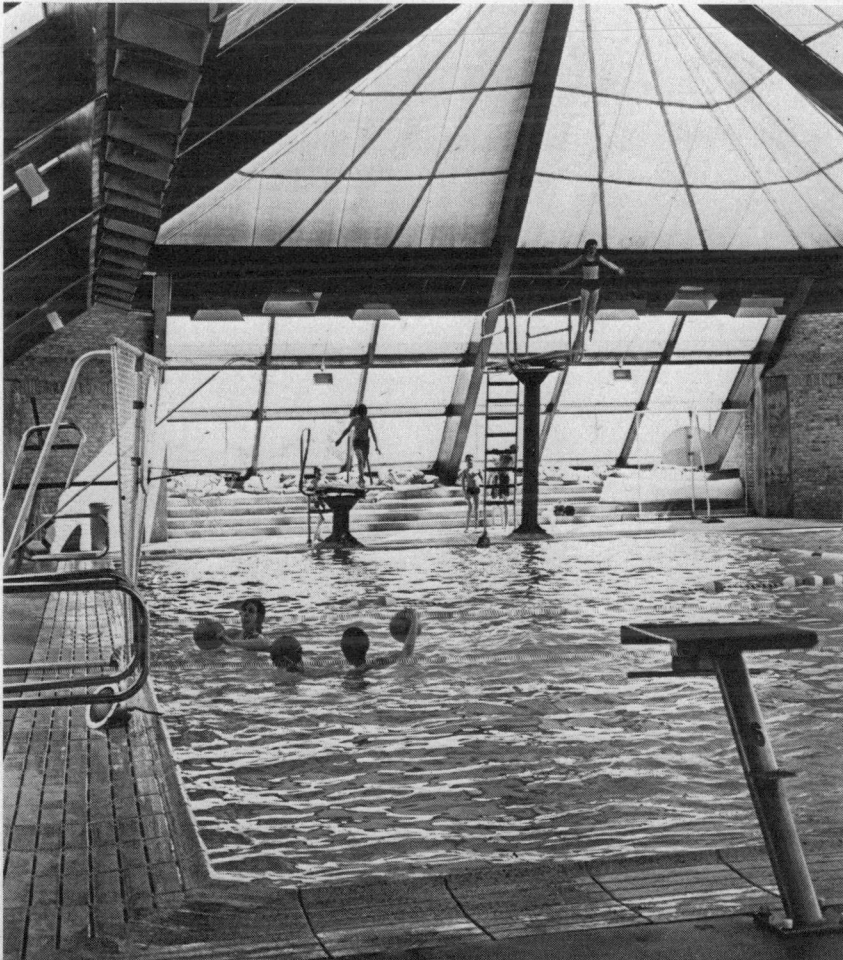

Like bicycling, the amount of work it takes for you to reach your training heart rate when swimming depends on these factors — stroke, speed, temperature and skill.

that position for 5-10 seconds. Then bend the trunk forward and down, flexing the knees, trying to touch the floor. Hold that position for 20-30 seconds and repeat several times.

Back Stretcher

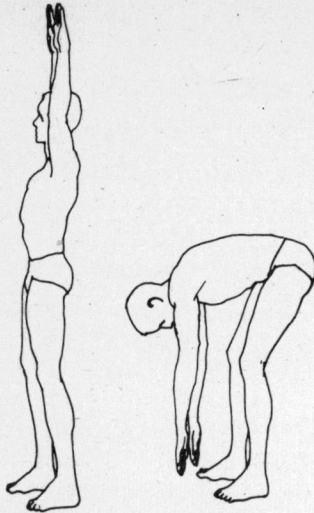

Alternate Toe Touch

Aquatic Flexibility Exercises

Increased flexibility work is performed more easily in water because of the lessening of gravitational pull. A person immersed to the neck in water experiences an apparent loss of 90 percent of his weight. This means that the feet and legs of a woman weighing 130 lbs. immersed in water only have to support a weight of 13 lbs. Thus, individuals and especially older people with painful joints or weak leg muscles will usually find it possible and comfortable to move in the water. It is much easier to do leg straddle or stride stretches in water than on the floor. Too, many individuals could do leg "bobbing" in the water who could never do so on land.

Through proper warm-up the body's deep muscle temperature will be raised and the ligaments and connecting tissues stretched, thereby preparing the body for vigorous work. This will help avoid injury and discomfort.

Alternate Toe Touch (hamstring muscles)
Standing, in waist-to-chest deep water, swimmer:

1. Raises left leg, bringing right hand toward left foot, looking back and left hand extended rearward.
2. Recovers to starting position.
3. Repeats.
4. Reverses.

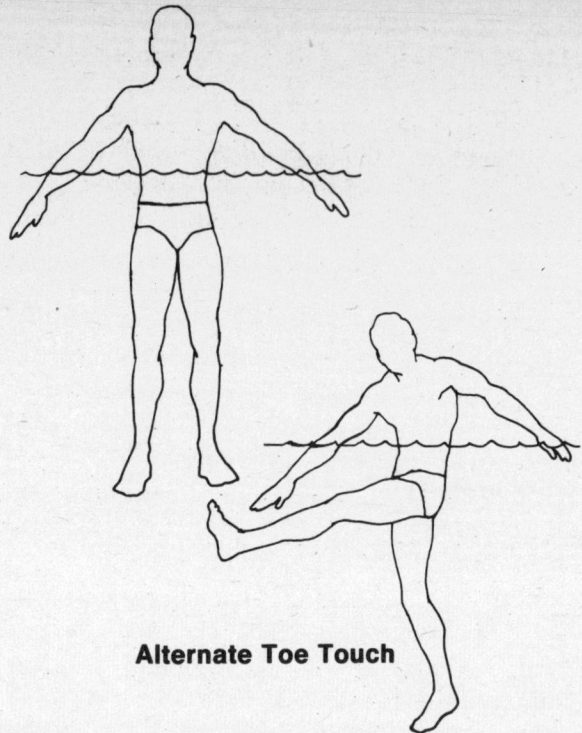

Side Bender (trunk muscles)
Standing in waist-deep water, with left arm at side and right arm over head, swimmer:

1. Stretches, slowly bending to the left.
2. Recovers to the starting position.
3. Repeats.
4. Reverses to right arm at side and left arm overhead.

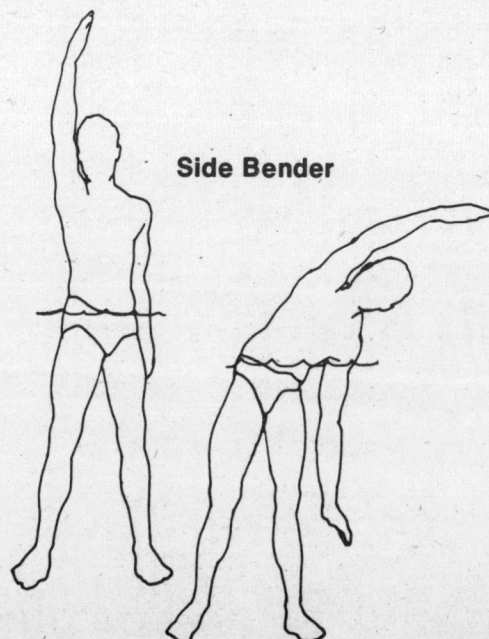

Side Bender

Toe Raises (lower leg muscles)
Standing in chest-deep water, swimmer:

1. Raises on toes.
2. Lowers to starting position.
3. Repeats.
4. Accelerates.

Toe Raises

Standing Crawl (shoulder, upper back and arm muscles)
Standing in waist-to-chest deep water, swimmer:

1. Simulates the overhand crawl stroke by:
   a. Reaching out with the left hand, getting a grip on the water, pressing downward and pulling, bringing the left hand through to the thigh.
   b. Reaching out with the right hand, etc.
2. Repeats.

Standing Crawl

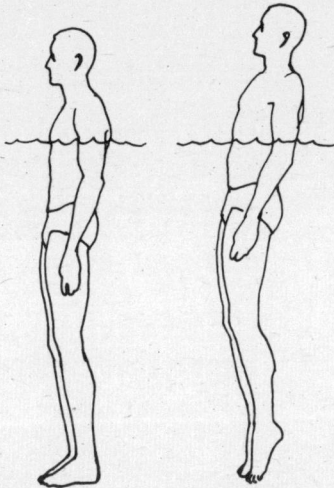

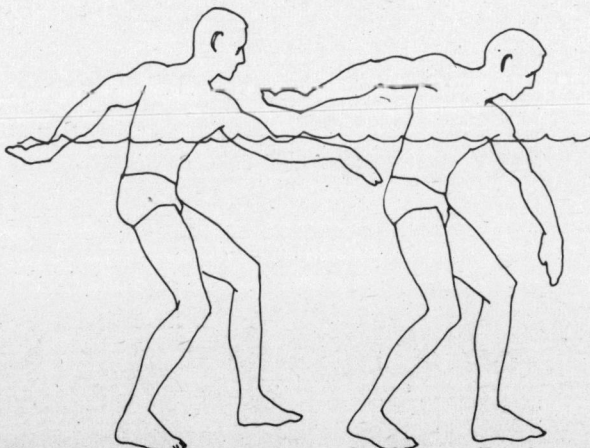

Walking Twists (lower back, trunk and leg muscles)
With fingers laced behind neck, swimmer:

1. Walks forward bringing up alternate legs, twisting body to touch knee with opposite elbow.
2. Repeats.

Walking Twists

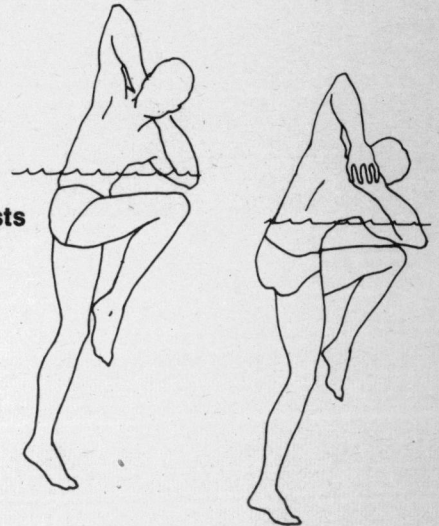

Stretch and Touch (upper back and arm muscles)
Standing, facing wall with arms extended and fingertips approximately 12 inches from wall, swimmer:

1. In chest-to-shoulder deep water, twists left and tries to touch wall with both hands.
2. Twists right and tries to touch wall with both hands.
3. Repeats.

Stretch and Touch

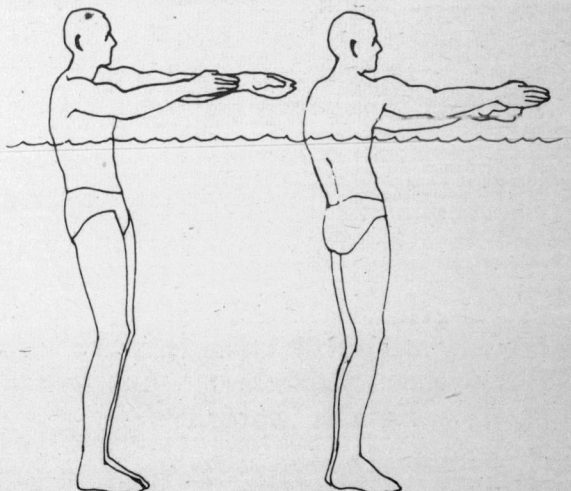

Flat Back (lower back muscles)
Standing at side of pool in waist-to-chest deep water, swimmer:

1. Presses back against wall, holding for six counts.
2. Relaxes to starting position.
3. Repeats.

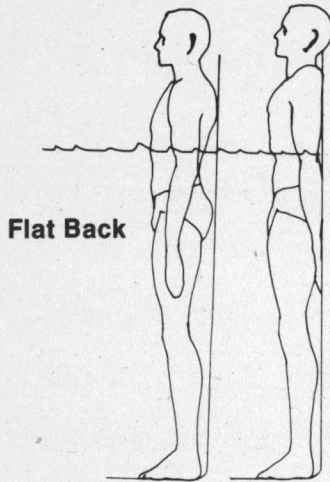

Flat Back

Leg Swing Outward (inner thigh)
Standing with back against poolside, and hands sideward holding gutter, swimmer:

1. Raises left foot as high as possible with leg straight.
2. Swings foot and leg to left side.
3. Recovers to starting position by pulling left leg vigorously to right.
4. Repeats.
5. Reverses to right leg.
6. Repeats.

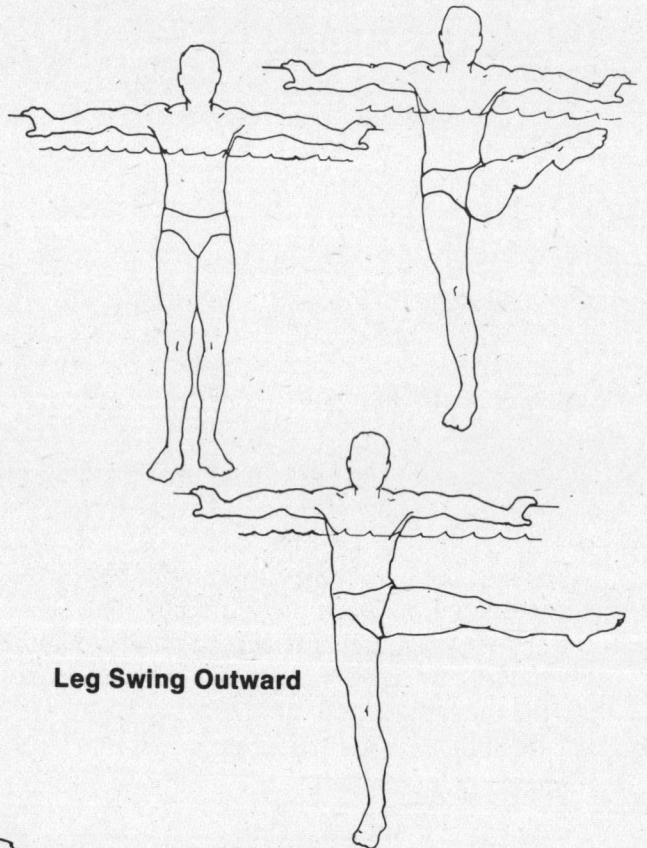

Leg Swing Outward

Leg Out (leg muscles)
Standing at side of pool with back against wall, swimmer:

1. Raises left knee to chest.
2. Extends left leg straight out.
3. Stretches leg.
4. Drops leg to starting position.
5. Repeats.
6. Reverses to right leg.

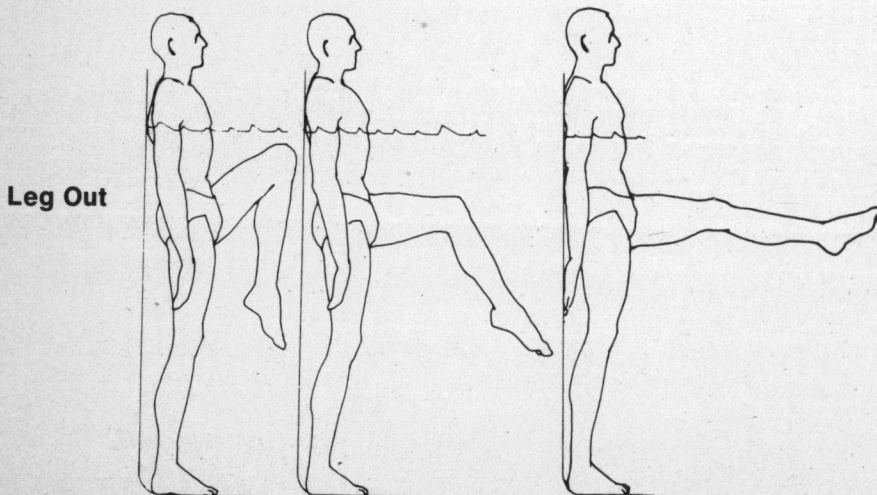

Leg Out

Twist Hips (trunk muscles)
Standing, holding on to pool gutter with hands, with back to wall, swimmer:

1. Twists hips to left as far as possible, keeping the upper trunk facing forward.
2. Recovers.
3. Twists hips to right.
4. Recovers.

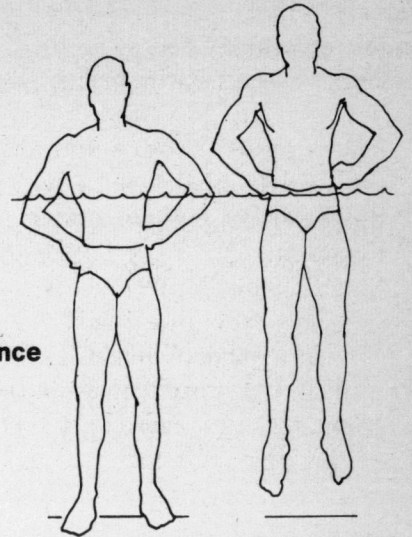

Toe Bounce

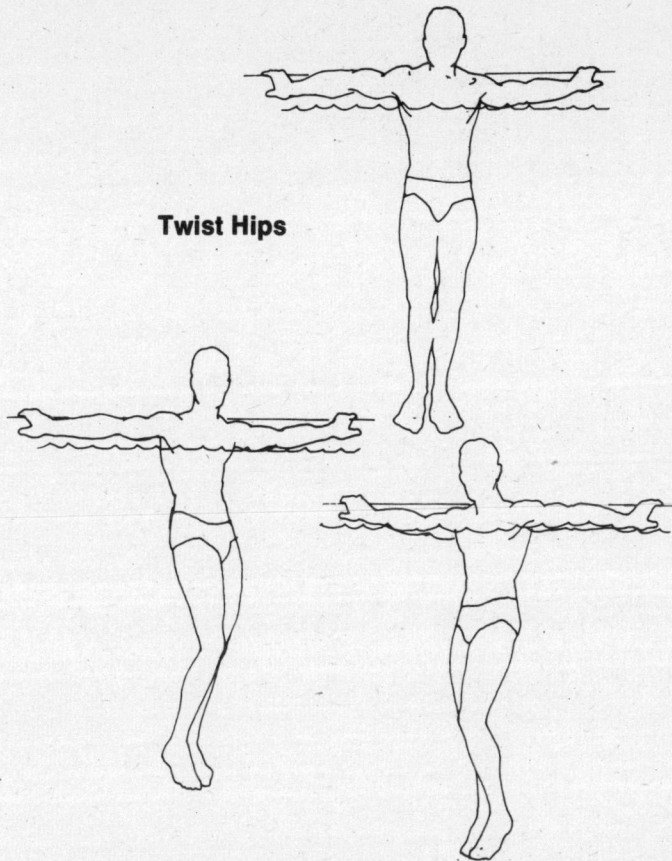

Twist Hips

Jogging in Place (upper and lower leg muscles)
Standing with arms bent in running position, swimmer:

1. Jogs in place.

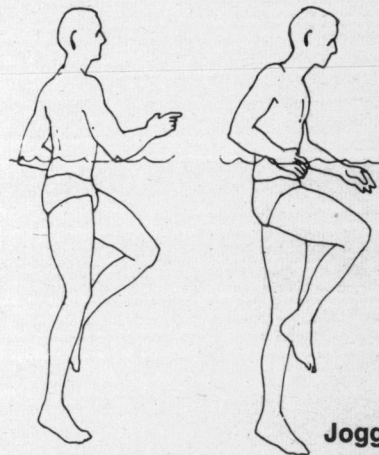

Jogging in Place

Aquatic Strength Exercises
Toe Bounce (lower leg muscles)
Standing in waist-to-chest deep water with hands on hips, swimmer:

1. Jumps high with feet together through a bouncing movement of the feet.
2. Repeats.

Front Flutter Kicking (leg muscles and back muscles)
Lying in a prone position and holding on to side of pool with hand(s), swimmer:

1. Kicks flutter style in which toes are pointed back, ankles are flexible, knee joint is loose but straight and the whole leg acts as a whip.

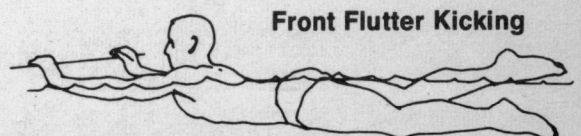

Front Flutter Kicking

High Bobbing

In water approximately 1 to 3 feet over the swimmer's head, swimmer:

1. Takes a vertical position, hands extended outward from the sides with palms turned downward. Legs are drawn in position for frog kick.
2. Simultaneously pulls hands sharply to thighs with legs executing frog kick.
3. Inhales at peak of height.
4. Drops with thrust of arms downward with palms turned upward until feet reach bottom of the pool and tucks to a squat position. Exhales throughout this action.
5. Jumps upward with power leg thrust at the same time pulling arms in a breast stroke position downward, causing the head and shoulders to rise high out of water. Exhales during (4) and (5).
6. Inhales and repeats cycles (4) and (5), etc.

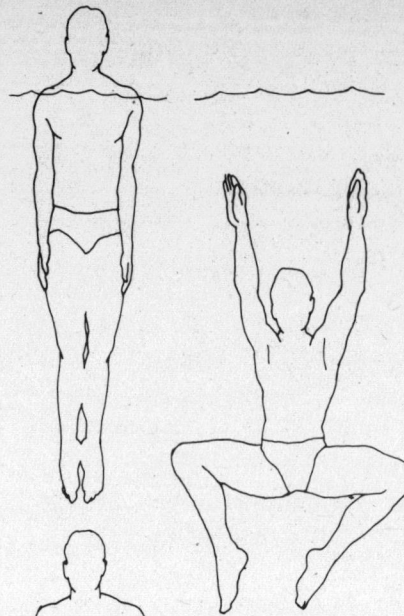

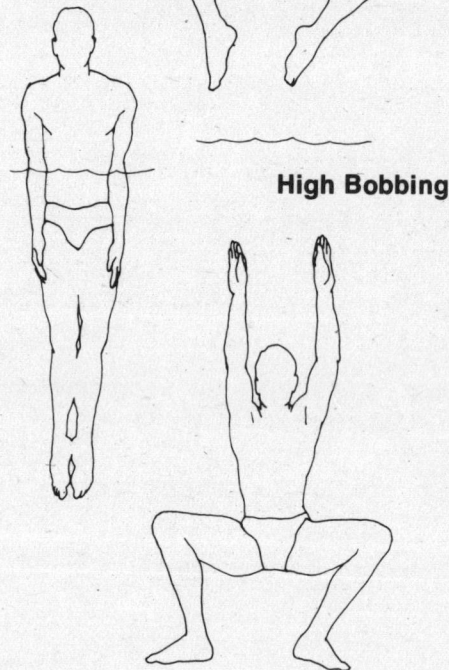

High Bobbing

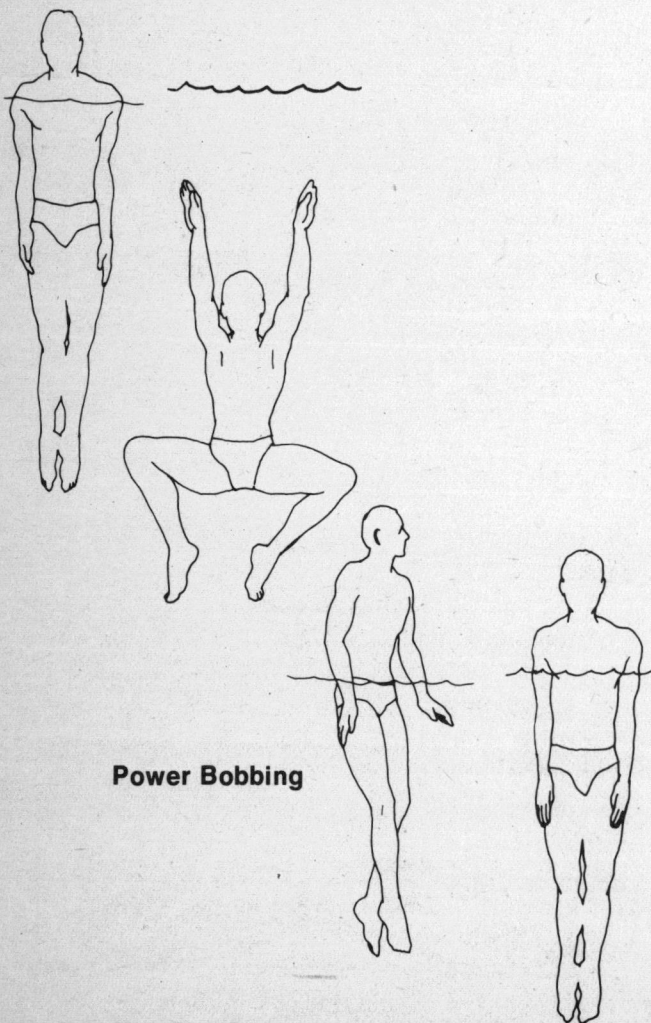

Power Bobbing

Power Bobbing (leg, arm and shoulder muscles)

Power bobbing is similar to "high bobbing" except that at the top of the upward thrust the hands scull vigorously as the legs flutter and kick. In "power bobbing" the swimmer will literally blast out of the water exposing all of the body to the hips. Bobbing is a well-rounded workout involving leg power, arm and shoulder work, heavy forced breathing, and rhythmical vigorous action.

Aquatic Cardiovascular Pulmonary Exercises

Crawl Stroke: The crawl stroke is the fastest of the swimming strokes. For the correct body position in crawl swimming, the body should be a streamlined whole with the body face down in the water and the legs extended and slightly below the surface. The arms move alternately so that as one ends its pull stroke, the other begins its pull stroke. The hand enters the water with the arm extended, elbow slightly bent and held high in the air. When the arm is pulling through the water, the shoulder should be over the elbow and the elbow over the wrist and hand. This position affords the greatest pulling power. As the palm hits the water, you press downward and backward with shoulder and arm muscles for the first third of the stroke, push downward in the

(Art courtesy American Red Cross, Mid-America Chapter.)

middle third and backward during final stroke. Do not push upward after final third—the arm should only be at about a 180-degree arc. As the arm comes out of the water, with the other arm beginning its pulling stroke, the elbow is bent and carried high in the air.

The legs are held fairly straight, with toes pointed and are kicked in a flutter motion. Breathing is done by turning the head to either side during the recovery of the overwater arm, with quick inhalation and then returning the face downward exhaling through the nose, mouth or both.

In performing the crawl, there should be no lateral movement or extreme arching of the back. This will cause imbalance, a decrease in speed and an increase fatigue.

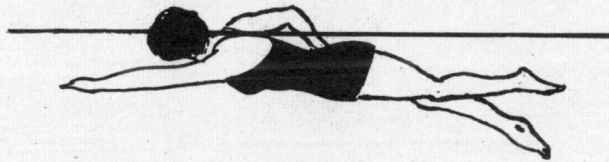

1

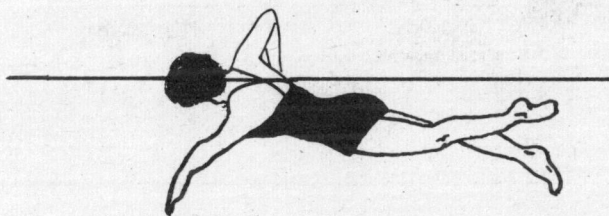

2

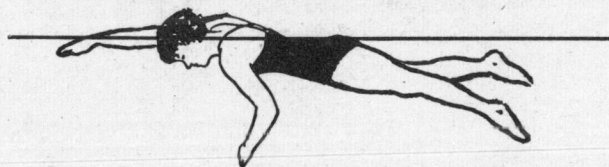

3

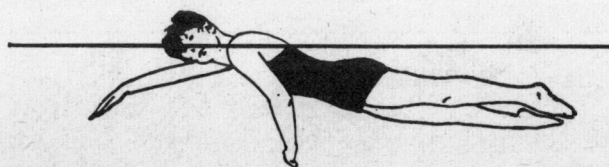

4

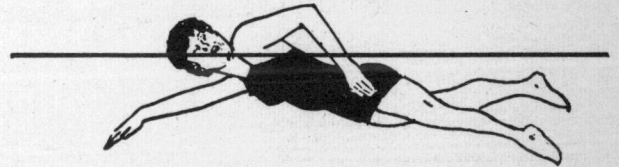

5

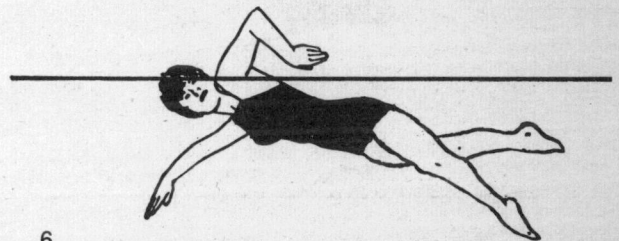

6

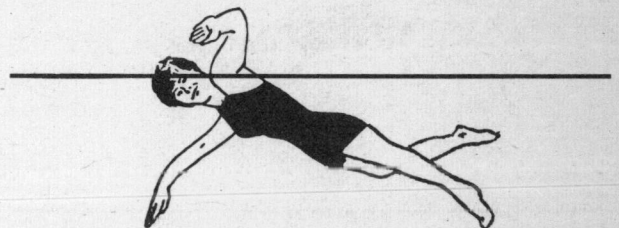

7

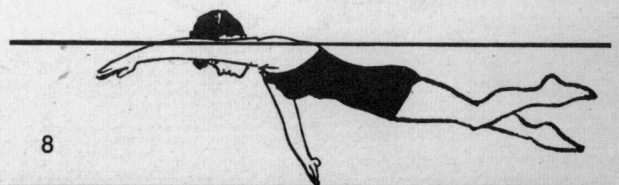

8

Chapter 4: Endurance

Breaststroke: The breaststroke and butterfly are very similar in form but differ primarily in arm action. In the breaststroke, the arms always remain beneath the surface of the water. The two hands are extended together in front of the body, palms facing outward and are pulled outward and backward until the arms are a little more than perpendicular to the body. At the point of maximum spread, the arms are brought together under the chest and extended again quickly.

The kick that accompanies the breaststroke can be of two types—the wedge (frog) kick or the whip kick. The whip kick is generally considered the more efficient of the two. Both are characterized by a "squeezing" action of the legs. The difference is that in the wedge the feet are drawn up to the body, knees bent, and are vigorously kicked outward to the fully extended position. The legs are then drawn together in a "squeezing" fashion. The whip kick is a much narrower kick with the knees kept much closer together and with the legs never reaching the fully extended position.

Breathing is accomplished by raising the head out of the water as the arms are completing their stroke and before they are being brought together underneath the chest.

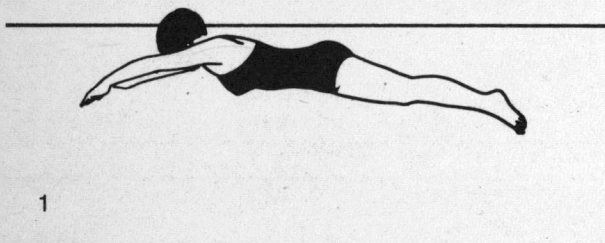

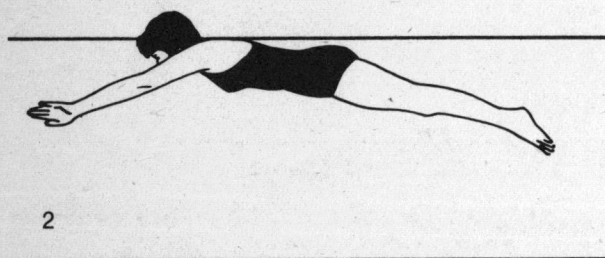

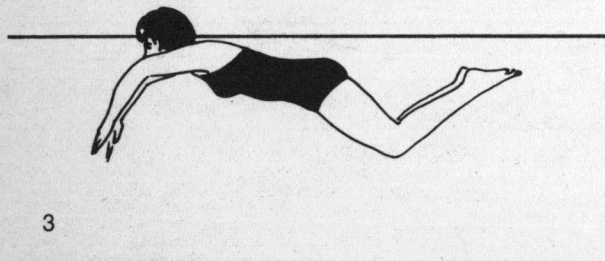

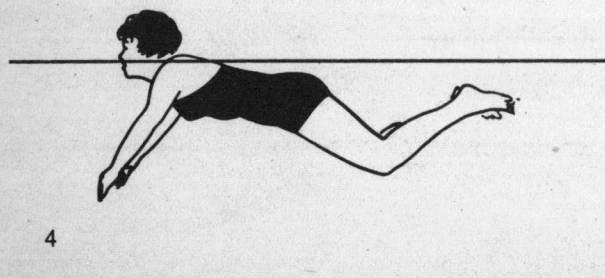

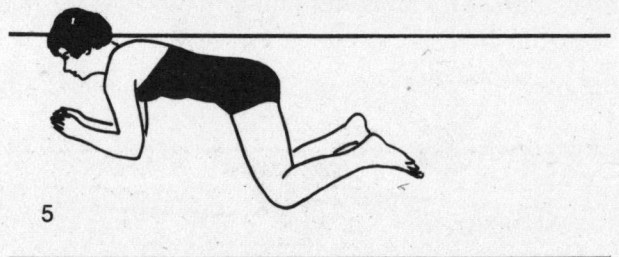

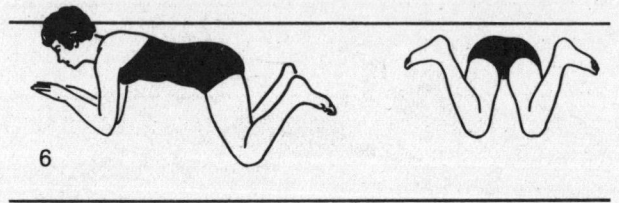

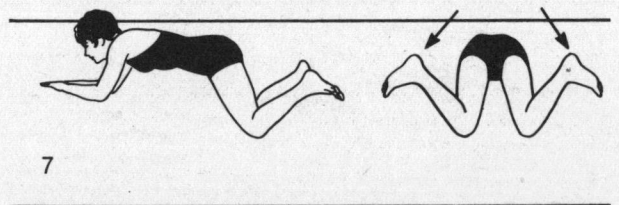

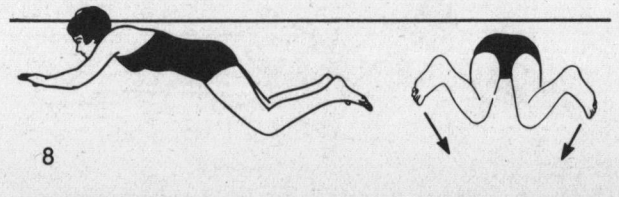

1

2

3

4

5

6

7

8

182

Butterfly: The butterfly is a competitive swimming stroke and is very strenuous and difficult to master. In the butterfly the arms are above water in the recovery stage, and in the propulsive stage are pressed downward and backward under the body all the way to the hips. They are then lifted in a rotary fashion out of the water, brought forward of body, in fully extended position with palms down, to begin the next stroke.

The kick used with the butterfly can be either the wedge kick or the dolphin or fishtail kick. The dolphin kick, however, must be used if swimming competitively. In the dolphin kick, the legs are kept together and simultaneously move up-and-down in a vertical plane.

Breathing during the butterfly takes place at the end of each stroke with the head raised out of the water for a quick breath and then lowered as the arms are brought forward again.

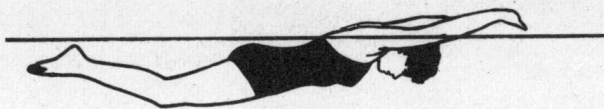

1

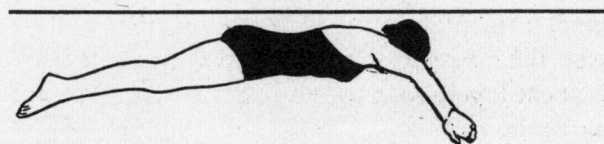

5

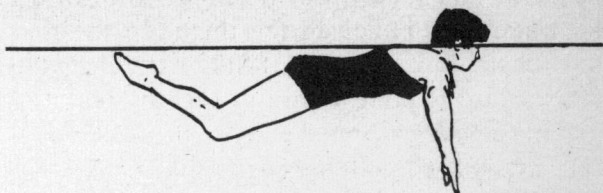

2

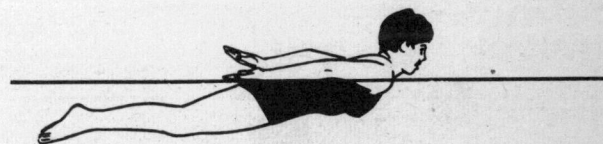

6

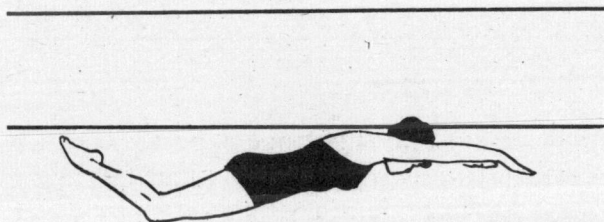

3

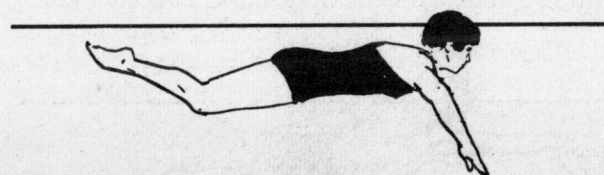

7

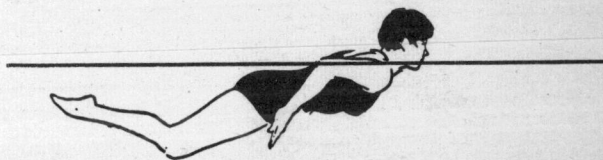

4

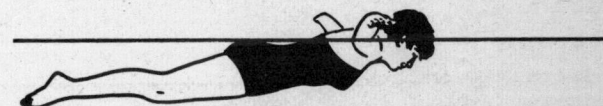

8

Backstroke: As in the sidestroke, the face in performing the backstroke is always out of the water. In performing the backstroke, keeping the body as streamlined as possible, with legs together and feet pointed is important. There should be a slight bend at the waist in order to get the maximum propulsion from the kicking action of the legs. But if the bend is too pronounced, it will create drag and will make the stroke less effective. Each arm alternately stretches above the head and enters the water directly above and in line with the shoulder with the palms facing outward. When the palm enters the water it is pulled to the thigh. In the first third of the pull, the arm is fully extended, the middle third is done with arm slightly bent and final third with arm in full extension.

The kick used with the backstroke is like that of the crawl stroke. Legs extended, toes pointed, legs moving in up-and-down flutter motion but with the emphasis on the up beat of the kick.

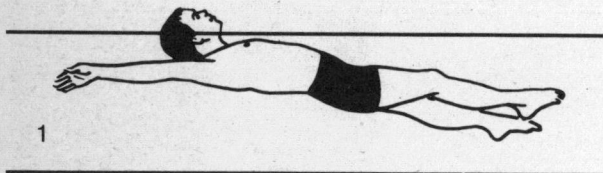

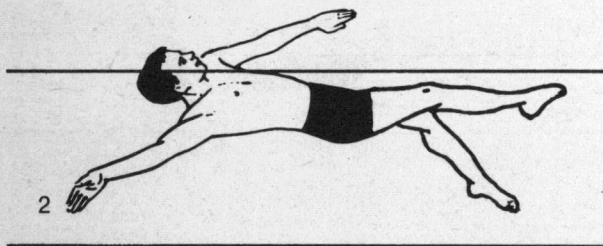

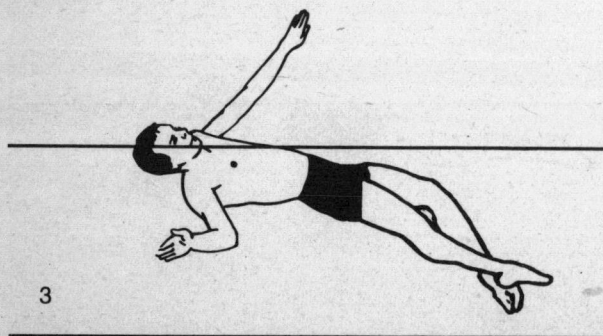

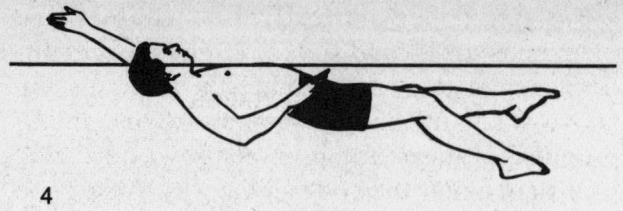

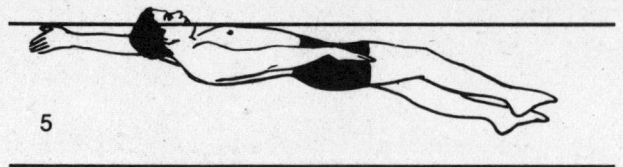

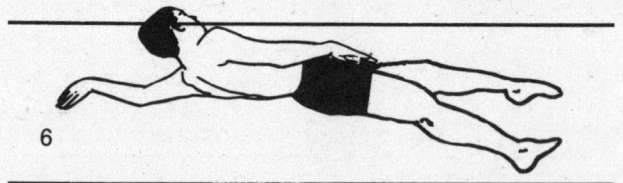

Sidestroke: The sidestroke is best known for its use in lifesaving situations and for many people is the preferred stroke for open water swimming because the face remains constantly above water. The body always remains on the side with the arms propelling the body alternately. The under arm begins from a fully extended position and pulls downward below the body to the waist, then bends upward and pushes forward to fully extended position. The upper arm pulls outside the body line, pulling from the chest to the thigh and is brought back to chest level close to the water surface but not above the surface.

The kick used with the sidestroke is the scissors kick. The legs open slowly by bending the knees, the underleg moving backward, the upper leg forward, and then are whipped together in a closing movement. The closing action is timed with finish of upper arm stroke.

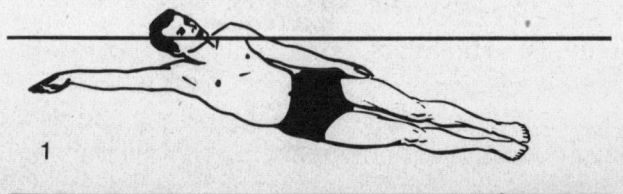

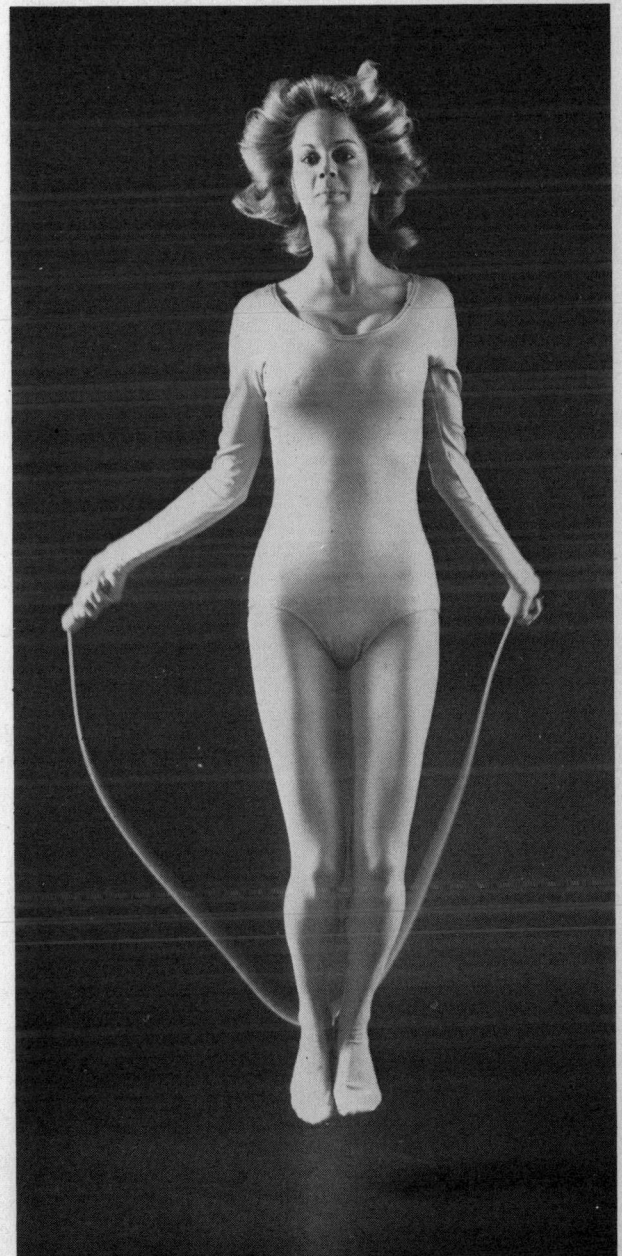

2

3

4

5

ROPE JUMPING

This is such a good exercise that it can be a full-time aerobic fitness activity. The equipment is inexpensive and easy to transport. You can skip rope anywhere, even in a hotel room. The exercise allows a wide range of exercise intensities, and research studies have equated 10 minutes of vigorous rope skipping in cardiovascular benefit to 20 to 30 minutes of jogging.

Rope length is important. It should reach the armpits when held beneath the feet. Commercial

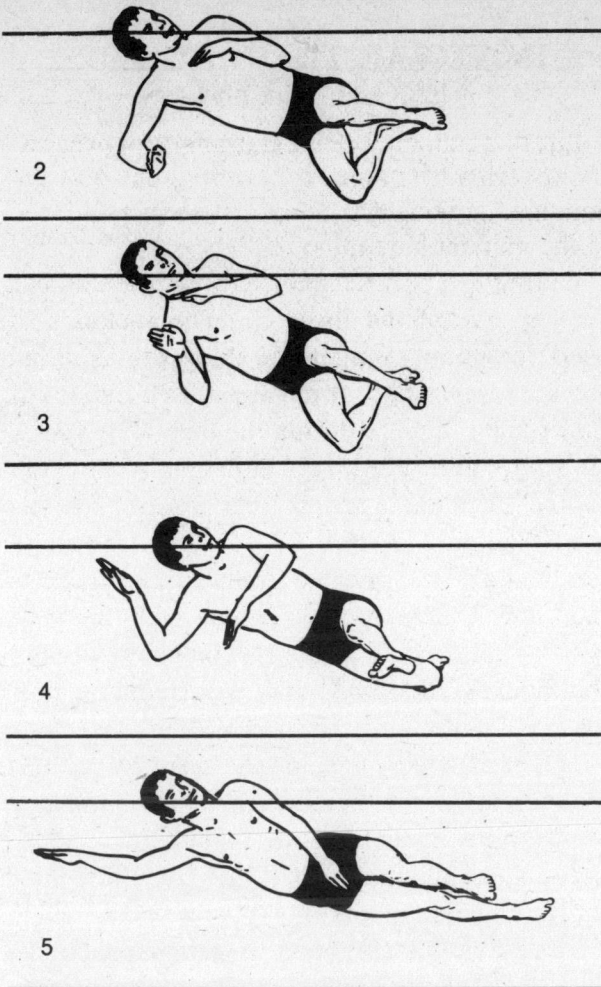

The Slow Progressive Build-Up

Swimming is unique in that age is no hindrance and individuals of varying exercise tolerance levels can utilize this activity to develop organic vigor and to improve flexibility, strength and the blood circulation.

Contrary to an old myth, swimming is compatible with training for other sports. It does not detract from the strength gained through other conditioning activities in the training regimen.

Obviously, individuals in poor condition must work slowly and progressively. It has taken many years for most adults to get out of shape. One should be patient and realize that rebuilding the heart, lungs and body may take a long period of time. A commitment to regularity and gradual build-up will pay off. There may be speed limits but no age limits for either sex. Daily workouts are recommended, but gains can be made with 30-40 minutes of water work 3-5 times per week. Train, don't strain!

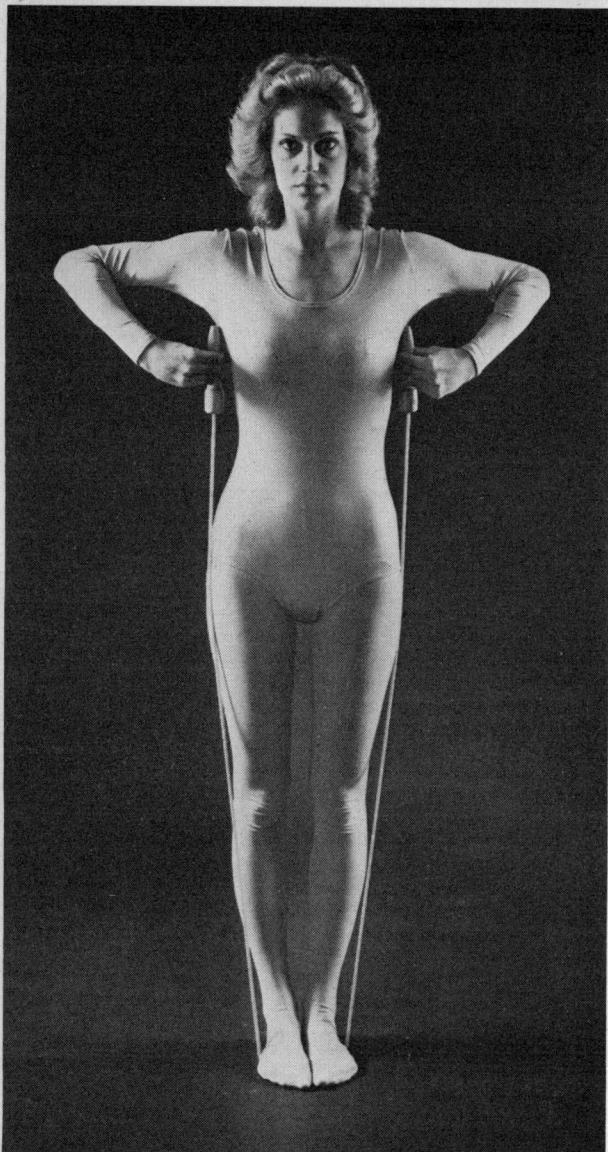

To test for proper rope length, stand heels down on the middle of the rope and bring handles up against body. The handle tips should just touch your armpits.

skip ropes with ball bearings in the handles are easier and smoother to use, but a length of #10 sash cord from your local hardware store serves quite well.

Rope skipping requires a degree of coordination, and if done inappropriately can quickly raise the heart rate above your training zone. If this happens, walk or jog in place slowly, then resume skipping.

Besides the aerobic benefits, rope skipping can improve your tennis, racquetball or handball, where rapid footwork is important.

INTERVAL TRAINING FOR AEROBIC FITNESS

Interval training is a good example of progressive overload. It aims at bettering physical endurance, increasing the capacity to respond well to the maximum load.

During the past decade, interval training has become one of the most common methods of conditioning for competition in events requiring physical endurance. It has been used by almost all distance runners during the past 10 years including such great athletes as Katherine Switzer, Francie Larrieu Lutz, Frank Shorter, John Walker, Filbert Bayi, Martin Liquori and Jim Ryun. The interval training approach is used universally for the training of swimmers, cyclists and rowers as well as members of soccer, hockey and basketball teams during preseason conditioning programs. Many coaches have contributed much of the tremendous improvement in the performance of endurance events in track and field and swimming to the increased use of interval training by athletes of both sexes and all ages and abilities.

Regardless of the type of physical activity used (running, swimming, cycling, bench stepping, etc.) interval training is simply repeated periods of physical stress interspersed with recovery periods during which activity of a reduced intensity or rest is performed. During the recovery periods, the individual usually keeps moving and does not completely recover before the next exercise interval. If running is the activity to be used, then the individual runs a specified distance at a pre-determined pace and then jogs or walks for a specified distance or time. This procedure is then repeated a certain number of times depending on the ability of the individual and the time available. The primary advantage of interval training over other forms of endurance conditioning is that with the interval approach a greater amount of work can be performed in a shorter period of time.

By alternating periods of vigorous physical activity with periods of light activity or recovery, a wide variety of training programs can be designed to meet the needs, ability and

Once achieving the level of fitness you want, you can switch to a maintenance program. (Photo courtesy of American Red Cross, Mid-America Chapter.)

interests of the individual and to fit within the available time and facilities. The total amount of exercise or work performed by an individual during interval training can be varied in several ways. They include variations in the (1) speed or intensity of the effort, (2) duration or distance of the effort, (3) the number of times the effort is repeated, (4) the length of the recovery period and (5) the nature of the activity during the recovery period.

Because of the ability to vary each of these components separately or together, the interval approach to training offers the possibility of unlimited variety and flexibility.

While interval training helps substantially to improve cardiovascular-respiratory condition, it contributes little to upper body muscular endurance, total body strength, flexibility, agility, balance or power.

MAINTAINING AEROBIC FITNESS

Once you've achieved the level of aerobic fitness that suits your personal needs as well as the work capacity needed for your job, you can switch to a maintenance program. Research indicates that you can maintain a given level of fitness with 2 or 3 days of activity a week. The activity must be at the same intensity and duration you employed to achieve fitness. Exercise of lesser intensity but longer duration achieves the same effect.

If a 40-year-old swims for several months to attain fitness, he or she can maintain that level with two or three workouts a week, or one swim a week and 2 hours of tennis, 4 or 5 days a week. A periodic recheck with the Step Test will tell you if you are, in fact, maintaining the fitness you worked so hard to achieve.

You're encouraged to seek activities you enjoy and to integrate them into your life-style. Before long you will find that exercise and training are no longer viewed as an obligation. When exercise becomes an enjoyable—even essential —part of your day, you'll have achieved the

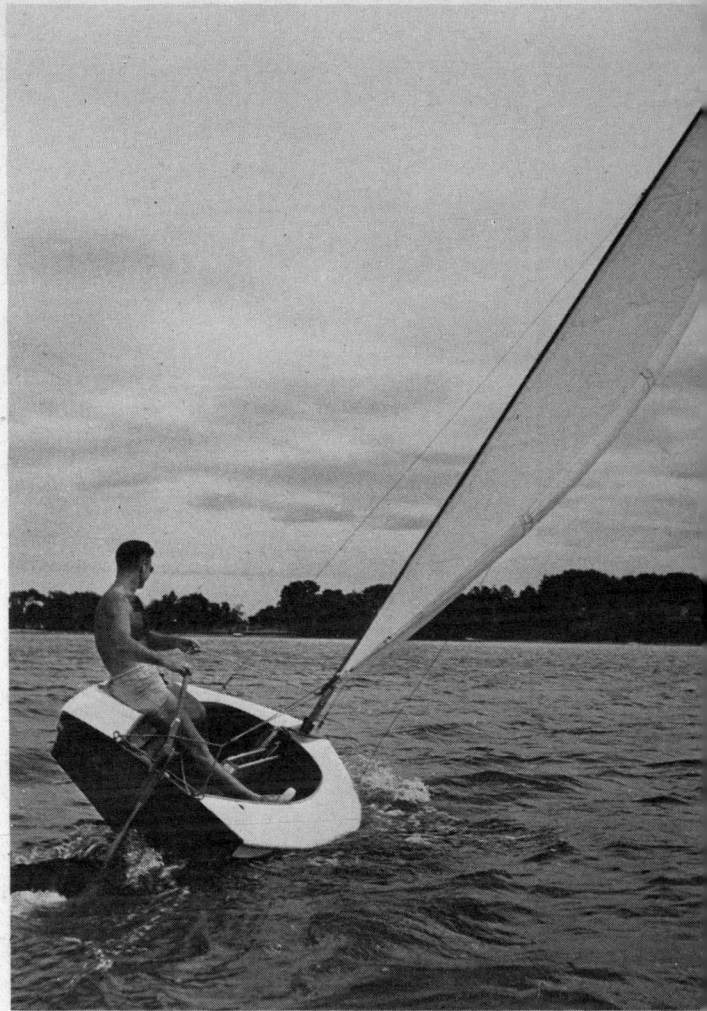

health, fitness, and work capacity needed to accomplish your job, and still have sufficient energy to enjoy leisure-time pursuits.

YEAR-ROUND ACTIVITY

Year-round activity is the ideal way to achieve and maintain fitness. It minimizes the pain and soreness associated with the return to activity. It keeps fitness at an optimal level and minimizes the problem of weight control. Take a moment to outline your current physical activity habits on a sheet of paper. Fill in the sports or activities you enjoy each season. When you find a blank spot consider a new activity, an exercise supplement, or an exercise to help you prepare for an upcoming season. This brief mental exercise will show how one activity might logically blend into the next, removing the need for extensive physical training.

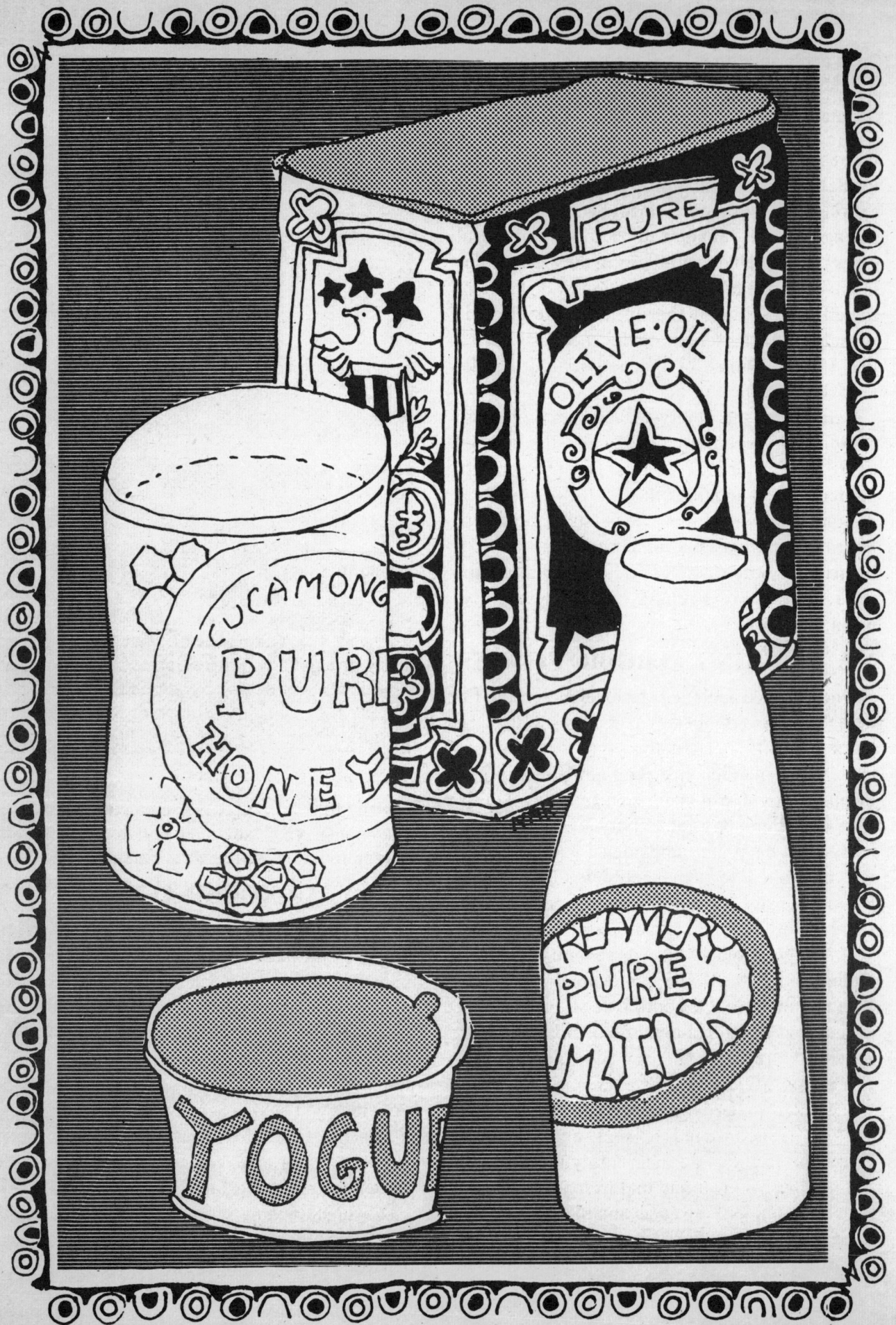

chapter 5

Nutrition & Weight

THE KEY TO effective weight control is keeping energy intake (food) and activity energy output (physical activity) in balance. This is true at all ages for both sexes. When the calories consumed in food equal those used to meet the body's needs, weight will remain about the same. When one eats more than this amount, one will put on fat unless physical activity is increased proportionately.

For years physicians have talked about the varying caloric needs of differing occupations and physical recreations. Yet in their attempts to lose excess fat, weight-watchers have often concentrated on counting the calories in their diets and have neglected the role of exercise. For those who are too fat, increasing physical activity can be just as important as decreasing food intake.

Weight depends not only on how many calories are taken in during the day, but also on how many are used up in physical activity. The overly fat person who merely cuts down his intake of food to lose weight will make slow progress since the number of calories needed to maintain the body is much smaller than most people think.

In fact, lack of exercise has been cited as the most important cause of the "creeping" obesity found in modern mechanized societies. Few occupations now require vigorous physical activity. Although there is more time available for recreation, many persons fail to fill this gap by choosing leisure time activities that give them exercise. Even among those who do exercise, their activity is often neither vigorous nor sustained.

Authorities point out that adding 30 minutes per day of moderate exercise to one's schedule can result in a loss of about 25 pounds in one year, assuming food consumption remains constant. To put it another way—just one extra slice of bread a day, or a soft drink, or any other food item that contains about 100 calories can add up to 10 extra pounds in a year if the amount of physical activity is not increased accordingly.

Recent studies seem to indicate that lack of physical activity is more often the cause of overweight than is overeating. These studies have compared the food intake and activity patterns of obese persons with those of normal weight. Several age levels—teenagers, adults, and older persons— have been studied. In each instance, the findings showed that the obese people did not consume any more calories than their normal-weighted agemates, but that they were very much less active.

The person who has a trim figure and wants to keep it should exercise regularly and eat a balanced, nutritious diet which provides sufficient calories to make up for the energy expended. The thin individual who wishes to gain weight should exercise regularly and increase the number of calories he consumes until the desired weight is reached. The overweight person should decrease the food intake and step up physical activity.

At this point let us dispel the myth that exercise increases a person's appetite. The idea that increased physical activity is useless as a means of losing weight because it always increases the appetite is fallacious.

It is true that a lean person in good condition may eat more following increased activity, but his exercise will burn up the extra calories he consumes. But the obese—the overly fat person—does not react the same way to exercise. Only when he exercises to excess will his appetite increase. Because he has large stores of fat, moderate exercise does not stimulate his appetite. This difference between the response to exercise of fat and lean people is important.

Laboratory tests on experimental animals have borne this out. When their exercise was moderate, food intake did not increase. In one experiment animals exercised 1 hour a day ate a smaller amount of food than those exercised less

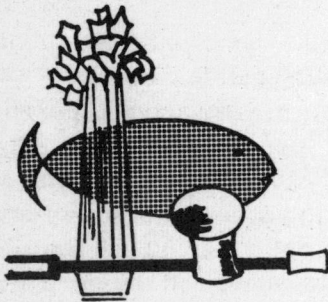

than an hour a day or not at all! On the other hand, when the animals were exercised vigorously over longer periods, they ate more but the extra activity kept their weight constant.

In other experiments, when the animals' activity was decreased, they continued to eat the same amount of food and became obese.

Similarly, a study of overweight adults showed that the start of their obesity corresponded with their decline in activity. Although their activity decreased, their appetites didn't. This is a common observation. When people finish school and go to work (especially if the job is a sedentary one), they tend to continue eating the same amount of food as before but, with their decline in activity, do not use all the calories they take in and gradually begin to gain weight.

Here are some guiding principles to acquaint you with sound, nutritional approaches to diet or caloric restriction:

- Don't starve and stuff. Eat three meals a day.

- Maintain minimal caloric intake equivalent to your basal energy expenditure.

- Eat a balanced diet, including adequate but not excessive vitamins and 1 to 2 grams of protein per kilogram of body weight per day (about ½ to 1 gram per pound per day). No more than 20 to 25 percent of your total caloric intake should be fats (reduce intake of saturated fats). The rest of your intake should be in carbohydrates (corn, rice, whole grains, potatoes, beans). Limit the sugar, soft drinks, cakes.

- Engage in regular moderate physical activity.

- Avoid an excessive caloric deficit (difference between intake and expenditure should not regularly exceed 1,000 calories).

- Practice behavior modification.

- Eat in only one room (dining or kitchen).

- Leave something on your plate.

- Slow your pace; pause between bites.

- Exercise before a meal.

- Engage in light exercise an hour or two after your main meal.

Now let's consider some basic things about food. Any food that's going to do anything for the human body must do the following three things:
1. Contribute body fuel to oxidation in the body to release energy.
2. Contribute material to build and sustain the body tissues.
3. Contribute materials that tend to regulate body processes.

Any sensible diet must give you foods that accomplish all three functions. If a food offers one or more of the above three things, it is a nutrient. There are six nutrients as far as class is concerned. They are fats, proteins, vitamins, carbohydrates, minerals and water—all essential to the body. Proteins, fats, and carbohydrates are combustible. Proteins, fats, minerals and water are part of our body composition, so we need them to preserve and build our body tissues.

Minerals and vitamins regulate body functions. Water is also important in regulating body functions because it holds elements in solution in our digestive juices as well as in our blood and tissues and helps to control body temperature, circulation and excretion.

The U.S. Department of Agriculture has indexed foods into four main groups—the Milk Group, the Meat Group, the Vegetable and Fruit Group and the Bread and Cereal Group.

The diet recommendations are:

Milk Group: At least two 8-ounce servings every day. Small children and teenagers are considered to require a quart or four 8-ounce servings. The group includes milk, cheese, ice cream and ice milk.

Meat Group: At least two 3-ounce servings every day. The group includes not only meat but fish, eggs, nuts and poultry. These foods are all high in protein, vitamins and iron.

Vegetable/Fruit Group: Four or more servings every day. Tomato or citrus fruit juice or the fruit itself should be a part of the daily diet, since they are the primary suppliers of Vitamin C. Fruits and vegetables also contribute important minerals and Vitamin A.

Bread/Cereal Group: Should be used at some time every week, an important source of B group vitamins and vitamin K.

Depending on the person, the servings may need to be increased to give enough calories for necessary energy.

The standard measurement of energy is the calorie.

But how many calories do you need to function properly? To start with, you need carbohydrates, and foods that have them in abundance include plain granulated sugar, cookies, candy, cake, jam, jelly, white bread, potatoes, rice, pasta and dry cereals.

Fats are another source of energy, useful when you aren't getting enough carbohydrates to fulfill your energy requirements.

On some reducing diets, you cut down on carbohydrates and fats, prompting the body to use up stored fats.

Caloric tables, accurately computed, will tell you exactly how many calories every common food contains, in a specific-size serving.

But the number of calories your body requires is by no means standard. The so-called "standard" man used in most computations is 5 feet, 7 inches tall and weighs about 150 pounds. Obviously, not everyone is " standard." Regardless of size, the energy calorie requirements of a person are determined by the number of square meters in the body surface area.

But to complicate things even more, this calorie requirement measurement is for the human body at complete rest.

Even minor activities such as dressing, standing up and sitting down add to the requirements. Even such sedentary pursuits as singing and piano playing add to the calories needed per hour.

And such activities as heavy exercise and sports participation add tremendously to the number of calories per hour used up. Such things as basketball, non-competitive swimming, jogging, bicycling at a moderate speed, handball, running and sprinting consume great quantities of calories per hour.

Consequently, it takes a real expert to tell you with any degree of accuracy the number of calories you need to ingest per day.

Ideally, you want a balance between intake and consumption of calories—in other words, you need a diet that will keep your weight where it is.

But many people are either too light or too heavy.

And that has created a giant industry—weight control. It's an industry containing many competent, reliable practitioners—along with some incompetent ones and a multitude of so-called "weight control pills," most of which are almost totally ineffective without proper diet, and some of which are definitely injurious to the health. Exercise alone won't reduce weight, in spite of what some exercise health spas advertise. A combination of lower calorie intake and higher calorie consumption is usually most effective.

Everyone who is overweight is, of course, looking for a quick, easy way to take off the desired number of pounds. As a rule-of-thumb, it is safer and better to take off weight slowly, always with a balance of the nutrients needed for good health.

It is quite true that there are ways to take off

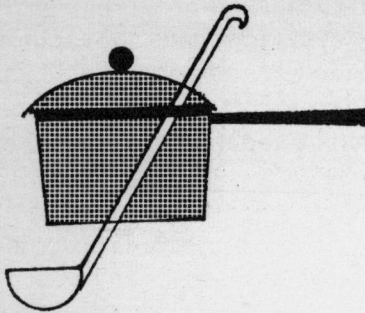

weight quickly. As a rule, these methods don't produce any lasting results or are injurious to the health.

Boxers who must make a certain weight before a match sometimes resort to steam baths to get off the required number of pounds, just before weigh-in. It's comparatively easy to take off a few pounds this way, but the weight will usually come back overnight, and the loss of water from the body is always debilitating.

A young lady of my acquaintance took off 20 pounds in a few weeks by the constant ingestion of amphetamines—and was such a nervous wreck as a result that she'd have been far better off to have retained the weight.

If you want to take off weight without endangering health, after getting a diet schedule from a reliable physician, you have to resign yourself to following a diet.

Even the items that are sold with the claims that they will lessen your appetite all carry a printed diet schedule of one kind or another, and some of the diets aren't very good ones.

Emotional stress of one kind or another causes many people to eat too much. Over-eating gives emotional satisfaction. A glandular malfunction is another cause.

Fad diets come and go, usually after making considerable money for their sponsors. Sometimes, according to doctors, they cause serious bodily harm. The sponsor of a new diet will always vouch for it, and sometimes the sponsor is a physician with a good record. But other doctors may disagree with him.

A high school girl who was grossly overweight went on a diet, eating less than the amount recommended. She began to get quick and drastic results. By the time her weight got down to the desired poundage, her stomach had shrunk to the point where she no longer wanted a healthful amount of food.

She developed a strange syndrome where she didn't want *any* food, and, when she was forced to eat, regurgitated the meal. She became almost a living skeleton, and the last I heard of her, doctors were afraid she was going to die of malnutrition.

Hers was a rare case of going to extremes. In contrast, many dieters "fudge" on the diet with snacks.

A housewife in our community who never seemed to overeat took on a big amount of surplus poundage and decided it must be the result of a glandular condition.

She wisely went to her doctor, who found nothing wrong with her glands but solved the problem, which he'd run across previously.

The woman was a good cook who fed her family well. She *liked* to cook. And while she was busy in the kitchen, she "tasted" enough of the food she was preparing to make anyone fat.

I've had fat friends describe their meals to me, and the meals certainly weren't excessive. But investigation showed that these people were chronic snackers who were eating something—or drinking it—almost all day long. One fellow admitted under questioning that he never ate less than three big candy bars during the working day.

Another took on enough calories every noon in pre-lunch cocktails to make anyone fat—and the cocktails gave him such a hearty appetite that his lunch contained far more calories than he should have had.

Some overweight people lack the willpower to limit their diet to a reasonable amount unless they have almost constant supervision.

For many such people, Weight Watchers and similar organizations have been an effective answer. Thrown into constant contact with other people who are in the same boat, they straighten up and fly right. There are others who need competition to spur them into doing anything well. They get it in these organizations.

Right now, I'm talking about obesity. Many people are a few pounds overweight without being obese. The obese person is one who is carrying too much body fat around with him. When a person reaches the point where he or she is from 15 to 20 percent heavier than the average for a height and age, that person must accept the fact that obesity is a problem.

And obesity is always a serious problem as far

as health is concerned.

Obese people usually get far too little exercise, and as a result have little or no endurance. They have a greater than normal tendency to hypertension and diabetes, along with other diseases. As far as heart trouble is concerned, obese men are twice as apt to die as lighter men of the same age. Also, with lack of sufficient exercise, they have a tendency toward arthritis, which compounds the inactivity problem.

The U.S. Department of Agriculture has published a table which lists approximate proper weight for men and women with small, medium and large frames, according to height.

Approximately Proper Weights
MEN

Height (barefoot)	Light Build	Medium Build	Heavy Build
5'3"	118	129	141
5'4"	122	133	145
5'5"	126	137	149
5'6"	130	142	155
5'7"	134	147	161
5'8"	139	151	166
5'9"	143	155	170
5'10"	147	159	174
5'11"	150	163	178
6'	154	167	183
6'1"	158	171	188
6'2"	162	175	192
6'3"	165	178	195

WOMEN

Height (barefoot)	Light Build	Medium Build	Heavy Build
5'	100	109	118
5'1"	104	112	121
5'2"	107	115	125
5'3"	110	118	128
5'4"	113	122	132
5'5"	116	125	135
5'6"	120	129	139
5'7"	123	132	142
5'8"	126	136	146
5'9"	130	140	151
5'10"	133	144	156
5'11"	137	148	161
6'	141	152	166

You'll notice that there's considerable latitude in average weights for different heights and small, medium and large frames. This leeway is as it should be.

My doctor thinks there are too many variants in body structure, age and basic metabolism to permit such a table to be completely accurate. He says to give yourself what he calls the "Gotcha" test to see if you're obese.

Here's how he describes it. "First, pinch yourself on the back of your upper arm, next on the lower side of your chest and finally just below the shoulder blades. Pinch fairly hard. If there's an inch or more of flabby flesh between your thumb and forefinger, you're obese and you better darned well do something about it if you want to stay alive and healthy."

He told me that American Medical Association statistics show the following relationship between overweight and death rate:

10 percent overweight—13 percent increase in death rates.
20 percent overweight—25 percent increase in death rates.
30 percent overweight—40 percent increase in death rates.

Even if you're a chronic gambler, you'd be foolish to gamble against such odds.

But before we get into a discussion of the basic food groups, it's astonishing how little most people know about the elements that go into foods. They don't know what proteins are, what vitamins are or what minerals are.

Protein is in essence the basis of life. It's what builds the body and maintains as well as repairs the tissues. You need protein to produce infection-fighting anti-bodies, enzymes and hormones. Protein isn't a single thing but many compounds called amino acids, of which 22 have been catalogued to date. Eight of these are essential to life and must be ingested as food, since the body can't create them. The best proteins with the most amino acid essentials are found in such foods as meat, poultry, seafood, milk, cheese and eggs.

Carbohydrates are the energy foods, including sugars and starches. The most universal problem in carbohydrates is ingesting too many rather than too few.

Cholesterol is not technically a fat but is a fatty

substance that forms vitamin D and some specific hormones. The more hydrogen a fat contains, the harder or stiffer it is.

Vitamins are chemical compounds which exist in small, almost minute quantities in foods. Vitamin A helps the human eye to adjust to changing light intensities and is an aid to avoiding night blindness. Good sources are dark yellow or orange fruits, dark green or yellow vegetables, whole milk, cream, butter, fortified margarine and liver. Since it can be stored in the body, overdoses of vitamin pills should be avoided.

There are about a dozen B vitamins, of which B_1, thiamine, B_2, riboflavin, and B_3, niacin, are the most important. Thiamine promotes good appetite, helps carbohydrate metabolism, and assists in keeping muscles, heart and nerves performing efficiently. Good sources are meat, especially pork, fish, poultry, enriched breads and cereals, dried peas and beans.

Riboflavin is required to utilize oxygen in the body and for enzyme function. The sources are the same as for thiamine.

Niacin is necessary for the proper use of oxygen and for healthy skin, tongue and digestive system. Lean meats, poultry, cereals, peanuts, dried peas and beans are good sources.

Vitamin C, ascorbic acid, helps to hold the body together. It also helps to heal wounds and stave off infection. Citrus fruits, such as cantaloupe and strawberries, or tomatoes, sweet green peppers, raw cabbage, kale and collards, broccoli and fresh potatoes are good sources.

Only vitamins B and C are damaged by cooking.

Vitamin D is needed for calcium metabolism and sound bones and teeth. Eggs, fish, liver oils, sardines, salmon, tuna and sunshine are good sources. Vitamin D can be stored in the body, and overdoses in vitamin pills can cause illness.

Vitamin E's primary benefit seems to be as an antioxidant in the body and in foods. Because it is so prevalent in foods we commonly eat, a vitamin E deficiency is only a remote possibility.

Among the minerals, calcium and phosphorous promote strong bones and teeth, good muscle tone and a good nervous system.

Iodine, required for normal thyroid function, is found in seafood and iodized salt.

Good sources for iron, essential for rich red blood, are organ meats, red meats, oysters, dark green leafy vegetables, eggs, dried fruits, and cereals.

Water isn't a food, but is certainly essential. Actually, the human body is about two-thirds water, and must have a supply of water to survive, to regulate body temperature, to help digestion and to carry off wastes. Six to eight glasses of water or liquid a day are usually recommended.

Following is a fairly complete list of foods containing the necessary nutrients for good health. We start with the Meat Group.

MEAT GROUP

There's a big difference in the number of calories in lean and fat meats, and it's virtually impossible to determine sharply how many calories are in a specific piece of meat.

Pot Roast: Taking both the lean and the fat into consideration, 3 ounces, which usually amounts to one thick slice or two thin ones, will be 245 calories. Taking the lean only, one thick or two thin slices will be 140 calories. Oven roasts vary so greatly in proportion of lean to fat that the same number of slices, one thick or two thin, may vary all the way from 375 down to 115 calories.

Steak: One thick or two thin slices of broiled steak, including both lean and fat, will be about 330 calories, where the same slices of lean meat only will be about 110 to 120 calories.

Hamburger: There's even a big difference in the number of calories in a 3-ounce hamburger: 245 for regular ground beef and 185 for lean ground beef.

Corned Beef: Three ounces of canned corned beef contain 185 calories. Surprisingly, the same weight of corned beef hash is about 150 calories.

Chipped Beef: Two ounces of dried chipped beef add up to 110 or 115 calories.

Meat Loaf: A slice of meat loaf about ½-inch

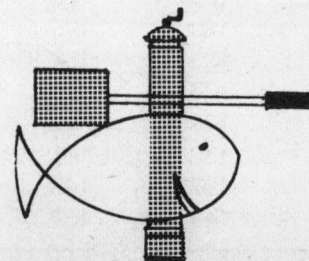

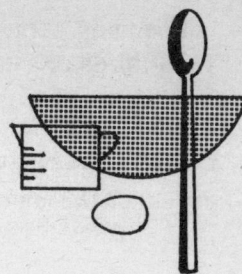

thick (2 ounces) is 115 calories, more or less, depending on the amount of fat left in it.

Beef Pot Pie: An 8-ounce beef pot pie contains a whopping 550 calories.

Veal Cutlet: A 3-ounce veal cutlet, broiled, is 175 to 185 calories.

Lamb Chop: A 4-ounce lamb chop, including both the lean and the fat, is 400 calories, while the lean only of the same size chop (about 2½ ounces) will contain only 140 calories. A thick slice of roast leg of lamb, containing both lean and fat, is 225 to 235 calories, while the same thickness of the lean meat only is 125 calories.

Pork Chops: A 2½-ounce pork chop, with both the lean and the fat, has 260 calories, while the same chop, with lean only, will weigh ½-ounce less and will contain about 150 calories.

Pork Loin Roast: The difference between a thick slice of roast loin of pork, depending on whether both the lean and fat or only the lean is eaten, is 300 calories or 175.

Ham: Three ounces of ham, a thick slice, with both lean and fat, has 245 calories and a 2½-ounce slice with lean only is about 125 calories.

Bacon: Two thin slices of bacon, broiled or fried, add up to 100 calories.

Bologna: Two slices of bologna sausage (about 2 ounces) offer 170 calories, and the same amount of liverwurst is approximately the same. Two ounces of canned Vienna sausages contain about 135 calories, but a 2-ounce patty of bulk pork sausage will run from 260 to 275 calories.

Beef Liver: Two ounces of fried beef liver is 125-135 calories, depending on the amount of fat used in frying it.

Beef Heart: Three ounces of braised beef heart, with most of the fat trimmed from it, will run about 215 calories, while the same amount of beef tongue, braised, will contain 160 calories.

Hot Dog: A frankfurter usually runs about 150 calories, unless it's one of the very large, plump ones.

Duck and Goose: Two ounces of duck or goose run to about 150 calories.

Bluefish: Baked bluefish, a 3-ounce piece, offers 135 calories.

Clams and Crabs: Three ounces of raw clams, shelled, considering meat only, contain 65 calories, while 3 ounces of canned clams and juice, including the juice has 45 to 50 calories.

Three ounces of canned crab meat is 85 calories.

Fish Sticks: On the other hand, fish sticks, which come breaded, cooked and frozen, with fat for frying, contain about 150 calories for 3 ounces.

Haddock: Three ounces of fried haddock, including fat for frying, will offer about 140 to 150 calories.

Mackerel: Three ounces of broiled mackerel contain 200 calories, while 3 ounces of canned mackerel will be about 150 calories.

Ocean Perch: Three ounces of fried ocean perch, including the egg and breadcrumb batter and frying fat, will be close to 200 calories.

Oysters: Half a cup of raw shucked oysters will contain about 75 to 85 calories.

Salmon: Four ounces of salmon, broiled or baked, will be about 200 calories, while 3 ounces of canned pink salmon, including the liquid, will be about 125 calories.

Sardines: Three ounces of drained canned sardines in oil will be at least 175 calories.

Shrimp: Three ounces of canned shrimp will be about 100 calories and 3 ounces of canned tuna fish, drained of oil, will be about 175 calories.

Eggs: A fried egg, including fat for frying, contains about 100 calories. On the other hand, a hard or soft-boiled egg of the same size will run from 75 to 80 calories. A large egg scrambled or in an omelet, including milk and cooking fat, will hit 110 to 115 calories. A poached egg is 75 to 80 calories.

THE MILK GROUP

Milk: Two cups of skimmed milk, buttermilk, or plain yogurt will hit 150 calories, while a cup and a half of only partly skimmed milk or yogurt will contain the same number.

Cottage Cheese: Two-thirds of a cup of creamed cottage cheese likewise will contain 150 calories.

Cheese: Two ounces of cheese contain from 150

to 200 calories, depending somewhat on the kind of cheese. Two-thirds of a cup of cottage cheese, uncreamed, contains the same number.

Ice cream, iced milk, milk shakes, etc., all contain milk to help meet the milk quota for a healthy diet.

BREAD AND CEREAL GROUP

Commercial bakery breads, buns and rolls vary greatly in caloric count. Some bakery breads are full of ingredients not found in homemade bread. One type of bakery bread that apparently appeals to some people is so puffed up with air that it can be compressed to less than half its size. We are talking here about good, standard homemade or high-class bakery bread.

Breads

Cracked Wheat: One slice of cracked wheat or raisin bread contains 60 calories, as does a slice of white.

Rye: A slice of rye bread or whole wheat bread is about 5 calories less. All the breads are rated by ½-inch slices.

Biscuits: A baking powder biscuit is 140 calories.

Buns: A hamburger bun or English muffin adds up to 150 calories.

Crackers, Pancakes/Waffles: Four large crackers will amount to 75 calories and a 4-inch waffle or pancake without butter or syrup will hit from 80 to 150 calories, depending on thickness.

Muffins: A plain muffin will be 140 calories, a bran muffin about 10 calories less, and a corn muffin about 10 calories more.

Cereals

Bran Flakes: A cup of bran flakes will contain about 100 calories. An ounce of corn flakes will be 110. A cup of Farina has about 100 calories.

Oatmeal: Three-fourths of a cup of oatmeal or rolled oats, cooked, have 100 calories.

Puffed Rice: A cup of puffed rice is just over 50 calories.

Noodles

Macaroni: Half a cup of macaroni and cheese has 235 calories and 3/4-cup of noodles, cooked, amount to 150 calories.

Spaghetti: Three-quarters of a cup of spaghetti

has 115 calories. In tomato sauce with cheese, it mounts to almost 200 calories.

VEGETABLE AND FRUIT GROUP

Vegetables

Potatoes: A medium-sized baked potato has 90 calories. Half a cup of diced, boiled potatoes is 50 calories. Ten 2-inch potato chips will run from 110 to 125 calories. Ten french fries contain about 150 calories. Half a cup of hashed brown potatoes is 225 calories, while half a cup of mashed potatoes is only 60 calories. Half a cup of pan-fried potatoes is about 225 calories.

Carrots: One raw carrot an inch in diameter will usually run about 25 calories. Half a cup of cooked carrots contains the same number.

Green Peas: Half a cup of cooked green peas will run from 60 to 70 calories.

Beets: Half a cup of cooked beets runs about 30 calories.

Beans: Half a cup of cooked or canned lima or green beans contains 75 calories, while half a cup of snap, green or wax beans, cooked or canned, will run about 20 calories.

Broccoli/Brussels Sprouts: Half a cup of broccoli or brussel sprouts, contain 20 calories.

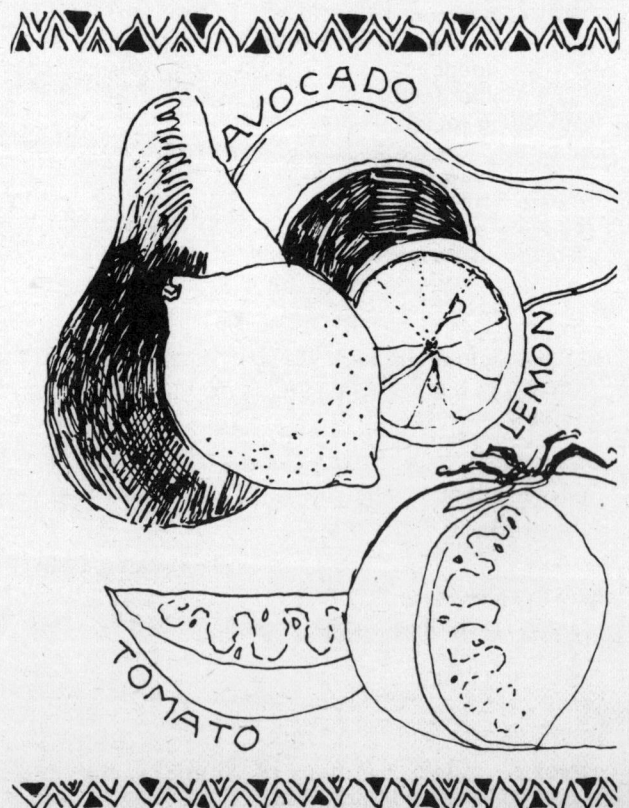

Calories Burned in Various Physical Activities*

ACTIVITY	Calories per minute	ACTIVITY	Calories per minute
Work Tasks		**Recreation**	
Carpentry	3.8	Archery	5.2
Chopping wood	7.5	Badminton (recreation-competition)	5.2-10.0
Cleaning windows	3.7	Baseball (except pitcher)	4.7
Clerical work	1.2-1.6	Basketball Half-full court (more for fastbreak)	6.0-9.0
Dressing	3.4		
Driving car	2.8	Bowling (while active)	7.0
Driving motorcycle	3.4	Calisthenics	5.0
Farming		Canoeing (2.5-4.0 mph)	3.0-7.0
Chores	3.8	Cycling (5-15 mph - 10-speed bicycle)	5.0-12.0
Haying, plowing with horse	6.7	Dancing	
Planting, hoeing, raking	4.7	Modern: moderate-vigorous	4.2-5.7
Gardening		Ballroom: waltz-rumba	5.7-7.0
Digging	8.6	Square	7.7
Weeding	5.6	Football (while active)	13.3
Hiking		Golf (foursome-twosome)	3.7-5.0
Road-field (3.5 mph)	5.6-7.0	Handball and squash	10.0
Snow: hard-soft (3.5-2.5 mph)	10.0-20.0	Horseshoes	3.8
Downhill: 5-10% grade (2.5 mph)	3.5-3.6	Judo and karate	13.0
Downhill: 15-20% grade (2.5 mph)	3.7-4.3	Mountain climbing	10.0
Uphill: 5-15% grade (3.5 mph)	8.0-15.0	Pool or billiards	1.8
40-lb pack: (3.0 mph)	5.0	Rowing (pleasure-vigorous)	5.0-15.0
40-lb pack: (1.5 mph) 36% slope	16.0	Running	
House painting	3.5	12-min mile (5 mph)	10.0
Ironing clothes	4.2	8-min mile (7.5 mph)	15.0
Making beds	3.4	6-min mile (10 mph)	20.0
Metal working	3.5	5-min mile (12 mph)	25.0
Mixing cement	4.7	Skating (recreation-vigorous)	5.0-15.0
Mopping floors	4.9	Skiing	
Pick-and-shovel work	6.7	Moderate to steep	8.0-12.0
Plastering walls	4.1	Downhill racing	16.5
Pulaski (depends on rate of work and other factors)	7.8	Cross-country (3-8 mph)	9.0-17.0
		Snowshoeing (2.5 mph)	9.0
Repaving roads	5.0	Soccer	9.0
Sawing		Swimming	
Chain saw	6.2	Pleasure	6.0
Crosscut saw	7.5-10.5	Crawl (25-50 yd/min)	6.0-12.5
Shining shoes	3.2	Butterfly (50 yd/min)	14.0
Shoveling (depends on weight of load, rate of work, height of lift)	5.4-10.5	Backstroke (25-50 yd/min)	6.0-12.5
		Breaststroke (25-50 yd/min)	6.0-12.5
(average)	8.0	Sidestroke (40 yd/min)	11.0
Showering	3.4	Skipping rope	10.0-15.0
Stacking lumber	5.8	Table tennis	4.9-7.0
Standing, Light activity	2.6	Tennis (recreation-competition)	7.0-11.0
Stone masonry	6.3	Volleyball (recreation-competition)	3.5-8.0
Sweeping floors	3.9	Water skiing	8.0
Tree felling (ax)	8.4-12.7	Wrestling	14.4
Truck and auto repair	4.2		
Walking			
Downstairs	7.1		
Indoors	3.1		
Upstairs	10.0-18.0		
Washing clothes	3.1		
Washing and dressing	2.6		
Washing and shaving	2.6		

*Calories burned depends on efficiency and body size. Add 10 percent for each 15 pounds above 150; subtract 10 percent for each 15 pounds under 150.

Cabbage: Half a cup of shredded raw cabbage is only 10 calories while half a cup of cole slaw has 60 calories.

Corn: An ear of corn on the cob, cooked, runs about 75 calories, while half a cup of corn kernels, cooked or canned, runs about 10 calories more than that.

Cucumber: Six slices of raw cucumber contain only 5 calories.

Lettuce: Four small leaves of lettuce add up to only 10 calories.

Greens: Half a cup of cooked chard is only 15 calories. The same amount of cooked collards is twice that. Half a cup of mustard greens is about 20 and half a cup of turnip greens, cooked, is slightly less than that.

Green Pepper: A medium-sized pepper, either raw or cooked, is about 10 calories, the same number as four pods of cooked okra.

Radishes: Four small radishes contain only 5 calories.

Fruit

Apples: One raw apple, around 1/3-pound, contains about 75 calories. Half a cup of canned apple juice has 60 calories. Half a cup of sweetened applesauce is 110 calories. If it's unsweetened, the calorie count is only 50.

Apricots: Three raw apricots are 55 calories, and a half a cup canned in heavy syrup has 110 calories.

Avocado: Five ounces of avocado runs about 180 calories.

Berries: Half a cup of blackberries, blueberries or raspberries contains about 40 calories, while the same amount of strawberries has 10 calories less, the same number as the same amount of cherries. Sweet cherries contain 10 calories more.

Cranberries: A tablespoon of sweetened cranberry sauce has 25 calories, and half a cup of cranberry juice cocktail has 80 calories.

Dates: Half a cup of pitted dates adds up to about 250 calories. Three medium figs are about 100.

Grapefruit: Half a grapefruit will run from 55 to 60 calories, while half a cup of grapefruit juice, either fresh or canned, contains about 50 calories.

Grapes: Half a cup of raw grapes will run from 45 to 50 calories, depending on whether they are sweet or not. Half a cup of grapejuice contains 80 calories.

Cantaloupe: Half a raw cantaloupe is about 60 calories, while a 2-inch wedge of honeydew melon is 50.

Prunes: Eight or nine cooked dried prunes run about 100 calories. If they're sweetened, the calorie count goes up to 250. Half a cup of canned prune juice is 250 calories.

Raisins: Half a cup of dried raisins is 100 calories.

Rhubarb: A cup of cooked, sweetened rhubarb is about 375 calories.

Tangerine: A medium-sized tangerine is under 50 calories.

Tomato: Half a cup of canned tomatoes is about 25 calories. A medium size raw tomato will run from 30 to 40 calories. Half a cup of tomato juice is only 20 calories.

Watermelon: A 2-pound wedge of watermelon contains 115 calories.

MISCELLANEOUS FOODS

Popcorn: A cup of popped popcorn with oil and salt added is 50 to 60 calories.

Olives: Four medium green olives or three small ripe olives are 15 calories.

Pickles: A big dill pickle is 15 calories, while a smaller sweet pickle is twice that number.

Soups: In soups, broth and consomme contain the fewest calories, about 30 to a cup. Oyster stew contains the most, about 200 to a cup. One of the most popular soups, tomato, has 90 calories to a cup. Vegetable beef soup runs about 5 calories less and beef noodle 10 calories fewer than vegetable beef.

Nuts: Two tablespoonfuls of shelled almonds, Brazil nuts, cashews, peanuts, pecans or walnuts all run in the neighborhood of 100 calories, with English walnuts the lowest, about 85.

SWEETS

Here we get into some high calorie counts.

Ice Creams: Real "no-nos" on a reducing diet are a chocolate milkshake, 520 calories, and a chocolate ice cream soda, 450 calories.

Caramels and Chocolates: An ounce of candy caramels contains 115 calories, as does an ounce of plain chocolate fudge, an ounce of hard candy and an ounce of peanut brittle. An ounce of chocolate creams is 10 calories more than that. A 1-ounce bar of milk chocolate, either with or without almonds, contains 150 calories. Gum drops and marshmallows run 100 calories to the ounce.

Cakes: A 2-inch slice of angelfood cake has 110 calories and the same size piece of butter cake with chocolate icing has 370 calories. The same size piece of chocolate cake with chocolate icing runs to 445 calories. A 2-inch cube of gingerbread has 115 calories.

Pies: Four inch cuts of pie run as follows: apple (345), cherry (350), custard (275), mince (300), pumpkin (275).

BEVERAGES

There are almost no calories in coffee and tea. The low-cal type of carbonated drinks contain about 10 calories per 8-ounce glass. Regular cola type drinks are close to 100 calories for the same size glass, and gingerale runs from 65 to 75. The same size glass of beer contains 100 calories.

One hundred-proof whiskey, gin and rum have 125 calories to a 1½-ounce jigger. At 80 proof, the calorie content drops to 100.

A 3-ounce glass of table wine contains about 75 calories, while the same size dessert wine jumps up to 125.

For a balanced diet from the standpoint of health, you should have the equivalent of 2 cups of milk a day. There should be four or more servings a day of fruits and vegetables, including one citrus fruit for Vitamin C. Also, there should be four or more servings a day of bread or cereals. Two or more servings of meat completes the balanced diet.

For those who are only a few pounds overweight and want to keep from getting fatter, here's a quick 5-day diet that averages about 1,800 calories a day and meets the requirements of balanced nourishment.

5 DAY "QUICKIE" DIET

Monday

Breakfast
 Half a cantaloupe or grapefruit
 1-ounce cold cereal with cup of skim milk
 2 pieces dry toast
 2 cups coffee or tea

Lunch
 1-cup vegetable beef soup
 1-cup skim milk or buttermilk
 Sardine, canned salmon or fried haddock
  sandwich
 Fresh fruit
Dinner
 3 ounces lean ground-round patty
 1-medium baked potato
 Tomato, lettuce salad, with 1-tsp. dressing
 2 slices bread
 1 pat butter
 2 cups coffee or tea

Tuesday
Breakfast
 ½-cup orange or grapefruit juice
 Boiled egg
 ½-ounce cold cereal with skim milk
 2 slices dry toast
 2 cups coffee or tea
Lunch
 1-cup bouillon
 5 fish sticks
 1-cup skim milk or buttermilk
 Sliced peach
Dinner
 3-ounces baked salmon
 Boiled potato
 ½-cup corn
 Vegetable salad, lemon dressing
 2 slices bread or toast with 1 pat butter
 ½-cup sherbet
 2 cups coffee or tea

Wednesday
Breakfast
 Half a grapefruit
 3/4-cup oatmeal or rolled oats with skim milk
 Bran muffin, with 1-tbsp. jelly
 2 cups coffee or tea

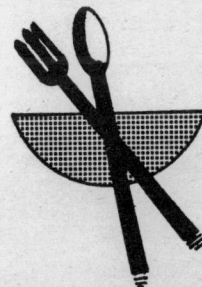

Lunch
1-cup tomato soup
1-cup skim milk
Lean beef sandwich
½-cup Rennet
Dinner
½-pound steak, lean
½-cup mashed potatoes
½-cup hot broccoli
Small vegetable salad
½-cup fresh fruit
2 cups coffee or tea

Thursday
Breakfast
½-cup cranberry juice
1-ounce cold cereal with 1-cup skim milk
2 slices dry toast
2 cups coffee or tea
Lunch
1-cup skim milk
1-cup minestrone soup
Lean ham sandwich
½-cup gelatine
Dinner
Broiled chicken breast
½-cup cauliflower
¼-cup peas
Small vegetable salad
½-cup sherbet
2 cups coffee or tea

Friday
Breakfast
Small wedge honeydew
Poached egg
2 slices dry toast, with jelly
2 cups coffee or tea
Lunch
1-cup clam chowder
Tunafish sandwich
1-cup skim milk
Sliced orange
Dinner
Broiled bluefish
Medium baked potato
½-cup diced beets
Small vegetable salad
½-cup lemon ice
2 cups coffee or milk

Anyone who regards this as a hardship diet is probably guilty of consistently overeating. A friend of mine who doesn't seem to me to be overweight at all goes on this 5-day diet during the last week of every month. He said that along with the vigorous exercise he gets all the time, he can eat rather heartily on the remaining weeks of the month and still maintain his weight just where he wants it.

It's not necessary to follow this diet on the specific days listed. Menus can be switched from Monday to any of the other four days. Also, foods in each category that don't contain more calories than the ones listed may be substituted. If you want a pre-dinner snack, to dull your dinner appetite, raw carrots, strips of green pepper and celery sticks aren't many calories. Even with a light dip, it's doubtful that you'll go over 150 calories.

With all of the diets that are on the market today, it is entirely outside the province of this book to recommend any one of them over any other.

Significantly, most doctors and dieticians steer clear of all these "special, new, miracle" diets.

Back when I was about 30 pounds overweight—thank goodness, a long time ago—I tried every new fad diet that came along, with no success and in several instances with slight damage to my health that would have become serious if I'd persisted in the diet.

When I finally went to my doctor and told him the difficulty I'd been having in losing weight, he observed, "You like certain foods more than others and some of the foods on the diets you've described you admit you almost dislike. You have lunch every day, 5 days a week, with business associates or clients at a restaurant or club—and the eating places you patronize don't cater to dieters. You eat about the same lunches that the others at your table are ordering—and I'd guess that lunch is preceded by a couple of cocktails with high caloric content.

"It would take a real magic diet to make up, in breakfast and dinner, for the calories you pack in at lunch. You're getting in that one meal amost the total number of calories you should have in a day—but you're not getting in that meal all of the nutrients your body should have. From what you've told me, you're definitely deficient in milk consumption and fruit intake, particularly.

"I'm going to prescribe the simplest diet you've ever tried, with whatever you want to eat on it. We'll call it the Think Thin diet."

THE THINK THIN DIET

He continued, "Thinking Thin isn't going to have any miraculous reducing effect. All it's going to do is get you in the proper frame of mind for the no-change diet I'm going to give you."

"If there's no change in my diet, I can't see how it could reduce my weight," I protested.

"There'll be no change in the foods you eat," he said, "but there *will* be a change in your diet. You'll eat no more than half of everything that's served to you at your business lunches. And at home, you'll eat no more than half of what's been a normal serving."

My first reaction was shock at the thought of paying for food and not eating it. When I was a child, every parent admonished his children to "clean your plate." Leaving any food on the plate was considered an almost unforgivable crime. And, like many others, I'd grown up with a guilt feeling about not licking my plate clean.

I told my doctor it seemed a shame to pay for food and not eat it.

"In most good restaurants," he told me, "you'd pay the same amount for a smaller portion. And by the end of a month, you'll have become so accustomed to the smaller portions you've been eating that you won't dish up more than you need."

Somewhat to my surprise, the Think Thin Diet worked for me. I took off weight without any real discomfort. I should add that my doctor had given me the basic requirements in each of the food groups and told me not to cut them at all.

As my weight went down, I felt so good that I realized all the excess poundage had been debilitating me. It had tired me, and kept me from getting the exercise I should have had. Exercising became easy and pleasant. I thought better. I slept better. I was more alert in every way.

Occasionally, I fudged, overeating fattening foods that I enjoyed. Invariably, my weight went up a little.

And before I tell you what took care of those lapses, I must say that my doctor had told me to get on the bathroom scale, stripped, every morning before I bathed and dressed. "If you don't,"

he explained, "the extra weight can get out of hand before you realize what's happening."

So when my weight would go up 2 or 3 pounds, which was usually on a Saturday or Sunday, I either had a light lunch or had a very light dinner or both. I never had to do that more than 2 days in a row to take off the extra blubber.

The head of Intermatic, Inc. in Wisconsin has found an effective way to control obesity among his employees. If any of them become seriously overweight, they're ineligible for advancement and pay increases until the obesity is corrected. Those who are slightly overweight are offered bonuses and extra vacation as rewards if they correct the problem. His whole work force is weight-conscious and "thinks thin." He says there's no question but what it has increased plant efficiency, and adds that the people feel better, are happier and contribute to higher plant morale. "Sick leaves" have dropped off sharply. The exercise recreation facilities he's installed on the grounds get heavy use.

DIET RESTAURANTS

Another solution for those who must eat their lunches in restaurants and those who eat a good many of their dinners away from home is the comparatively new diet restaurant, as distinguished from the health food bar. Apparently, they started on the West Coast and other parts of the country are beginning to copy them because of their success.

In Chicago, there's even a diet Chinese restaurant, the Hong Kong Garden. Fran Situ went on a Weight Watchers program about 5 years ago and has lost 80 pounds. She and her husband, Gordon Situ, own the Hong Kong Garden. It now lists both Chinese and American dishes that are "legal"—the Weight Watcher designation for foods that are acceptable.

The diet menu has different kinds of chop suey and war mein without fat, sweet-and-sour chicken prepared with a sugar substitute, shrimp cantonese and Hong Kong Garden steak with 8 ounces of filet and snow peapods. The prices are moderate for today's standards and with all of the food prepared to order, any diet restriction from low-cal to low sodium and low cholesterol can be produced. There are numerous other attractive entrees, all served with ½-cup of rice.

There's even a freezer of low-cal cookies, breads and desserts, including pineapple cheesecake, spice cake, banana bread, raisin loaf and Rice Krispie muffins.

To make things even simpler for dieters, there's a prepared-on-the-premises array of diet frozen dinners, and now a bakery and snack shop under the same name—The Skinny Gourmet—has opened in Niles, Illinois.

Even more surprisingly, one of the deluxe gourmet restaurants in the Lettuce Entertain You group of Chicago gourmet restaurants, is offering a diet menu.

One of the partners, Rich Melman, visited the West Coast and saw the growing popularity of diet restaurants. As he tells it, "I wasn't sure if Chicago was ready for a diet restaurant, so I decided to try a diet section in one of our dining rooms, and Jonathan Livingston Seafoods seemed to be a good place to start. George Bay, one of the chefs at the group's Pump Room in the Ambassador East Hotel who had lost about 50 pounds through diet worked out the recipes. He used little fat, some sugar substitutes, fruit juices and unthickened sauces made from natural juices. The menu includes a lot of seafood and chicken. Two rotating diet menus are offered at dinner and another at lunch. A four-course dinner could easily contain less than 600 calories. A typical dinner begins with a complimentary tray of sliced raw vegetables: mushrooms, zucchini and green peppers, served with a diet Thousand-Island dip. Among the appetizers, there's chopped chicken liver paté (148 calories) melon slice with proscuitto ham (80 calories) and a 40-calorie sesame salad as well as a 50-calorie Caesar salad.

There's a choice of three dinner entrees. For example, the poached salmon with walnut sauce offers a large portion of fresh fish and a sauce made with artificial whipped cream, horseradish sauce and walnuts. It's only 302 calories. The chicken with barbecue sauce contains only 313 calories.

The group is now planning to put diet sections in other restaurants. Plans even call for diet pastas at Lawrence of Oregano and an ultra-sophisticated diet lunch for the Pump Room.

For anyone who needs or wants more information, there's the *Goldberg's Diet Catalog,* authored by Larry Goldberg, who once weighed

320 pounds and was, he admits, "a foodaholic, a mainliner on Mallomars and a Chunky junkie" as a boy. He weighed 200 pounds by the time he entered the sixth grade.

His advice to the overweight is, "Find what works for you. Any diet that will help you lose weight must fit into your life plan." The book describes hundreds of diets, diet systems, scales, over-the-counter medications, exercise equipment, mind-control therapy, diet cookbooks and diet groups. The book is published by Collier Macmillan and is not only comprehensive but entertaining.

"FAD" DIETS

Fad diets persist, as I've indicated, because overweight people want some quick, easy way to lose weight. Most fad diet followers quickly gain back the weight they've gotten rid of as soon as the diet is over.

And that should tell every would-be reducer something. Reverting to previous eating habits that put the weight onto your body will do it again. What most people who are overweight really need is a change in eating habits that remains for the rest of that person's life. The money spent on magic diet aids in 1977 is estimated at somewhere in the neighborhood of 10 billion dollars. And the money often brings quick results—but results that last only briefly.

Dieters don't want to accept the medical advice to consume fewer calories than the body burns up—by eating fewer high calorie foods and exercising more. And no diet should eliminate any one nutrient, which some fad diets do. A sensible weight-reducing diet isn't as fast as a fad diet, with about 3 weeks needed before results begin to show.

Maybe new discoveries will come up with a truly magic solution to the problem. The farther out an idea is, the quicker most dieters will embrace it.

Sarfaraz Niazi, a researcher at the University of Illinois, says he has discovered a chemical that will coat the intestinal lining and thus keep food from being absorbed into the body. He says he has 7,000 volunteers for experimentation with the drug and will start tests on human beings as soon as he gets permission from the Food and Drug Administration.

The name of the drug? Perfluorooctyl

bromide. The researcher says it blocks food absorption without any harmful side effects and should enable people to lose from 5 to 7 pounds a week.

Another research discovery by Dr. John D. Davis, a psychology professor at the University of Illinois Circle Campus in Chicago, is that a natural fatty substance, glycerol, can control the appetites of animals. His explanation is that fat cells produce glycerol, and that the substance becomes a signal to the brain that the body is overweight, resulting in a loss of appetite. If glycerol is injected into the blood stream, Dr. Davis says, it reaches the brain and shuts down the appetite. For it to be practical in weight control, he thinks, a way will have to be found to take it orally and still be effective.

The so-called liquid protein diet in which 300 to 400 calories of protein extract are the only sustenances ingested has been associated with more than 50 deaths. The FDA says that for women on this diet the chance of suffering a fatal heart attack is increased by 30 times, and the FDA is asking for warning labels to be placed on liquid protein products stating that a liquid protein diet be followed only on advice of a doctor and under his supervision. The diet causes alterations in electrolytes, like sodium and potassium, which help to maintain the human body's fluid balance, a possible cause of cardiac arrest. The danger may become greater when the dieter starts to eat normal foods again, because the metabolism is maladjusted to digest them.

One-food diets that allow only grapefruit or rice or some other food must almost inevitably lead to serious lacks of nutrients.

Taking diuretics to lose weight, as mentioned, have no lasting effect and may be dangerous. Thyroid hormones, like amphetamines, speed up calorie consumption but also speed up other bodily functions, making them extremely dangerous for anyone with a tendency toward heart trouble.

One of the most drastic treatments for overweight that has ever been offered is the gastric bypass. It is a surgical operation in which most of the stomach is locked off from the intestine by a surgical staple, so that food can pass only into the small stomach space. The tiny stomach, which doesn't grow, stops patients from overeating. If they do, they simply throw up. People who have the operation start out still trying to overeat, but

quickly learn that the consequences are altogether too undesirable.

Among the newer diet books is *The Nine-Day Wonder Diet,* by Dr. Seymour Isenberg and Dr. L. M. Elting, published by St. Martin's Press. It's a 7-day diet of high-protein menus with low carbohydrates, and 2 days of fasting. The authors say it's safe and should produce a 15-pound weight loss in 9 days. Critics of the diet say most of the weight loss is water and that the 2-day fast could cause serious trouble for diabetics.

An unusual new diet book is *Dr. Bahr's Acu-Diet,* published by William Morrow & Co. It maintains that a slight up-and-down pressure on the hollow groove in the upper lip for a few seconds before every meal will interrupt the appetite passageway to the brain and stop hunger pangs. The author, Dr. Frank Bahr, a German acupuncture specialist, says the idea gets results through acupressure, based on acupuncture. He adds that the pressure movement also is a reminder to eat less.

A more conservative diet book is *The Right Diet,* by Dr. Bessie Dituri, published by Quadrangle. In the same vein is *The Thin Game,* by Edwin Bayard, published by Newsweek Books. Both espouse a low-calorie, balanced, slow, but permanent weight loss.

The Water Pik manufacturers put out a reducing plan complete with a machine to control the speed with which you eat. It is based on observations that overeaters eat more quickly. It instructs dieters to chew their food with a controlled rhythm and to chew each bite a certain number of times before swallowing it. When I was trying to lose weight, I read something in a newspaper about this theory, which made sense to me, so I began chewing every bite of food far more thoroughly than I ever had before. As a result, it took me much longer to eat a meal than it previously had, but I didn't eat nearly as much before feeling that I'd had enough. I still follow the practice of eating slowly, and it not only works but I enjoy my meals more.

An idea based on somewhat the same theory is to lay down your fork between bites.

Doctors are completely frustrated by the ongoing success of fad diets. There is an anti-medical attitude on the part of reducers, and promoters of fad diets, and diet aids take full advantage of it, particularly when there's no scientific evidence to support the efficacy of what's being sold.

Summing up, our own advice on reducing:

1. Have a well-balanced diet containing all the necessary nutrients, every day.
2. Cut down on caloric intake, depending on the amount of calories you consume, your age, your weight and your metabolism.
3. Eat slowly, chewing every bite of food until it is ready to digest.
4. Don't try to go on a diet of foods you don't like, because you probably won't stick with it. Instead, eat less than you normally do of foods you like.
5. Avoid snacking and "tasting" between meals.
6. Do your food shopping *after* eating, not before when you're hungry.
7. Get plenty of exercise.

DIET AND EMOTIONAL HEALTH

In 1974, Dr. E. Cheraskin, Chairman of the Department of Oral Medicine at the University of Alabama, Dr. W. M. Ringsdorf, Jr., Associate Professor of Medicine at the same school, and Arlene Brecher, an expert medical writer, wrote a book entitled, *Psychodietetics,* published by Stein and Day, New York, which set up the premise and proved it to the satisfaction of many that diet has much to do with a person's moods. They claim that: Diet deficiencies can cause alcoholism and replacement of those deficiencies can eliminate the cause; that diet of the wrong kind can drive you crazy; that hypoglycemia can cause a bad disposition and can be cured; and that most cases of schizophrenia, caught early enough, can be rectified by a change in diet. They even make a good case for a psychodietic approach to sexual inadequacy, hyperactivity, senility and allergy.

They present an optimal diet for mental health and offer the disturbing conclusion that some of the balanced diets recommended by most health authorities specializing in nutrition can be quite wrong by offering food choices in each of the four categories that could be bad for a specific person's mental health.

Their clinical studies indicate that vitamin B^3, niacin, can be of great help to most hard-core alcoholics. In a follow-up on 507 original patients, only 70 were lost through insobriety or death.

The B^3 treatment doesn't allow a true alcoholic to return to moderate drinking, but definitely aids in keeping a patient from returning to alcohol.

One mental health center director, Dr. David R. Hawkins, reported to the authors of the book that most of the 600 alcoholics he treated since 1966 have fully recovered.

Doctors have come up with a pill in which vitamins are basic that could be called a "sober" pill, because it reduces intoxication time by speeding up the body's use of the alcohol and lowering the alcohol levels in the blood. A test made on California policemen in which half received healthy amounts of vitamin B complex showed that this half felt less intoxicated and tested substantially higher on perception and mental acuity tests than the others.

If you feel that alcohol is becoming or has become a problem, it would behoove you to investigate what seems to be the simplest approach to the difficulty yet discovered.

Schizophrenia is not confined to any one age. Babies can be born with it. It's been estimated that one out of every 100 people has it, and it's not confined to any particular society, culture, ethnic group or social class. For one reason or another, the schizophrenic's metabolism doesn't handle nutrients, hormones and enzymes normally.

Huge doses of vitamin B^3 have, in clinical tests, cured an amazing 93 percent of one group's schizophrenic patients who had suffered less than 2 years. The authors of *Psychodietetics* point out that other forms of therapy are used in *addition* to the daily doses of vitamins.

Hypoglycemia, the opposite of diabetes, still often precedes that disease. In hypoglycemia, too much insulin circulates in the bloodstream, lowering blood-sugar below normal and bringing on a craving that amounts to an obsession for sweets.

Headaches, fatigue, drowsiness, narcolepsy, muscle pains, insomnia, irritability, worry and depression, allergies, loss of sex drive and loss of appetite are some of the symptoms. Many hypoglycemics are called "cranks" and "complainers." Sweetened snack foods, white-flour products and sweetened soft drinks are the worst things a hypoglycemic can have. Some common drugs can add to the problem. The disease is caused by not only what we eat but how we eat.

Frankly, I didn't believe that sugar could be such a great cause of irritability when I read *Psychodietetics*. However, my wife seemed to me to be constantly complaining about how cross I was. I attributed what I thought of as mild irritability to business pressures.

However, I decided to go "on the wagon" as far as sweets were concerned, and the only sugar I got from then on was what was contained in prepared food products such as catsup and canned vegetables.

To my utter astonishment, my wife said to me a few weeks later, "I don't know what's happened to you, but your disposition has certainly improved. You've actually become pleasant."

The psychodietetics approach to curing sexual impotency or lack of virility is complicated enough so that anyone with such a problem should get the book, read it, and then consult a doctor who knows what he's doing. The authors say that even a degenerating prostate can be brought back to health.

They cite tests to show what proper approaches can do to halt senility.

They frankly admit that some hidden non-dietetic factors can cause mental problems.

And I'm pleased to note that in those cases where proper diet is part of their solution to problems, they agree that plenty of vigorous, healthful exercise will speed and aid recovery.

The authors also point out that some vitamins may have annoying side effects for some people. They helpfully suggest a booklet, *Megavitamin Therapy,* published by Karpat Publishing Co., P.O. Box 5348, Cleveland, Ohio 44101, which is most informative on the subject.

Psychodietetics contains numerous questionnaires which the reader may answer to satisfy himself that he does or does not need help on any mental health problem.

A PERSONAL WORD

We hope the information presented in this chapter has helped you gain a greater appreciation of the value of exercise and proper nutrition in maintaining proper weight. More important, if you have a weight problem, we hope you have been motivated to do something about it.

Instead of sitting around worrying about why you are gaining weight, or cannot lose it, do something about it. With your doctor's advice, find some type of regular vigorous physical activity you can enjoy and a diet that you can live with.

Each of us deep down inside has some feelings about his own self-image and what he wants it to be. Each person in these intimate aspects of life has to answer mainly to himself. So make up your mind to begin your program now and stay with it.

It won't be easy—especially at the start. But as you begin to feel better, look better and enjoy a new zest for life, you will be rewarded many times over for your effort.

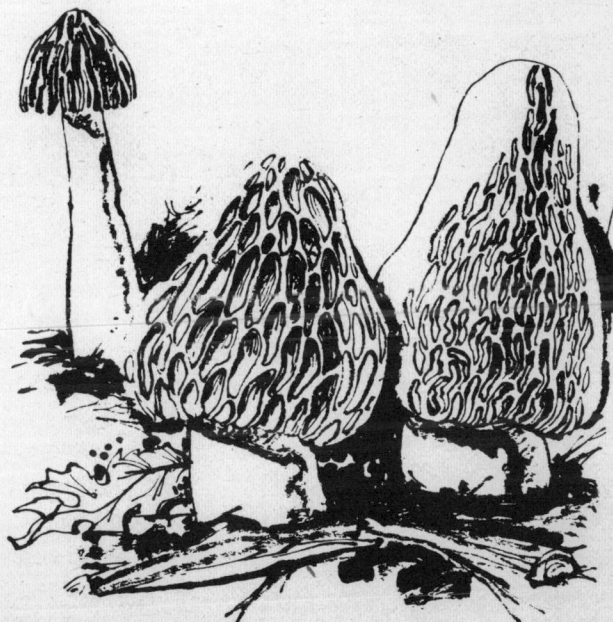

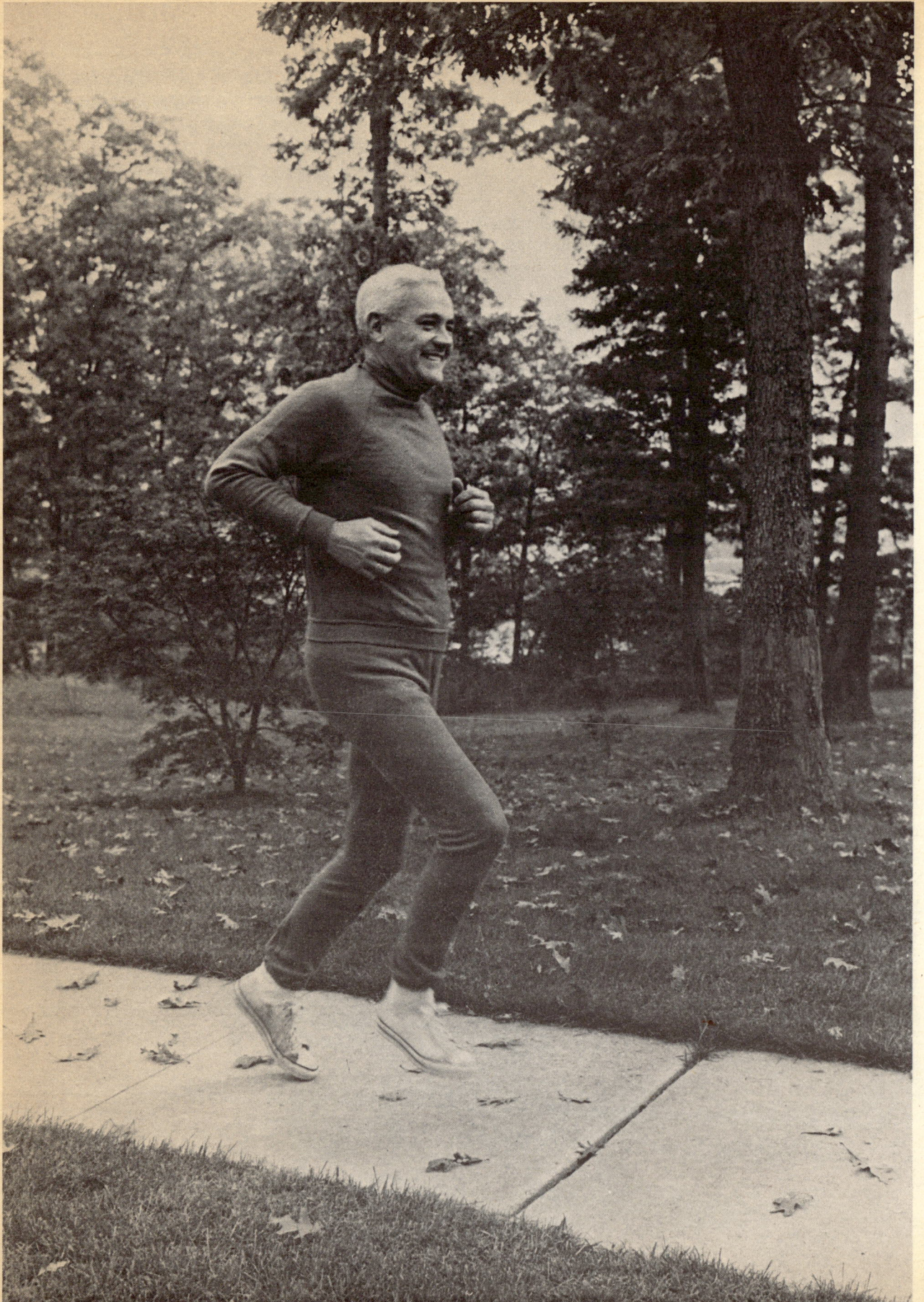

chapter 6

Programs

THIS CHAPTER IS divided into four sections—Developmental Exercise Programs, Total Physical Fitness Programs, Personalized Exercise Programs and Corrective Exercise Programs. The Developmental Exercise section will give you programs for specifically developing flexibility, strength and cardiovascular endurance. They are *not* complete programs but are merely supplements to help you improve your fitness in specific areas. The Total Physical Fitness Programs are, as the name implies, complete progressive programs for each level of fitness—poor, average and excellent—and for every age group —child, adult and senior citizen. For the working woman, corporate executive, for the family who enjoys exercising together, there are the Personalized Exercise Programs. Though not total fitness programs, they are excellent supplements. The Corrective Programs are designed to help correct problem areas of the body—sore back, arthritic joints—or to help test for potential problem areas.

DEVELOPMENTAL EXERCISE PROGRAMS

A QUICK FLEXIBILITY EXERCISE ROUTINE

This routine is recommended for preventing or relieving sore muscles. As a preventive, three times a week is ample.

1. Do *stationary running* long enough to perspire lightly. This will help warm your muscles so they can more easily be stretched.
2. *Wall Stretch* (lower leg muscles)
   a. Stand on a 2-inch thick book that is 2 feet away from a wall. Stand facing the wall, with only the ball of the foot flat on the outer edge of the book.
   b. Lean forward, resting the palms of your hands on the wall. Bend the elbows as far as you can to make the leaning movement as pronounced as possible. Hold the position for a count of 30.
   c. Maintaining the position, drop your heels slowly as far as possible toward the floor. Hold the position for a count of 30 and then bring the heels back up until you're standing on tiptoe. Hold that position for a count of 30. Repeat the routine four times.
3. *Squat* (leg muscles)
   a. Standing with the feet about 2½ feet apart, bend your knees slowly and go into a squat, hands touching the floor between the knees.
   b. Hold the position for a count of 20 and slowly move back to standing position. Repeat four times.
4. Do the Hatha Yoga *Triangle* exercise (see

Chapter 2, page 64) four times on each side.

5. *Trunk Pull* (trunk and back muscles)
    a. Bend the upper body forward so it's parallel to the floor. Clasp hands behind neck.
    b. Rotate the upper body from the torso to the left, as far behind you as possible. Hold for a count of 30.
    c. Then rotate to the right as far as possible and hold for a count of 30. Repeat five times.

6. *Neck Twist* (neck muscles)
    a. Twist your neck as far to the right as it will go and hold the position for a count of 10, feeling the muscles stretch.
    b. Then make the same movement to the left. Repeat four times.

7. *Half Back Bend* (abdominal muscles)
    a. Face up on the floor, clasp hands behind neck and bring feet back up as close to buttocks as possible.
    b. Try to lift both the buttocks and the shoulders from the floor, so that weight is supported on the back of neck. Hold the position for a count of five. Repeat three times.

8. *Shoulder Stretch* (shoulder muscles)
    If arms or shoulders are sore, stretch them both back and forward alternately, holding the maximum stretch until you feel a strong pull on the muscles. Repeat four times.

If any particular part of your body has aching muscles, concentrate on a stretching exercise for that particular part of the anatomy (see Chapter 2 for alternate flexibility exercises). Flexibility exercises are usually needed more by elderly people than by the young, who keep their muscles flexible through constant use.

One caution that the medical profession gives is not to stretch the back too far in either direction, to avoid serious spinal damage.

A DUMBBELL EXERCISE PROGRAM FOR MUSCLE STRENGTH AND ENDURANCE

For most beginners, 5-pound dumbbells are heavy enough. Women and children should start with 2- or 3-pound bells. This routine includes exercises for the neck, the shoulders and arms, the chest, abdomen and the legs. To increase strength, increase weight lifted; to increase endurance, increase number of repetitions.

Exercise 1 (biceps and shoulder muscles): Standing with the feet about 4 inches apart, hold dumbbells in the hands, which are hanging at the sides. Bend the arm, flexing muscles until the bells are brought to shoulder level and the arms are bent at the elbow as far as possible. Raise elbows to shoulder level. Repeat 6-8 times for strength development. Repeat a minimum of 15 times for endurance development.

Exercise 2 (triceps and shoulder muscles): Body erect, heels together, bend arms at the elbows and let the dumbbells rest lightly against the shoulders. With one arm held in this position, thrust the other straight up over the head. Let that arm drop slowly to the starting position and thrust the other arm up. Alternate arms until each one has done the exercise at least 15 times for endurance. Repeat 6-8 times for strength.

Exercise 3 (shoulder muscles): With arms extended straight out in front of body, a dumbbell grasped in each hand, raise the arms straight overhead and then bring slowly back to the starting position. Repeat about 15 times for endurance, 6-8 times for strength.

Exercise 4 (back muscles and chest muscles): With arms holding dumbbells hanging at sides, lean slightly forward and then swing the bells upward while bending the head and upper body backward. Return to starting position and repeat 6-8 times for strength, 15 times for endurance.

Exercise 5 (upper back and tricep muscles): With arms holding bells hanging at sides, draw the arms upward and backward, forcing the shoulders as far back as possible. Repeat 15 times for endurance, 6-8 times for strength.

Exercise 6 (arm muscles): Standing erect, heels a few inches apart, toes turned out, bend the arms at the elbows until the bells are in front of the body at the waist. Then step out as far as possible with the left foot while striking up and out with the right arm as if aiming a blow. Return to starting position and repeat with the right foot and left arm. Alternately, aim a blow with each arm and leg 6-8 times for strength, 15 times for endurance.

Exercise 7 (abdominal muscles): For strength development, do 6-8 situps while holding the dumbbells above the head, then behind the neck and then on the chest. For endurance, do the same exercise but for a minimum of 15 repetitions. Most people must work for several weeks before they can do the situps with the arms holding the bells on the chest.

Exercise 8 (leg muscles): Do half knee bends from standing position while holding the dumbbells at about the hips. Repeat 6-8 times for strength, a minimum of 15 times for endurance.

Exercise 9 (leg muscles): Sitting in a straight-back chair, with dumbbell strapped to right ankle, lift right leg from floor to straight out position, hold momentarily and return it slowly to the floor. Do this 6-8 times with each leg for strength development and 15 times or more for endurance.

AN INTERVAL TRAINING ROUTINE FOR CARDIOVASCULAR ENDURANCE

The basic idea of interval training is to put the body through short but repeated periods of intense exercise broken up by recovery periods or intervals where the intensity of the exercise is reduced. It is aimed first at cardiovascular pulmonary endurance and is a good example of progressive overload, increasing the capacity of the body to respond well to a greater maximum load.

It adds to other programs that include the variable of repetition, intensity and duration, a fourth variable—a recovery or rest interval which is decreased in length as endurance levels are increased.

You consider the following things in setting up an interval training routine:

1. Number or repetitions of the exercise.
2. Distance and duration of the exercise (in most cases, running or swimming).
3. Time or speed of an exercise.
4. Duration of the recovery or rest intervals.
5. Type of rest activity (usually walking or jogging).
6. Intensity of the activity during the rest interval.

Interval training has much to recommend it. The program doesn't require constant supervision. The recovery intervals minimize build-up

of fatigue. The exercise periods are short and there's a challenge to accomplish specific goals in a specific time frame.

Interval Training Swimming Routine

1. Swim the length of the pool at about two-thirds maximum speed.
2. Get out of the water and jog back to starting point on the pool deck at a moderate speed.
3. Swim two lengths at the same speed.
4. Jog back for one length.
5. Continue by adding to the number of lengths swimming, but keep the jogging distance the same as endurance levels rise.

Interval Training Running Routine

1. Jog a block and back without stopping.
2. Run a block and back at half-speed without stopping.
3. Run a block at full speed and do five pushups.
4. Run a block and a half and back at two-thirds speed and do five pushups.
5. Run the same distance at full speed and do eight pushups.
6. Run two blocks and back at full speed and do 10 pushups and five situps.
7. Work up to running three blocks and back at two-thirds speed and then do 10 pushups, 10 situps and five jumping jacks.
8. Run three blocks and back at full speed and do 10 pushups, 10 situps, and 10 jumping jacks.

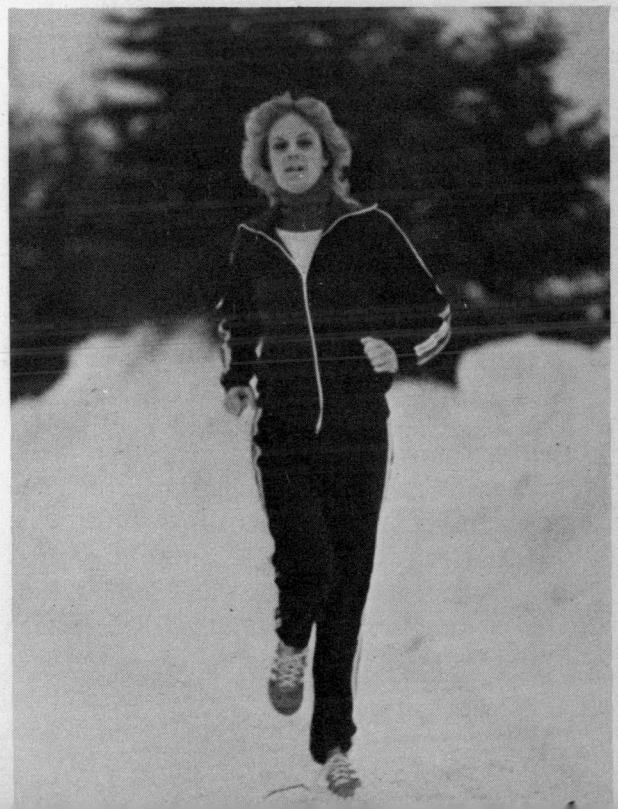

TOTAL PHYSICAL FITNESS PROGRAMS

ADULT PHYSICAL FITNESS PROGRAMS/MEN AND WOMEN

About the Programs

They assume that you have not been engaging recently in consistent, vigorous, all-round physical activity—even though, in daily routines, you have put some muscles to extensive use. Your Personal Physical Fitness Evaluation Chart scores in Chapter 1 will tell you what your present state of physical fitness is. Unless you are in excellent condition, you should begin with the Orientation Program and progress through all the exercise levels.

The Physical Fitness Programs for men and women are basically the same with but two exceptions: the knee pushup for women is replaced by the standard pushup for men; and the number of exercise repetions and distances for circulatory activities is greater for men.

What the Exercises are for

There are four general types—*warm-up* exercises, *conditioning* exercises, *circulatory* activities, and *cool-down* exercises.

The *warm-up* exercises stretch and limber up the muscles and speed up the action of the heart and lungs, thus preparing the body for greater exertion and reducing the possibility of unnecessary strain.

The *conditioning* exercises are systematically planned to tone up abdominal, back, leg, arm and other major muscles.

The *circulatory* activities produce contractions of large muscle groups for relatively longer periods than the conditioning exercises—to stimulate and strengthen the cardio-circulatory and respiratory systems.

The *cool-down* exercise period helps gradually to bring your cardiovascular system back down to its normal functioning rate and also helps stretch muscles to reduce soreness. The same cool-off exercises outlined in the Orientation Program will be used after each exercise session and throughout the five levels.

When it comes to the circulatory activities,
you choose one each workout. Alternately running and walking, skipping rope or running in place. All are effective. You can choose running and walking on a pleasant day, one of the others for use indoors when the weather is inclement. You can switch about for variety.

How You Progress

A sound physical conditioning program should take into account your individual tolerance—your ability to execute a series of activities without undue discomfort or fatigue. It should provide for developing your tolerance by increasing the work load so you gradually become able to achieve more and more with less and less fatigue and with increasingly rapid recovery.

As you move from level to level, some exercises will be modified so they call for increased effort.

Others will remain the same but you will build more strength and stamina by increasing the number of repetitions.

You will be increasing your fitness another way as well.

At the Orientation Level your objective is to complete all the exercises without a breathing spell in between. If you cannot complete the exercises without taking a breathing spell, stay with the Orientation Program until you can. Then move to Level 1. Also, the first six exercises of the Orientation Program will be used as warm-up exercises throughout the graded levels (Levels 1 thru 5).

At Level 1, your objective will be gradually to reduce, from workout to workout, the "breathing spells" between exercises until you can do the seven conditioning exercises without resting. You will proceed in the same fashion with the more difficult exercises and increased repetitions at succeeding levels.

You will find the program designed—the progression carefully planned—to make this feasible. You will be able to proceed at your own pace, competing with yourself rather than with anyone else—and this is of great importance for sound conditioning.

Note: Gradually speeding up, from workout to workout, the rate at which you do each exercise will provide greater stimulation for the circulatory and respiratory systems and also help to keep your workouts short. However, the seven conditioning exercises should not be a race against time. Perform each exercise correctly to insure maximum benefit.

Choosing Your Goal

There is no need to pick the level to which you want to go—now.

Many of you will be able to advance through the first three levels. While the fourth is challenging, some of you will be able to achieve it. The fifth is one which only extremely vigorous, well-conditioned individuals will reach.

The level of fitness you can reach depends upon your age, your body's built-in potential capacity and previous conditioning. It also depends upon your state of mind; as you know, when you want to do something and believe you can, it is much easier to do than otherwise.

While there will be no dramatic overnight changes, gradually over the next weeks and months, as you progress through the first levels, you will begin to notice a new spring in your step, a new ease with which you accomplish your ordinary daily activities. You will find yourself with more energy left at the end of the working day and a new zest for recreation in the evening. Quite likely, you will be sleeping more soundly than you have slept for many years and waking more refreshed in the morning.

After completing the early levels, you may come to realize that you can—and want to—go further. Go as far as you can.

The important point is that, no matter what level you choose as your goal, you will improve your fitness, and you will be able to maintain the improvement and to enjoy the benefits.

When and How Often to Workout

To be the most beneficial, exercise should become part of your daily routine—as much so as bathing or dressing.

Five workouts a week are called for throughout the program.

You can choose any time that's convenient. Preferably, it should be the same time every day—but it doesn't matter whether it's upon arising, at some point during the morning or afternoon, or in the evening.

How Long at Each Level

Your objective at each level will be to reach the point where you can do all the exercises called for, for the number of times indicated, without resting between exercises.

But, start slowly.

It cannot be emphasized enough that by moving forward gradually you will be moving forward solidly, avoiding sudden strains and excesses that could make you ache and hold you back for several days.

If you find yourself at first unable to complete any exercises—to do continuously all the repetitions called for—stop when you encounter difficulty. Rest briefly, then take up where you left off and complete the count. If you have difficulty at first, there will be less and less with succeeding workouts.

Stay at each level for at least 3 weeks. If you have not passed the prove-out test at the end of that time, continue at the same level until you do. The prove-out test calls for performing—in three consecutive workouts—the seven conditioning exercises without resting and satisfactorily fulfilling the requirement for one circulatory activity.

A Measure of Your Progress

You will, of course, be able to observe the increase in your strength and stamina from week to week in many ways—including the increasing facility with which you do the exercises at a given level.

In addition, by taking the 4-minute Step Test (Chapter 1, page 14) you can measure and keep a running record of the improvement in your cardiovascular pulmonary efficiency, one of the most important aspects of fitness.

The immediate response of the cardiovascular

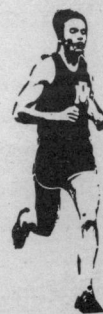

system to exercise differs markedly between well-conditioned individuals and others. The test measures the response in terms of pulse rate taken shortly after a series of steps up and down onto a bench or chair. Although it does not take long, it is necessarily vigorous. Stop if you become overly fatigued while taking it.

Your Progress Records

Charts are provided for the Orientation Program and for each of the five levels.

They list the exercises to be done and the goal for each exercise in terms of number of repetitions, distance, etc.

They also provide space in which to record

**FITNESS CAN NEITHER BE BOUGHT NOR BESTOWED
LIKE HONOR IT MUST BE EARNED**

---

your progress: (1) in completing the recommended 15 workouts at each level; (2) in accomplishing the three prove-out workouts before moving on to a succeeding level; and (3) in the results as you take the Step Test from time to time.

You do the warm-up exercises and the conditioning exercises along with one circulatory activity for each workout. Following the circulatory activity period, you do the five cooling-off exercises.

Check off each workout as you complete it. The last three numbers are for the prove-out workouts, in which the seven conditioning exercises should be done without resting. Check them off as you accomplish them.

You are now ready to proceed to the next level.

As you take the Step Test—at about 2-week intervals—enter your pulse rate.

When you move on to the next level, transfer the last pulse rate from the preceding level. Enter it in the margin to the left of the new progress record and circle it so it will be convenient for continuing reference.

212

ORIENTATION PROGRAM

1. *Bend and Stretch*
Starting position: Stand erect, feet shoulder-width apart.
Action: Count 1. Bend trunk forward and down, flexing knees. Stretch gently in attempt to touch fingers to toes or floor. Count 2. Return to starting position.
Note: Do slowly, stretch and relax at intervals rather than in rhythm.

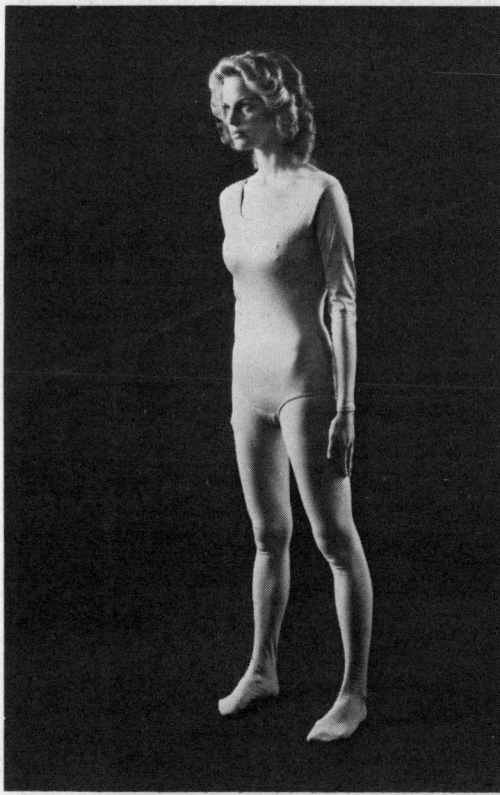

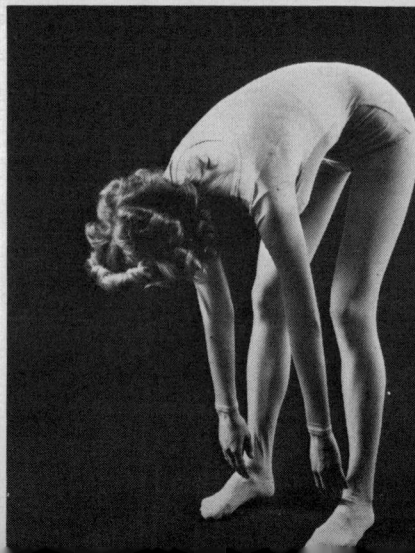

2. *Knee Lift*
Starting position: Stand erect, feet together, arms at sides.
Action: Count 1. Raise left knee as high as possible, grasping leg with hands and pulling knee against body while keeping back straight. Count 2. Lower to starting position. Counts 3 and 4. Repeat with right knee.

3. *Wing Stretcher* (See Chapter 2, page 40.)

4. *Half Knee Bend* (See Chapter 2, page 35.)

5. *Arm Circles*
Starting position: Stand erect, arms extended sideward at shoulder height, palms up.
Action: Describe small circles backward with hands. Keep head erect. Do 15 backward circles. Reverse, turn palms down and do 15 small circles forward.

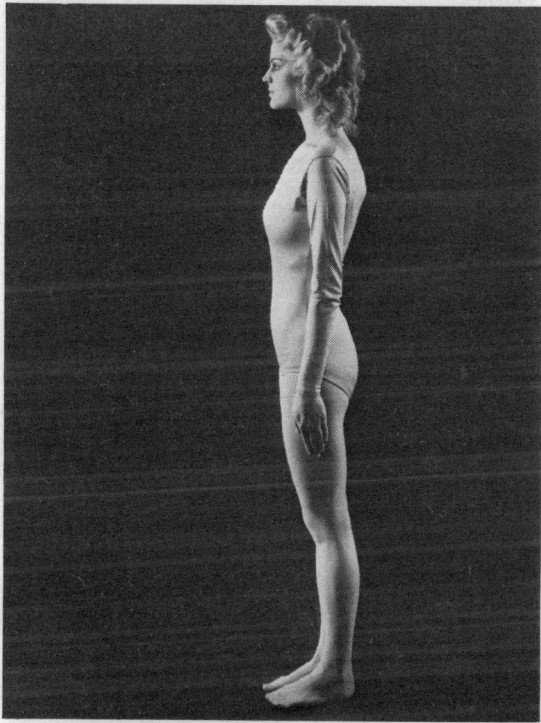

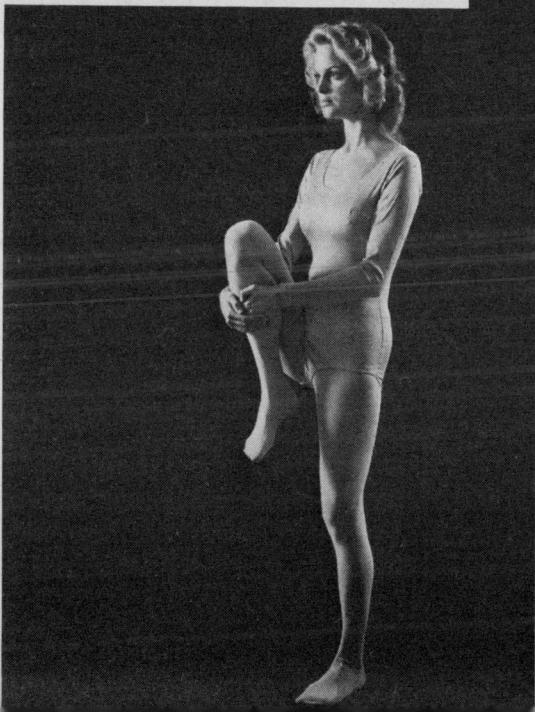

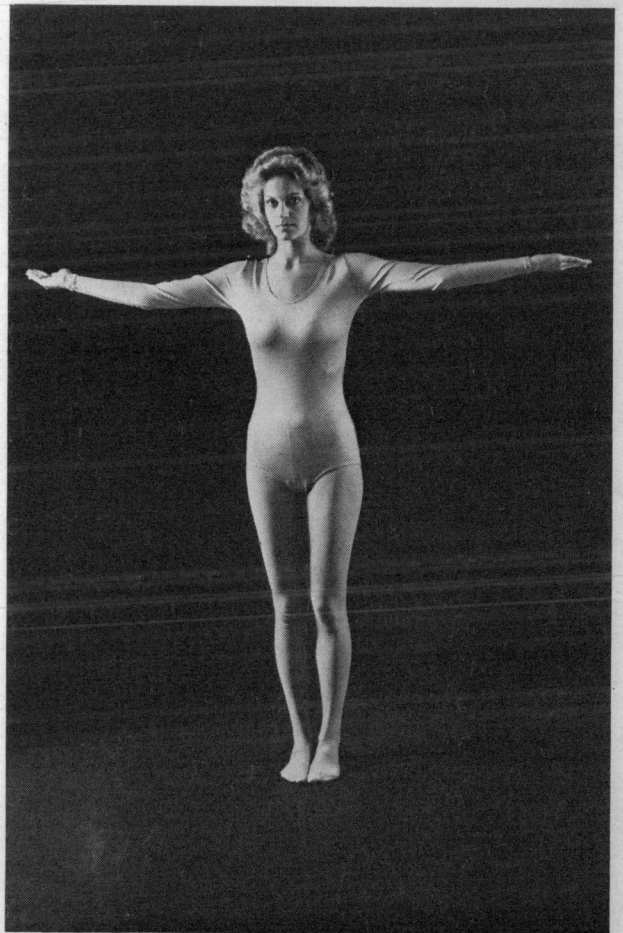

6. *Body Bender*

Starting position: Stand, feet shoulder-width apart, hands behind neck, fingers interlaced.

Action: Count 1. Bend trunk sideward to left as far as possible, keeping hands behind neck. Count 2. Return to starting position. Counts 3 and 4. Repeat to the right.

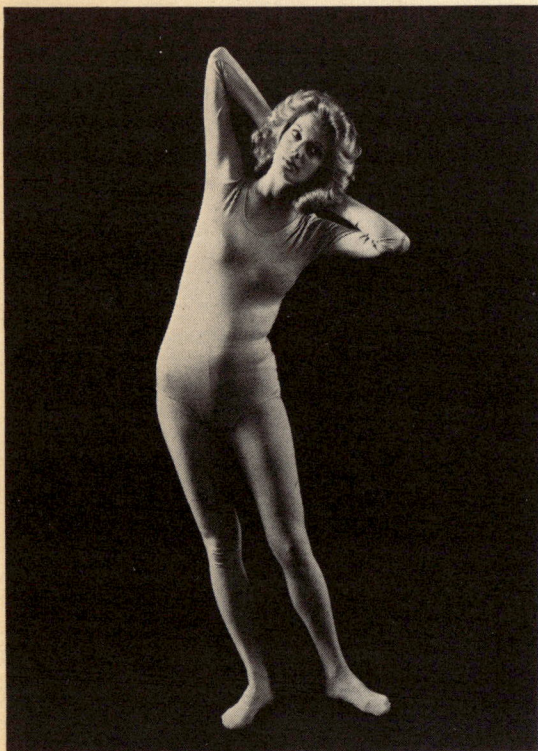

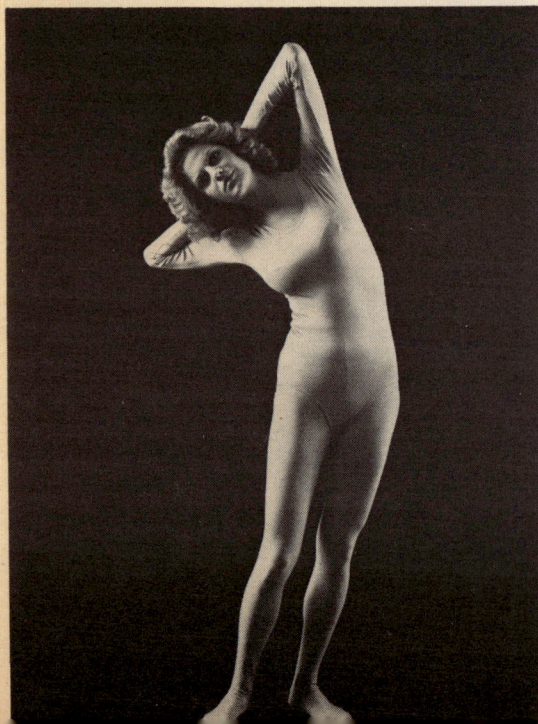

7. *Prone Arch* (See Chapter 3, page 102.)

8. *Knee Pushup* (Men and Women)

Starting position: Lie on floor, face down, legs together, knees bent with feet raised off floor, hands on floor under shoulders, palms down.

Action: Count 1. Push upper body off floor until arms are fully extended and body is in straight line from head to knees. Count 2. Return to starting position.

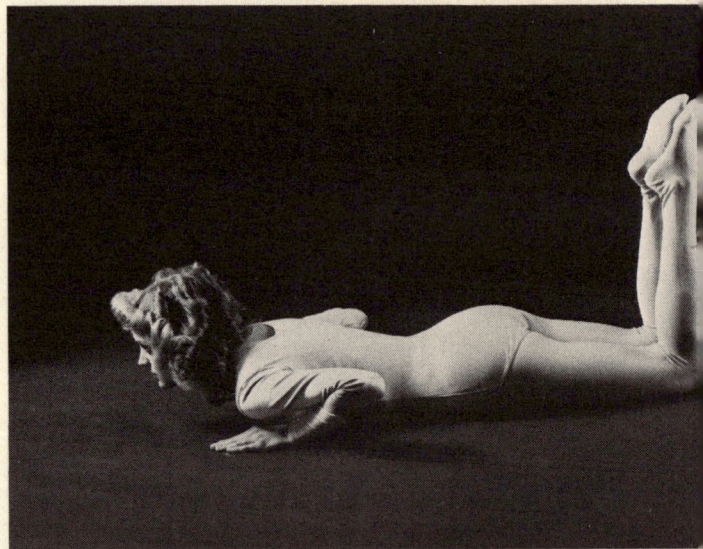

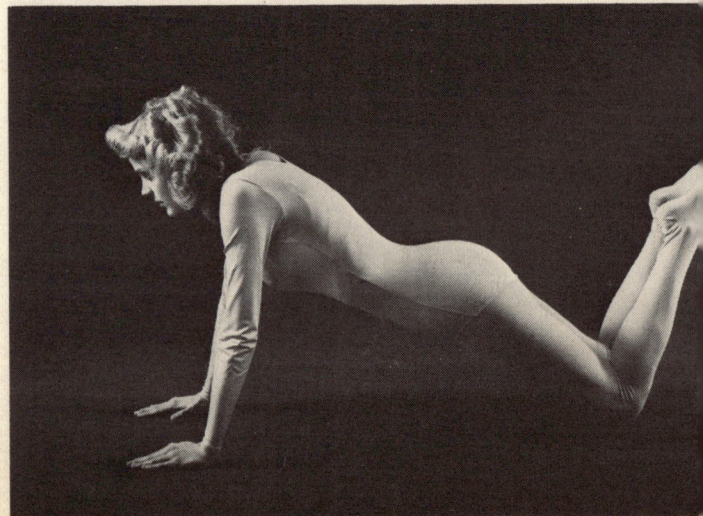

9. *Head and Shoulder Curl*

Starting position: Lie on back, hands tucked under small of back, palms down.

Action: Count 1. Tighten abdominal muscles, lift head and pull shoulders and elbows off floor. Hold for four seconds. Count 2. Return to starting position.

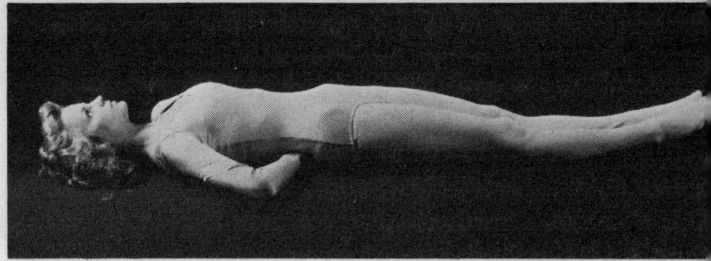

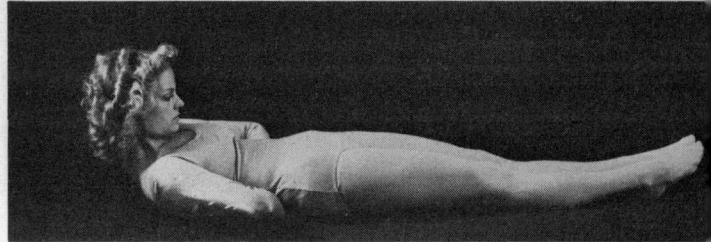

10. *Lower Leg Stretch* (See Chapter 2, page 33.)

Circulatory Activities

Walking: Step off at a lively pace, swing arms and breathe deeply.

Rope: Any form of skipping or jumping is acceptable. Gradually increase the tempo as your skill and condition improve.

ORIENTATION PROGRAM   GOAL

Conditioning Exercises   Repetitions

*1. Bend and Stretch	10
*2. Knee Lift	10 left, 10 right
*3. Wing Stretcher	20
*4. Half Knee Bend	10
*5. Arm Circles	15 each way
*6. Body Bender	10 left, 10 right
7. Prone Arch	10
8. Knee Pushup	6
9. Head and Shoulder Curl	5
10. Lower Leg Stretch	15

Circulatory activity   (choose one each workout)

Walking	½ mile
Rope (skip 15 sec.; rest 60 sec.)	3 series

Cooling-off exercises

(See Chapter 2, pages 60 to 68 for all cooling-off exercises.)

†1. Neck Roll
†2. Triangle
†3. Chest Stretch
†4. Hand-to-Foot
†5. Forward Back Bend

*The first six exercises of the Orientation Program will be used as warm-up exercises throughout the graded levels. *Step Test Record* — After completing the Orientation Program, take the 4-minute Step test (as described in Chapter 1, page 14). Record your pulse rate here: _____. This will be the base rate with which you can make comparisons in the future.

†The five cooling-off exercises will be used throughout the graded levels.

THE FIVE FITNESS LEVELS

LEVEL 1

Conditioning Activities.

1. *Toe Touch*
Starting position: Stand at attention.
Action: Count 1. Bend trunk forward and down, keeping knees slightly flexed, touching fingers to ankles. Count 2. Bounce and touch fingers to top of feet. Count 3. Bounce and touch fingers to toes. Count 4. Return to starting position.

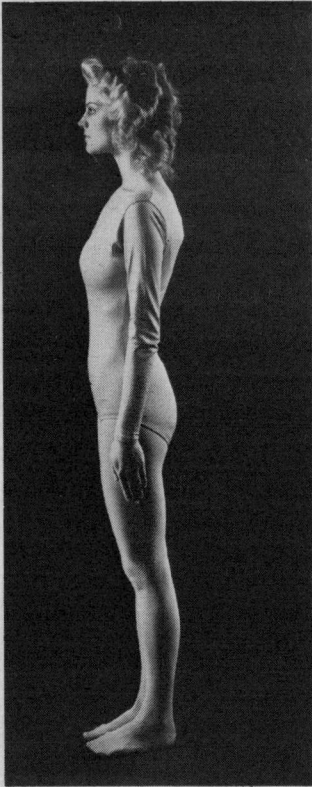

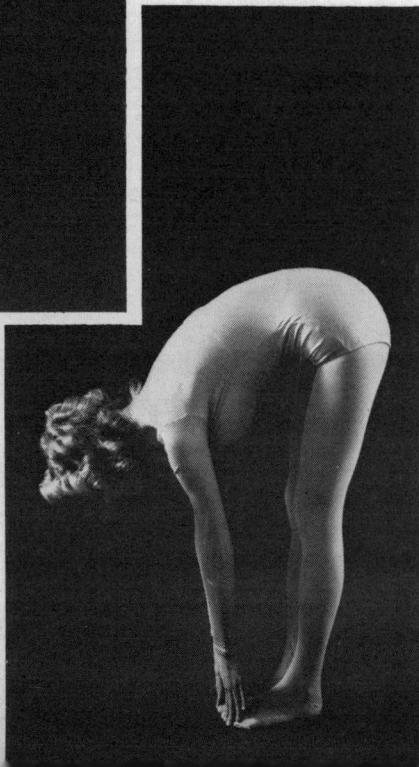

2. *Sprinter*
Starting position: Squat, hands on floor, fingers pointed forward. Extend left leg fully to rear.
Action: Count 1. Reverse position of feet in bouncing movement, bringing left foot to hands, extending right leg backward—all in one motion. Count 2. Reverse feet again, returning to starting position.

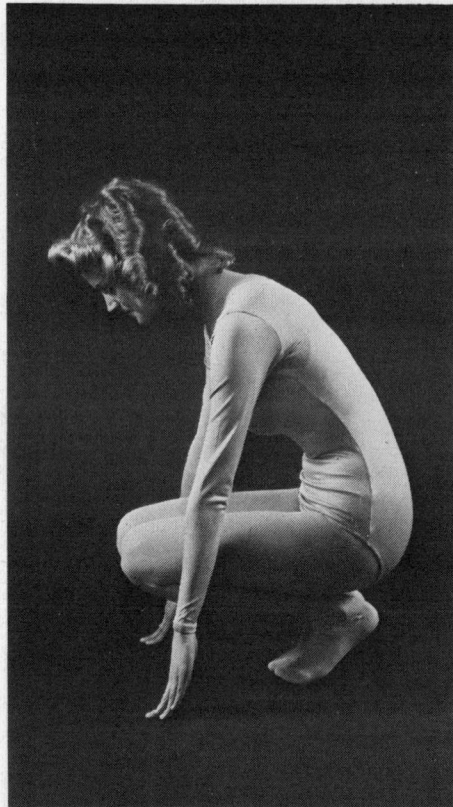

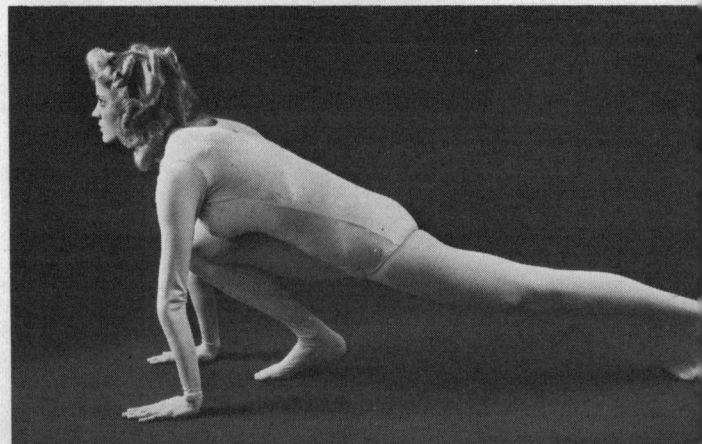

3. *Sit and Stretch* (See Chapter 2, page 43.)

4. *Knee Pushup:* Women (See Orientation Program.)

4. *Pushup:* Men
Starting position: Lie on floor, face down, legs together, hands on floor under shoulders with fingers pointing straight ahead.
Action: Count 1. Push body off floor by extending arms so that weight rests on hands and toes. Count 2. Lower the body until chest touches floor.
Note: Body should be kept straight, buttocks should not be raised, abdomen should not sag.

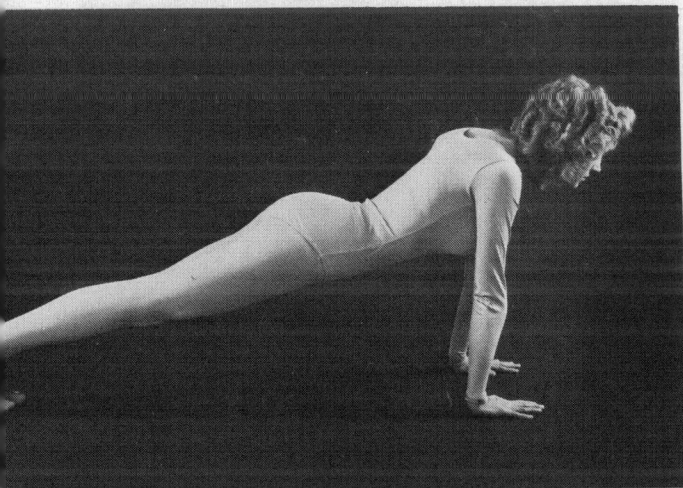

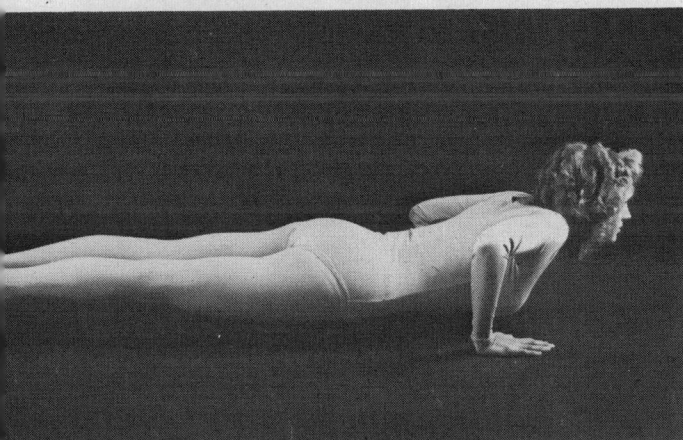

5. *Situp* (Arms Extended)
Starting position: Lie on back, legs straight and together, arms extended beyond head.
Action: Count 1. Bring arms forward over head, roll up to sitting position, sliding hands along legs, grasping ankles. Count 2. Roll back to starting position.

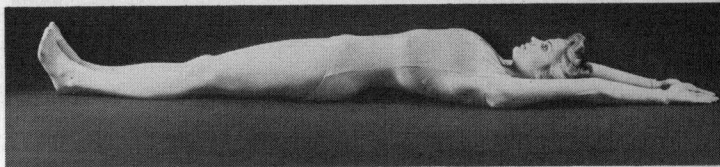

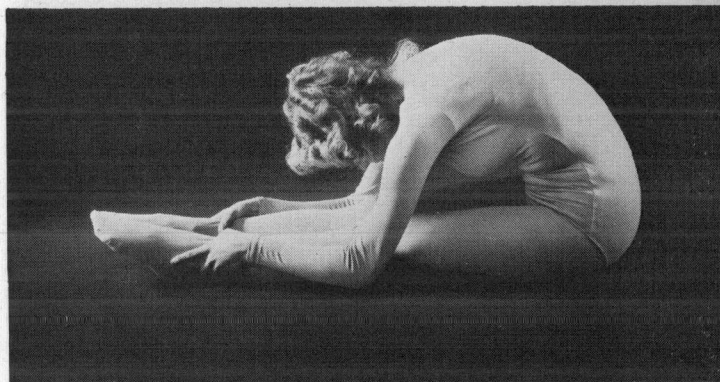

6. *Leg Raiser*
Starting position: Right side of body on floor, head resting on right arm.
Action: Lift leg about 24 inches off floor, then lower it. Do required number of repetitions. Repeat on other side.

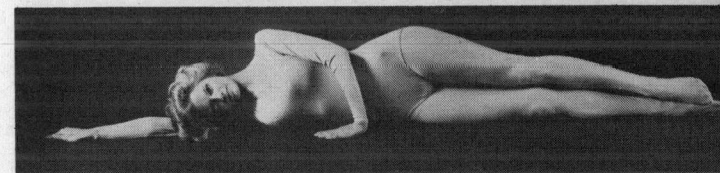

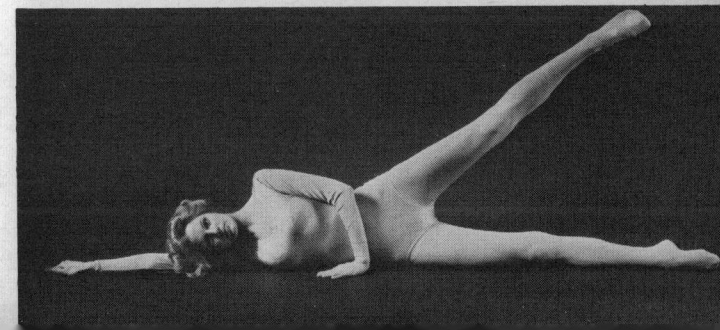

7. *Flutter Kick*

Starting position: Lie face down, hands tucked under thighs.

Action: Arch the back then flutter kick continuously, moving the legs 8-10 inches apart. Kick from hips with knees slightly bent. Count each kick as one.

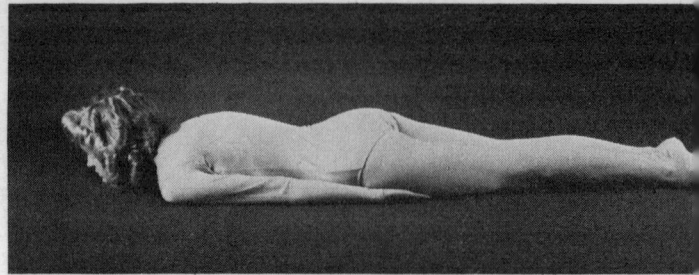

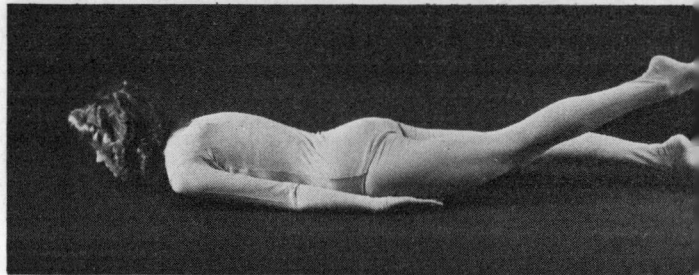

Circulatory Activities

Walking: Maintain a pace of 120 steps per minute for a distance of ½-mile. Swing arms and breathe deeply.

Rope: Skip or jump rope continuously using any form. See Level 1 chart for specified times and repetitions.

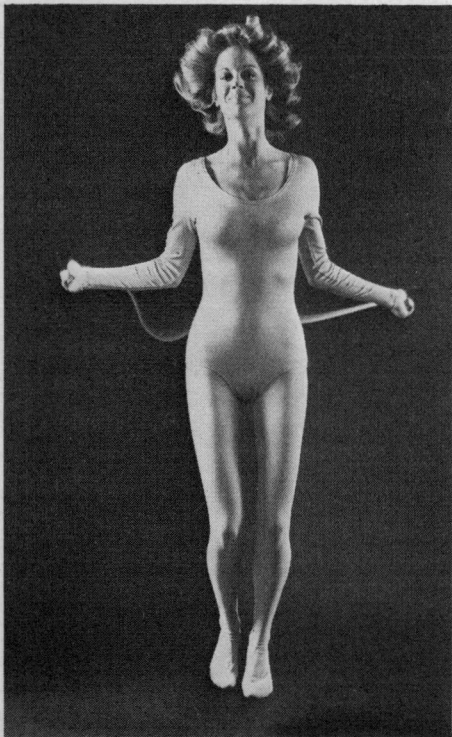

Run in place: Raise each foot at least 4 inches off the floor and jog in place. Count 1 each time left foot touches floor. Complete number of running steps called for in chart, then do specified number of straddle hops. Complete two cycles of alternate running and hopping for time specified on chart.

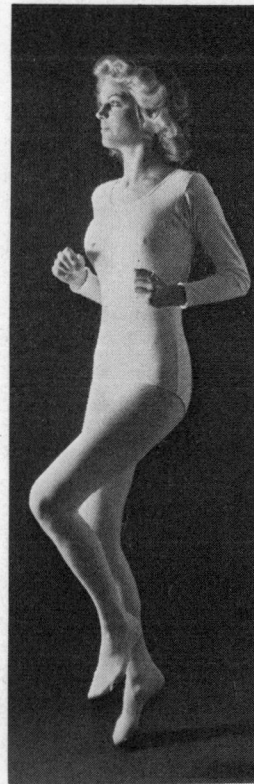

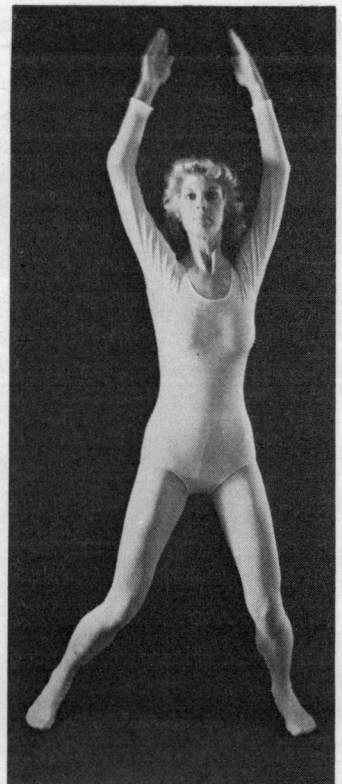

Straddle hop

Starting position: At attention.

Action: Count 1. Swing arms sideward and upward, touching hands above head (arms straight) while simultaneously moving feet sideward and apart in a single jumping motion. Count 2. Spring back to starting position. Two counts in one hop.

WOMEN: LEVEL 1   GOAL

Warm-up Exercises	Exercises 1-6 of Orientation Program

Conditioning Exercises	Uninterrupted repetitions
1. Toe Touch	5
2. Sprinter	8
3. Sit and Stretch	10
4. Knee Pushup	8
5. Situp (Arms Extended)	5
6. Leg Raiser	5 each leg
7. Flutter Kick	20

Circulatory activity (choose one each workout)

Walking (120 steps a minute)	½ mile
Rope (skip 30-secs.; rest 60 secs.)	2 series
Run in place (run 50; straddle hop 10 — 2 cycles)	2 minutes

Cooling-Off Exercises	See Orientation Program

Your progress record 1 2 3 4 5 6 7 8 9 10 11 12 | 13 14 15 Prove-out workouts

Step Test (pulse)

MEN: LEVEL 1   GOAL

Warm-up Exercises	Exercises 1-6 of Orientation Program

Conditioning Exercises	Uninterrupted repetitions
1. Toe Touch	10
2. Sprinter	12
3. Sit and Stretch	12
4. Pushup	4
5. Situp (Arms Extended)	5
6. Leg Raiser	12 each leg
7. Flutter Kick	30

Circulatory activity (choose one each workout)

Walking (120 steps a minute)	1 mile
Rope (skip 30-secs.; rest 30 secs.)	2 series
Run in place (run 60; straddle hop 10 — 2 cycles)	2 minutes

Cooling-Off Exercises	See Orientation Program

Your progress record 1 2 3 4 5 6 7 8 9 10 11 12 | 13 14 15 Prove-out workouts

Step Test (pulse)

LEVEL 2
Conditioning Activities

1. *Toe Touch* (See Level 1.)

2. *Sprinter* (See Level 1.)

3. *Sit and Stretch* (See Chapter 2, page 43.)

4. *Knee Pushup:* Women (See Orientation Program.)

4. *Pushup:* Men (See Level 1.)

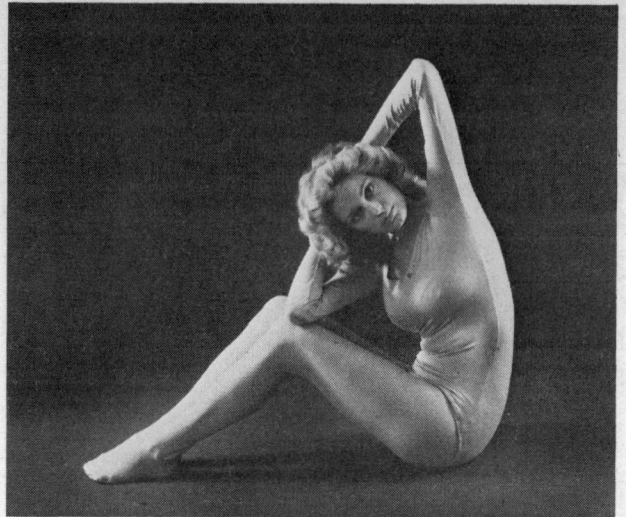

5. *Situp* (Fingers Laced)
Starting position: Lie on back, with knees bent fingers laced behind neck.
Action: Count 1. Curl up to sitting position and turn trunk to left. Touch right elbow to left knee. Count 2. Return to starting position. Count 3. Curl up to sitting position and turn trunk to right. Touch left elbow to right knee. Count 4. Return to starting position. Score one situp each time you return to starting position.

6. *Leg Raiser* (See Level 1.)

7. *Flutter Kick* (See Level 1.)

Circulatory Activities
Jog-Walk: Jog and walk alternately for number of paces indicated on chart for distance specified.

Rope: Skip or jump rope continuously using any form. See Level 2 chart for specified times and repetitions.

Run in place: Raise each foot at least 4 inches off floor and jog in place. Count 1 each time left foot touches floor. Complete number of running steps called for in chart, then do specified number of straddle hops. Complete two cycles of alternate running and hopping for time specified on chart.

Straddle Hop
Starting position: At attention.
Action: Count 1. Swing arms sideward and upward, touching hands above head (arms straight) while simultaneously moving feet sideward and apart in a single jumping motion. Count 2. Spring back to starting position. Two counts in one hop.

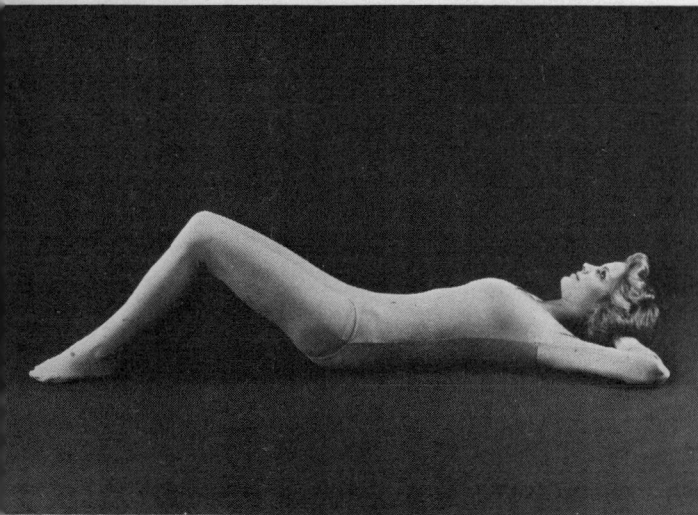

WOMEN: LEVEL 2   GOAL

Warm-up Exercises	Exercises 1-6 of Orientation Program

Conditioning Exercises	Uninterrupted repetitions
1. Toe Touch	10
2. Sprinter	12
3. Sit and Stretch	15
4. Knee Pushup	12
5. Situp (Fingers Laced)	10
6. Leg Raiser	10 each leg
7. Flutter Kick	30

Circulatory activity (choose one each workout)

Jog-walk (jog 50; walk 50)	½ mile
Rope (skip 30-secs.; rest 60 secs.)	3 series
Run in place (run 80; hop 15 — 2 cycles)	3 minutes

Cooling-Off Exercises	See Orientation Program

Your progress record	1 2 3 4 5 6 7 8 9 10 11 12	13 14 15 Prove-out workouts
Step Test (pulse)		

MEN: LEVEL 2   GOAL

Warm-up Exercises	Exercises 1-6 of Orientation Program

Conditioning Exercises	Uninterrupted repetitions
1. Toe Touch	20
2. Sprinter	16
3. Sit and Stretch	18
4. Pushup	10
5. Situp (Fingers Laced)	20
6. Leg Raiser	16 each leg
7. Flutter Kick	40

Circulatory activity (choose one each workout)

Jog-walk (jog 100; walk 100)	1 mile
Rope (skip 1 min.; rest 1 min.)	3 series
Run in place (run 95; hop 15 — 2 cycles)	3 minutes

Cooling-Off Exercises	See Orientation Program

Your progress record	1 2 3 4 5 6 7 8 9 10 11 12	13 14 15 Prove-out workouts
Step Test (pulse)		

LEVEL 3
Conditioning Activities

1. *Toe Touch* (See Level 1.)

2. *Sprinter* (See Level 1.)

3. *Sit and Stretch* (See Chapter 2, page 43.)

4. *Knee Pushup:* Women (See Orientation Program.)

4. *Pushup:* Men (See Level 1.)

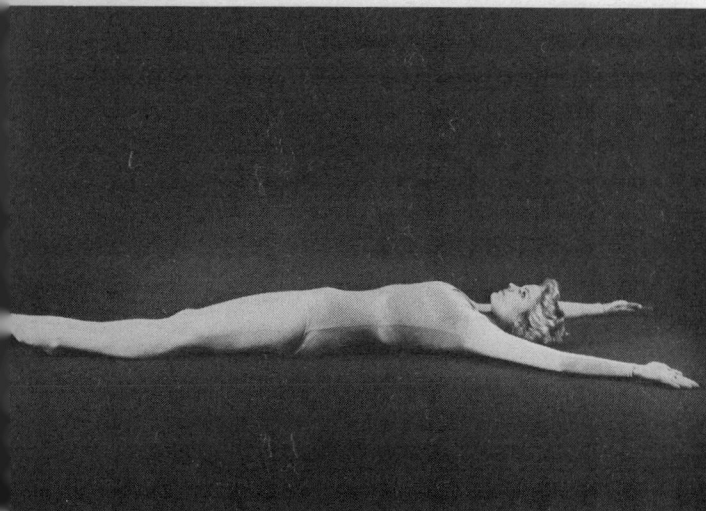

5. *Situp* (Arms Extended, Knees Up)
Starting position: Lie on back, legs straight, arms extended over head.
Action: Count 1. Sit up, reaching forward with arms encircling knees while pulling them tightly to chest. Count 2. Return to starting position. Do this exercise rhythmically, without breaks in movement.

6. *Leg Raiser* (See Level 1.)

7. *Flutter Kick* (See Level 1.)

Circulatory Activities
Jog-Walk: Jog and walk alternately for number of paces indicated on chart for distance specified.

Rope: Skip or jump rope continuously using any form. See Level 3 chart for specified times and repetitions.

Run in place: Raise each foot at least 4 inches off floor and jog in place. Count 1 each time left foot touches floor. Complete number of running steps called for in chart, then do specified number of straddle hops. Complete 2 cycles of alternate running and hopping for time specified on chart.

Straddle Hop
Starting position: At attention.
Action: Count 1. Swing arms sideward, touching hands above head (arms straight) while simultaneously moving feet sideward and apart in a single jumping motion. Count 2. Spring back to starting position. Two counts in one hop.

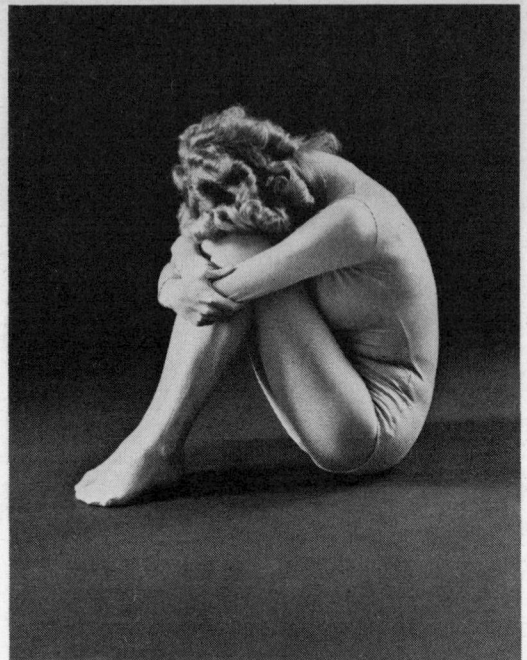

WOMEN: LEVEL 3   GOAL

Warm-up Exercises	Exercises 1-6 of Orientation Program

Conditioning Exercises	Uninterrupted repetitions
1. Toe Touch	20
2. Sprinter	16
3. Sit and Stretch	15
4. Knee Pushup	20
5. Situp (Arms Extended, Knees Up)	15
6. Leg Raiser	16 each leg
7. Flutter Kick	40

Circulatory activity (choose one each workout)

Jog-walk (jog 50, walk 50)	¾ mile
Rope (skip 45 secs.; rest 30 secs.)	3 series
Run in place (run 110; hop 20 — 2 cycles)	4 minutes

Cooling-Off Exercises	See Orientation Program

Your progress record 1 2 3 4 5 6 7 8 9 10 11 12 | 13 14 15 **Prove-out workouts**

Step Test (pulse)

MEN: LEVEL 3   GOAL

Warm-up Exercises	Exercises 1-6 of Orientation Program

Conditioning Exercises	Uninterrupted repetitions
1. Toe Touch	30
2. Sprinter	20
3. Sit and Stretch	18
4. Pushup	20
5. Situp (Arms Extended, Knees Up)	30
6. Leg Raiser	20 each leg
7. Flutter Kick	50

Circulatory activity (choose one each workout)

Jog-walk (jog 200; walk 100)	1½ miles
Rope (skip 1 min.; rest 1 min.)	5 series
Run in place (run 135; hop 20 — 2 cycles)	4 minutes

Cooling-Off Exercises	See Orientation Program

Your progress record 1 2 3 4 5 6 7 8 9 10 11 12 | 13 14 15 **Prove-out workouts**

Step Test (pulse)

LEVEL 4
Conditioning Activities

1. *Toe Touch* (Twist and Bend)

Starting position: Stand, feet shoulder-width apart, arms extended overhead, fingers touching.

Action: Count 1. Twist trunk to right and touch ankle. Count 2. Twist trunk to right and touch floor inside right foot with fingers of both hands. Count 3. Touch floor outside toes of right foot. Count 4. Touch floor outside heel of right foot. Count 5. Return to starting position, sweeping trunk and arms upward in a wide arc. On the next five counts, repeat action to left side.

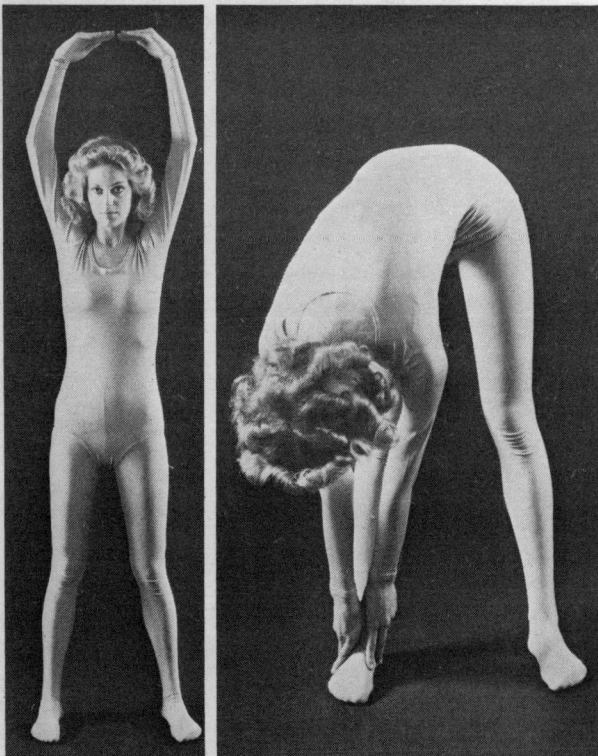

2. *Sprinter* (See Level 1.)

3. *Sit and Stretch* (Alternate)

Starting position: Sit, legs spread apart, fingers laced behind neck, elbows back.

Action: Count 1. Bend forward to left, touching forehead to left knee. Count 2. Return to starting position. Counts 3 and 4. Repeat to right. Score one repetition each time you return to starting position. Knees may be bent if necessary.

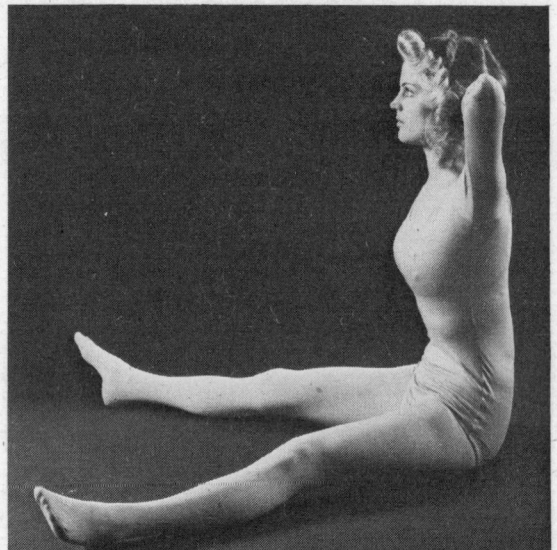

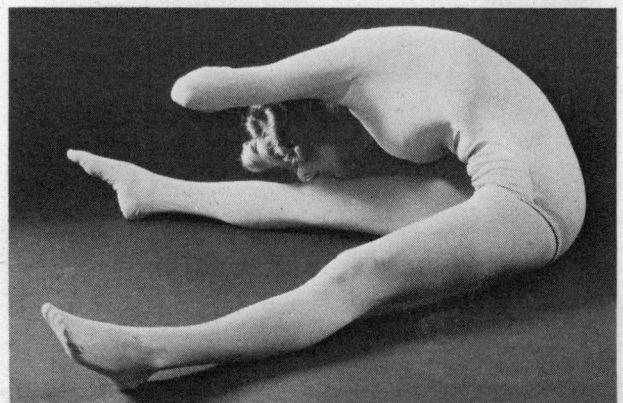

4. *Pushup:* Women (See Pushup: Men Level 1.)

4. *Pushup:* Men (See Level 1.)

5. *Situp* (Arms Crossed, Knees Bent)
Starting position: Lie on back, arms crossed on chest, hands grasping opposite shoulders, knees bent, feet flat on floor.
Action: Count 1. Curl up to sitting position. Count 2. Return to starting position.

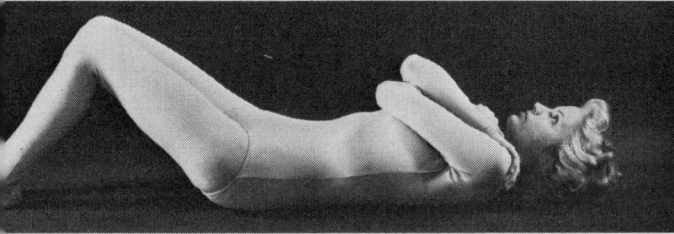

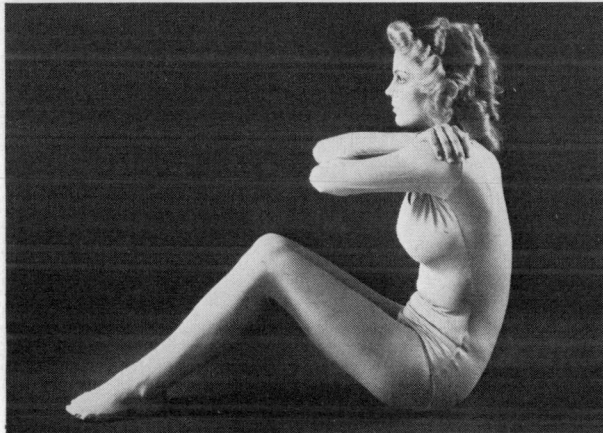

6. *Leg Raiser* (Whip)
Starting position: Right side of body on floor, right arm supporting head.
Action: Whip left leg up and down rapidly lifting as high as possible off the floor. Reverse position and whip right leg up and down.

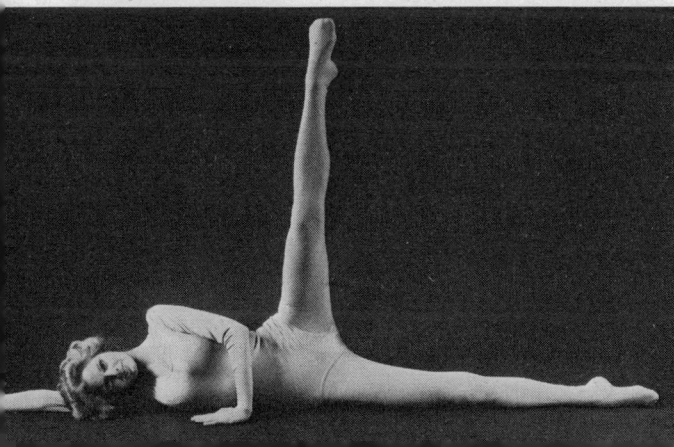

7. *Prone Arch* (Arms Extended)
Starting position: Lie face down, legs straight and together, arms extended at shoulder level.
Action: Count 1. Arch the back, bringing arms, chest and head up, and raising legs as high as possible. Count 2. Return to starting position.

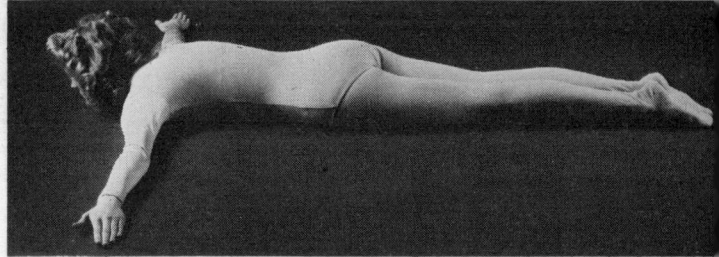

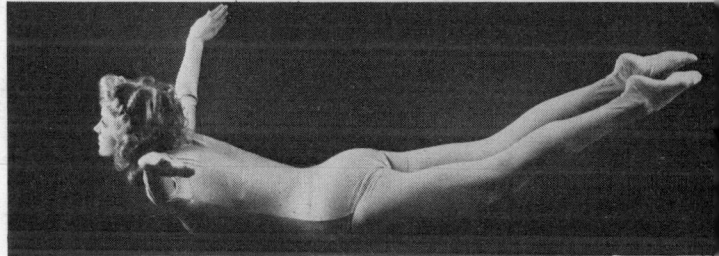

Circulatory Activities

Jog-Walk: Jog and walk alternately for number of paces indicated on chart for distance specified.

Rope: Skip or jump rope continuously using any form. See Level 4 chart for specified times and repetitions.

Run in place: Raise each foot at least 4 inches off floor and jog in place. Count 1 each time left foot touches floor. Complete number of running steps called for in chart, then do specified number of straddle hops. Complete 2 cycles of alternate running and hopping for time specified on chart.

Straddle Hop
Starting position: At attention.
Action: Count 1. Swing arms sideward and upward, touching hands above head (arms straight) while simultaneously moving feet sideward and apart in a single jumping motion. Count 2. Spring back to starting position. Two counts in one hop.

WOMEN: LEVEL 4   GOAL

Warm-up Exercises	Exercises 1-6 of Orientation Program

Conditioning Exercises	Uninterrupted repetitions
1. Toe Touch (Twist and Bend)	15 each side
2. Sprinter	20
3. Sit and Stretch (Alternate)	20
4. Pushup	8
5. Situp (Arms Crossed, Knees Bent)	20
6. Leg Raiser (Whip)	10 each leg
7. Prone Arch (Arms Extended)	15

Circulatory activity (choose one each workout)

Jog-walk (jog 100; walk 50)	1 mile
Rope (skip 60 secs.; rest 30 secs.)	3 series
Run in place (run 145; hop 25 — 2 cycles)	5 minutes

Cooling-Off Exercises	See Orientation Program

Your progress record	1 2 3 4 5 6 7 8 9 10 11 12	13 14 15
Step Test (pulse)		**Prove-out workouts**

MEN: LEVEL 4   GOAL

Warm-up Exercises	Exercises 1-6 of Orientation Program

Conditioning Exercises	Uninterrupted repetitions
1. Toe Touch (Twist and Bend)	20 each side
2. Sprinter	28
3. Sit and Stretch (Alternate)	24
4. Pushup	30
5. Situp (Arms Crossed, Knees Bent)	30
6. Leg Raiser (Whip)	20 each leg
7. Prone Arch (Arms Extended)	20

Circulatory activity (choose one each workout)

Jog	1 mile
Rope (skip 90 secs.; rest 30 secs.)	3 series
Run in place (run 180; hop 25 — 2 cycles)	5 minutes

Cooling-Off Exercises	See Orientation Program

Your progress record	1 2 3 4 5 6 7 8 9 10 11 12	13 14 15
Step Test (pulse)		**Prove-out workouts**

LEVEL 5
Conditioning Activities

1. *Toe Touch* Twist and Bend (See Level 4.)

2. *Sprinter* (See Level 1.)

3. *Sit and Stretch* Alternate (See Level 4.)

4. *Pushup:* Women (See Pushup: Men Level 1.)

4. *Pushup:* Men (See Level 1.)

5. *Situp* (Fingers Laced, Knees Bent)
Starting position: Lie on back, fingers laced behind neck, knees bent, feet flat on floor.
Action: Sit up, turn trunk to right, touch left elbow to right knee. Count 2. Return to starting position. Count 3. Sit up, turn trunk to left, touch right elbow to left knee. Count 4. Return to starting position. Score one each time you return to starting position.

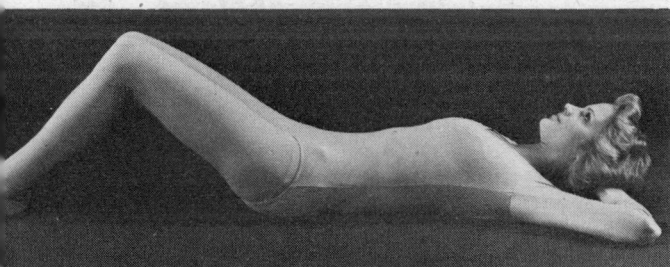

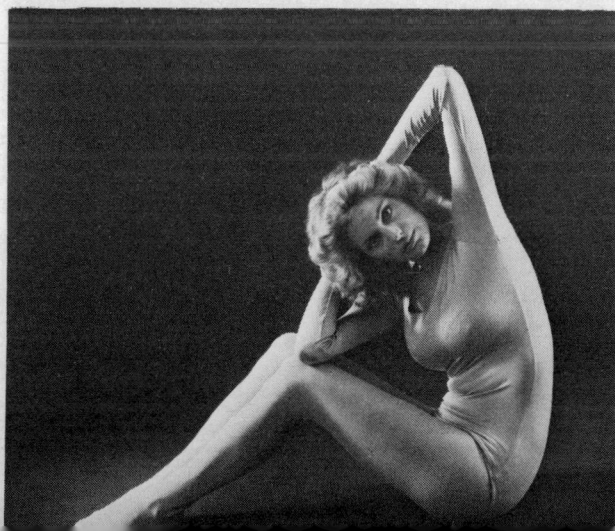

6. *Leg Raiser* (On Extended Arm)
Starting position: Body rigidly supported by extended right arm and foot. Left arm is held behind head.
Action: Count 1. Raise left leg high. Count 2. Return to starting position slowly. Repeat on other side. Do required number of repetitions.

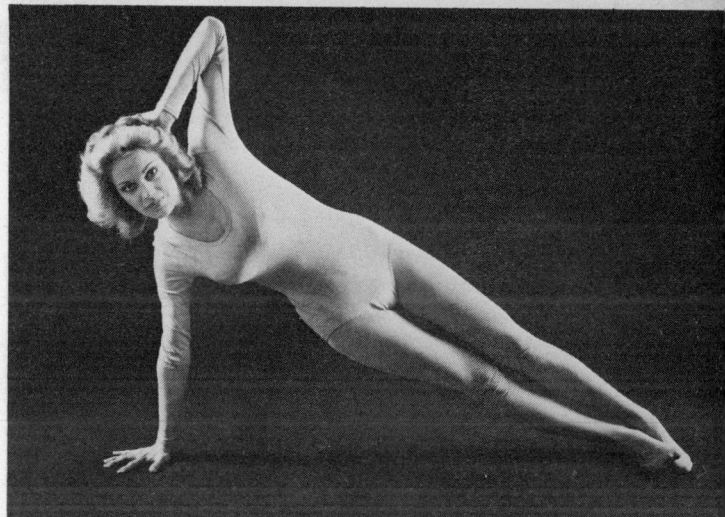

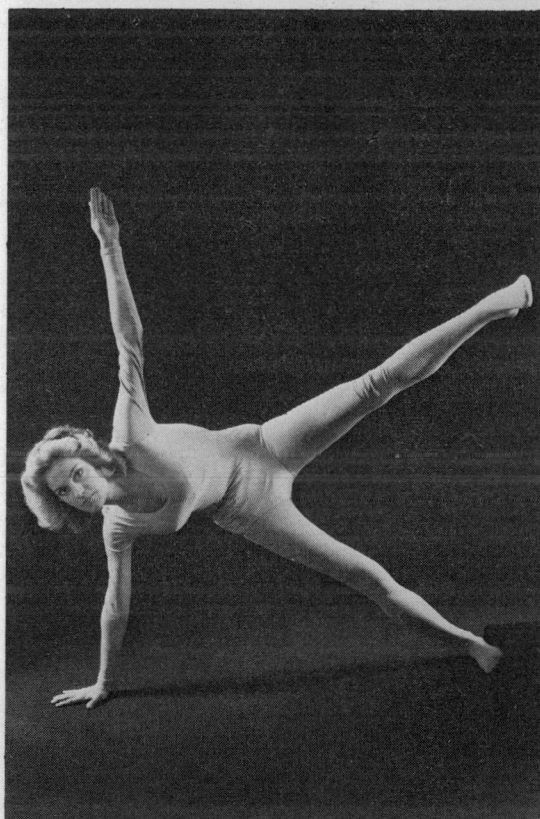

7. *Prone Arch* (Fingers Laced)

Starting position: Lie face down, fingers laced behind neck.

Action: Count 1. Arch back, legs and chest off floor. Count 2. Extend arms fully forward. Count 3. Return hands to behind neck. Count 4. Flatten body to floor.

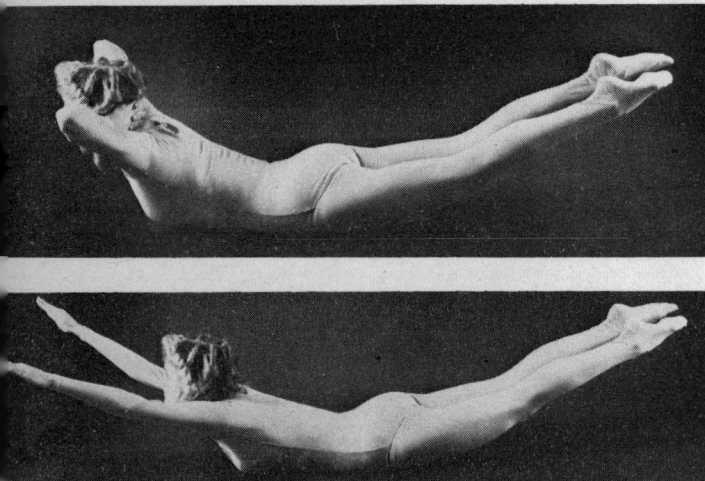

Circulatory Activities

Jog-Run: Jog and run alternately for distance specified on chart.

Rope: Skip or jump rope continuously using any form. See Level 5 chart for specified times and repetitions.

Run in place: Raise each foot at least 4 inches off floor and jog in place. Count 1 each time left foot touches floor. Complete number of running steps called for in chart, then do specified number of straddle hops. Complete 2 cycles of alternate running and hopping in time specified on the chart.

Straddle Hop

Starting position: At attention.

Action: Count 1. Swing arms sideward, touching hands above head (arms straight) while simultaneously moving feet sideward and apart in a single jumping motion. Count 2. Spring back to starting position. Two counts in one hop.

ALTERNATE WATER ACTIVITIES

The water exercises described on page 230 can be used as replacements for the circulatory activities of the basic program—jog-walk, jog-run, rope skipping and running in place. The goals for each of the five levels are shown in the chart below.

Swimming is one of the best physical activities for people of all ages—and for many of the handicapped.

With the body submerged in water, blood circulation automatically increases to some extent; pressure of water on the body also helps promote deeper ventilation of the lungs; and with well-planned activity, both circulation and ventilation increase still more.

WOMEN

Level	1	2	3	4	5
Bobs	10	15	20	50	100
Swim	5 min.	10 min.	15 min.	—	—
Interval Swimming	—	—	—	25 yds. (Repeat 10 times)	25 yds. (Repeat 20 times)

MEN

Level	1	2	3	4	5
Bobs	10	15	25	75	125
Swim	5 min.	10 min.	15 min.	—	—
Interval Swimming	—	—	—	25 yds. (Repeat 20 times)	50 yds. (Repeat 20 times)

WOMEN: LEVEL 5   GOAL

Warm-up Exercises	Exercises 1-6 of Orientation Program

Conditioning Exercises	Uninterrupted repetitions
1. Toe Touch (Twist and Bend)	25 each side
2. Sprinter	24
3. Sit and Stretch (Alternate)	26
4. Pushup	15
5. Situp (Fingers Laced, Knees Bent)	25
6. Leg Raiser (On Extended Arm)	10 each side
7. Prone Arch (Arms Extended)	25

Circulatory activity (choose one each workout)

Jog-run	1 mile
Rope (skip 2 mins.; rest 45 secs.)	2 series
Run in place (run 180; hop 30 — 2 cycles)	6 minutes

Cooling-Off Exercises	See Orientation Program

Your progress record 1 2 3 4 5 6 7 8 9 10 11 12 | **13 14 15**

Step Test (pulse) | **Prove-out workouts**

MEN: LEVEL 5   GOAL

Warm-up Exercises	Exercises 1-6 of Orientation Program

Conditioning Exercises	Uninterrupted repetitions
1. Toe Touch (Twist and Bend)	30 each side
2. Sprinter	36
3. Sit and Stretch (Alternate)	30
4. Pushup	50
5. Situp (Fingers Laced, Knees Bent)	40
6. Leg Raiser (On Extended Arm)	20 each side
7. Prone Arch (Fingers Laced)	30

Circulatory activity (choose one each workout)

Jog-run	3 miles
Rope (skip 2 mins.; rest 30 secs.)	3 series
Run in place (run 216; hop 30 — 2 cycles)	6 minutes

Cooling-Off Exercises	See Orientation Program

Your progress record 1 2 3 4 5 6 7 8 9 10 11 12 | **13 14 15**

Step Test (pulse) | **Prove-out workouts**

Bobbing
  Starting position: Face out of water.
  Action: Count 1. Take a breath. Count 2. Submerge while exhaling until feet touch bottom. Count 3. Push up from bottom to surface while continuing to exhale. Three counts to one bob.

Swimming
  Use any one of the five strokes described in Chapter 4, page 181. Swim continuously for the time specified.

Interval Swimming
  Use any type of stroke. Swim moderately fast for distance specified (30 yards a minute is recommended). You can then either swim back slowly to the starting point or get out of pool and walk back. Repeat specified number of times.

ADULT WALK-JOG-RUN PROGRAMS

Your fitness prescription gives you a great deal of freedom to tailor a personal fitness program to meet your specific fitness or recreation goals. You have a wide choice of exercises, and there are many options as far as the length of time you want to exercise and the intensity of that activity. Some of you, particularly those with a new-found interest in fitness, may prefer a more detailed, step-by-step approach. For this reason, some walk-jog-run programs are included.

We'll describe programs for three levels of ability: a *Starter Program* for those in *poor* fitness categories; an *Intermediate Program* for those in the *average* fitness category, and an *Advanced Program* for those in the *excellent* fitness category.

Before you begin any of the walk-jog-run activities, you should do a series of warm-up exercises. Use the warm-up exercises outlined in the Adult Physical Fitness Programs for Men and Women. If, after completing those exercises, your heart beat rate is not at your training level, run in place or jump rope until you achieve your heart beat training level.

After you complete a walk-jog-run session, follow it with a cooling-off period using the exercises outlined in the Adult Physical Fitness Programs. A gradual cooldown after your aerobic exercise is as important as the warm-up. Complete rest immediately after exercise causes blood to pool in the veins and slows the removal of metabolic waste products. Soreness, cramps or more serious cardiovascular complications may follow. Walking or easy jogging continues the pumping action of the muscles, promoting circulation and speeding recovery. A few minutes spent stretching also helps avoid soreness.

Never rush from a vigorous workout into a hot shower! The flow of blood to recently exercised muscles combined with the flow to the skin to dissipate heat may result in inadequate flow to the brain or heart. *Always* cool down after a workout.

STARTER PROGRAM

Take the *Walk Test* to determine your exercise level.
Walk Test
The object of this test is to determine how many minutes (up to 10) you can walk at a brisk pace, on a level surface, without undue difficulty or discomfort.

If you can't walk for 5 minutes, begin with **Walking Program A.**

If you can walk more than 5 minutes, but less than 10, begin with the **third week** of **Walking Program A.**

If you can walk for the full 10 minutes, but are somewhat tired and sore as a result, start with **Walk-Jog Program B.** If you can breeze through the full 10 minutes, you're ready for bigger things. Wait until the next day and take the 10-minute Walk-Jog Test.

Walk-Jog Test
In this test you alternately walk 50 steps (left foot strikes ground 25 times) and jog 50 steps for a total of 10 minutes. Walk at the rate of 120 steps a minute (left foot strikes the ground at 1-second intervals). Jog at the rate of 144 steps a minute (left foot strikes ground 18 times every 15 seconds).

If you can't complete the 10-minute test, begin

3 Jog 10 seconds (25 yards). Walk 1 minute (100 yards). Do 12 times.

4 Jog 20 seconds (50 yards). Walk 1 minute (100 yards). Do 12 times.

When you've completed Week 4 of Program B, begin at Week 1 of Program C.

Jogging Program C

Week	Activity (five times a week)
1	Jog 40 seconds (100 yards). Walk 1 minute (100 yards). Do 9 times.
2	Jog 1 minute (150 yards). Walk 1 minute (100 yards). Do 8 times.
3	Jog 2 minutes (300 yards). Walk 1 minute (100 yards). Do 6 times.
4	Jog 4 minutes (600 yards). Walk 1 minute (100 yards). Do 4 times.
5	Jog 6 minutes (900 yards). Walk 1 minute (100 yards). Do 3 times.
6	Jog 8 minutes (1,200 yards). Walk 2 minutes (200 yards). Do 2 times.
7	Jog 10 minutes (1,500 yards). Walk 2 minutes (200 yards). Do 2 times.
8	Jog 12 minutes (1,760 yards). Walk 2 minutes (200 yards). Do 2 times.

INTERMEDIATE PROGRAM (JOG-RUN)

If you've followed the Starter Program or are already reasonably active, you're ready for the Intermediate Program. You're able to jog 1 mile slowly without undue fatigue, rest 2 minutes, and do it again.

You're ready to increase both the intensity and the duration of your runs. You'll begin jogging 1 mile in 12 minutes, and when you finish this program, you may be able to complete 3 or more miles at a pace approaching 8 minutes a mile. Each week's program includes three phases—the basic workout, longer runs (overdistance), and shorter runs (underdistance). If a week's program seems too easy, move ahead; if it seems too hard, move back a week or two. Remember to make a warm-up and a cooling-off part of every exercise session.

---

at the **third week** of **Program B.** If you can complete the 10-minute test, but are tired and winded as a result, start with the **fourth week** of **Program B** before moving to Program C. If you can perform the 10-minute Walk-Jog Test without difficulty, start with **Program C.**

Walking Program A

Week	Activity (every other day at first)
1	Walk at a brisk pace for 5 minutes, or for a shorter time if you become uncomfortably tired. Walk slowly or rest for 3 minutes. Again walk briskly for 5 minutes, or until you become uncomfortably tired.
2	Same as Week 1, but increase pace as soon as you can walk 5 minutes without soreness or fatigue.
3	Walk at a brisk pace for 8 minutes, or for a shorter time if you become uncomfortably tired. Walk slowly or rest for 3 minutes. Again walk briskly for 8 minutes, or until you become uncomfortably tired.
4	Same as Week 3, but increase pace as soon as you can walk 8 minutes without soreness or fatigue.

When you've completed Week 4 of Program A, begin at Week 1 of Program B.

Walk-Jog Program B

Week	Activity (four times a week)
1	Walk at a brisk pace for 10 minutes, or for a shorter time if you become uncomfortably tired. Walk slowly or rest for 3 minutes. Again, walk briskly for 10 minutes, or until you become uncomfortably tired.
2	Walk at a brisk pace for 15 minutes, or for a shorter time if you become uncomfortably tired. Walk slowly for 3 minutes.

Week 1

Basic Workout (Monday, Thursday)

1 mile in 11 minutes; active recovery (walk). Run twice.

Underdistance (Tuesday, Friday)

¼ to ½ mile slowly.
½ mile in 5 minutes 30 seconds. Run twice (recovery between repeats).
¼ mile in 2 minutes 45 seconds. Run 4 times (recover between repeats).
Jog ¼ to ½ mile slowly.

Overdistance (Wednesday, Saturday or Sunday)

2 miles slowly. (Use the talk test: Jog at a pace that allows you to converse.)

Week 2

Basic Workout (Monday, Thursday)

1 mile in 10 minutes 30 seconds; active recovery. Run twice.

Underdistance (Tuesday, Friday)

¼ to ½ mile slowly.
½ mile in 5 minutes.
¼ mile in 2 minutes 30 seconds. Run 2 times (recover between repeats).
¼ mile in 2 minutes 45 seconds. Run 2 times (recover between repeats).
220 yards in 1 minute 20 seconds. Run 4 times (recover between repeats).
¼ to ½ mile slowly.

Overdistance (Wednesday, Saturday or Sunday)

2¼ miles slowly.

Week 3

Basic Workout (Monday, Thursday)

1 mile in 10 minutes, active recovery. Run twice.

Underdistance (Tuesday, Friday)

¼ to ½ mile slowly.
½ mile in 4 minutes 45 seconds.
¼ mile in 2 minutes 30 seconds. Run 4 times (recover between repeats).
220 yards in 1 minute 10 seconds. Run 4 times (recover between repeats).
100 yards in 30 seconds. Run 4 times (recover between repeats).
¼ to ½ mile slowly.

Overdistance (Wednesday, Saturday or Sunday)

2½ miles slowly.

Week 4

Basic Workout (Monday, Thursday)

1 mile in 9 minutes 30 seconds; active recovery. Run twice.

Underdistance (Tuesday, Friday)

¼ to ½ mile slowly.
½ mile in 4 minutes 45 seconds. Run twice (recover between repeats).
¼ mile in 2 minutes 20 seconds. Run 4 times (recover between repeats).
220 yards in 1 minute. Run 4 times (recover between repeats).
¼ to ½ mile slowly.

Overdistance (Wednesday, Saturday or Sunday)

2¾ miles slowly.

Week 5

Basic Workout (Monday, Thursday)
1 mile in 9 minutes; active recovery. Run twice.

Underdistance (Tuesday, Friday)

¼ to ½ mile slowly.
½ mile in 4 minutes 30 seconds.
¼ mile in 2 minutes 20 seconds. Run 4 times (recover between repeats).
220 yards in 60 seconds. Run 4 times (recover between repeats).
100 yards in 27 seconds. Run 4 times (recover between repeats).
¼ to ½ mile slowly.

Overdistance (Wednesday, Saturday or Sunday)

3 miles slowly.

Week 6

Basic Workout (Monday, Thursday)

1½ miles in 13 minutes 30 seconds; active recovery. Run twice.

Underdistance (Tuesday, Friday)

¼ to ½ mile slowly.
½ mile in 4 minutes 30 seconds. Run twice (recover between repeats).
¼ mile in 2 minutes 10 seconds. Run 4 times (recover between repeats).
220 yards in 60 seconds. Run 4 times (recover between repeats).
100 yards in 25 seconds. Run twice (recover between repeats).
¼ to ½ mile slowly.

Overdistance (Wednesday, Saturday or Sunday)

3 miles slowly; *increase pace* last ¼ mile.

Pace Guide for Gauging Speed Over Various Distances

	Pace	1 Mile	½ Mile	¼ Mile	220 Yards	100 Yards	50 Yards
				(in minutes and seconds)			
Slow Jog	10 cal/min. (120 cal/mile)*	12:00	6:00	3:00	1:30	0:40	0:20
Jog	12 cal/min (120 cal/mile)*	10:00	5:00	2:30	1:15	0:34	0:17
Run	15 cal/min (120 cal/mile)*	8:00	4:00	2:00	1:00	0:27	0:13
Fast Run	20 cal/min (120 cal/mile)*	6:00	3:00	1:30	0:45	0:20	0:10

*Depends on efficiency and body size; add 10 percent for each 15 pounds over 150; subtract 10 percent for each 15 pounds under 150.

Week 7

Basic Workout (Monday, Thursday)

1½ miles in 13 minutes; active recovery. Run twice.

Underdistance (Tuesday, Friday)

¼ to ½ mile slowly.
½ mile in 4 minutes 15 seconds. Run twice (recover between repeats).
¼ mile in 2 minutes. Run 4 times (recover between repeats).
220 yards in 55 seconds. Run 4 times (recover between repeats)
¼ to ½ mile slowly.

Overdistance (Wednesday, Saturday or Sunday)

3½ miles slowly; always increase pace near finish.

Week 8

Basic Workout (Monday, Thursday)

1 mile in 8 minutes; active recovery; run 1 mile in 8 minutes 30 seconds; active recovery; repeat (total of 3 miles).

Underdistance (Tuesday, Friday)

¼ to ½ mile slowly.
½ mile in 4 minutes. Run twice (recover between repeats).
¼ mile in 1 minute 50 seconds. Run 4 times (recover between repeats).
220 yards in 55 seconds. Run 4 times (recover between repeats).
100 yards in 23 seconds. Run 4 times (recover between repeats).
¼ to ½ mile slowly.

Overdistance (Wednesday, Saturday or Sunday)

3¾ miles slowly.

Week 9

Basic Workout (Monday, Thursday)

1 mile in 8 minutes. Run 3 times (recover between repeats).

Underdistance (Tuesday, Friday)

¼ to ½ mile slowly.
½ mile in 3 minutes 30 seconds.
¼ mile in 1 minute 45 seconds. Run 4 times (recover between repeats).
220 yards in 50 seconds. Run 4 times (recover between repeats).
100 yards in 20 seconds. Run 4 times (recover between repeats).
50 yards in 10 seconds. Run 4 times (recover between repeats).
¼ to ½ mile slowly.

Overdistance (Wednesday, Saturday or Sunday)

4 miles slowly.

Week 10

Basic Workout (Monday, Thursday)

1½ miles in 12 minutes. Run twice (recover between repeats).

Underdistance (Tuesday, Friday)

¼ to ½ mile slowly.
½ mile in 3 minutes 45 seconds. Run 3 times (recover between repeats).
¼ mile in 1 minute 50 seconds. Run 6 times (recover between repeats).
220 yards in 45 seconds. Run twice (recover between repeats).
¼ to ½ mile slowly.

Overdistance (Wednesday, Saturday or Sunday)

4 miles; increase pace last ½ mile.

Week 11

Basic Workout (Monday, Thursday)

1 mile in 7 minutes 30 seconds. Run 3 times (recover between repeats).

Underdistance (Tuesday, Friday)

¼ to ½ mile slowly.
½ mile in 3 minutes 50 seconds. Run 4 times (recover between repeats).
¼ mile in 1 minute 45 seconds. Run 4 times (recover between repeats).
220 yards in 45 seconds. Run 2 times (recover between repeats).
¼ to ½ mile slowly.

Overdistance (Wednesday, Saturday or Sunday)

Over 4 miles slowly (more than 400 calories per workout).

Week 12

Basic Workout

1½ miles in 11 minutes 40 seconds.

You've achieved the fitness standard of excellent. Proceed to the advanced aerobic fitness program.

ADVANCED PROGRAM

This section is for the well-trained runner. We'll provide some suggestions for advanced training, but keep in mind there is no single way to train. If you enjoy underdistance training, by all means use it. If you find that you prefer over-distance, you'll like the suggestions offered here.

Long, slow distance running seems to be the ideal way to train. It combines the features of overdistance and underdistance with a minimum of discomfort. Simply pick up the pace as you approach the end of a long run, and you'll receive an optimal training stimulus. Moreover, since the speed work is limited to a short span near the end of the run, discomfort is brief.

Consider the following suggestions:
- Always warm-up before your run.
- Use the high fitness heart rate training zone.
- Vary the location and distance of the run day by day (long-short; fast-slow; hilly-flat; hard-easy).
- Set distance goals:

    Phase 1: 20 miles a week
    Phase 2: 25 miles a week (ready for 3- to 5-mile road races)
    Phase 3: 30 miles a week
    Phase 4: 35 miles a week (ready for 5- to 7-mile road runs)
    Phase 5: 40 miles a week
    Phase 6: 45 miles a week (ready for 7- to 10-mile road races)
    Phase 7: More than 50 miles a week (consider longer races such as the marathon — 26.2 miles)

- Don't be a slave to your goals, and don't increase weekly mileage unless you enjoy it.
- Run 6 days a week if you enjoy it; otherwise, try an alternate day schedule with longer runs.
- Try one long run (not over one-third of weekly distance) on Saturday or Sunday.
- Try two shorter runs if the long ones seem difficult—5 + 5 instead of 10.
- Keep records if you like—you'll be surprised! Record data, distance, comments. Note resting pulse, body weight. At least annually, check your performance over a measured distance to observe progress (use a local road race or the 1½-mile-run test). Check your fitness score on the Step Test several times a year.
- Don't train with a stopwatch. Wear a wristwatch so you'll know how long you've run.
- Increase speed as you approach the finish of a run.
- Always cool down after a run.

CHILDREN'S PHYSICAL FITNESS PROGRAM

Warm-Up Activities: Ages 6-9

Young children love to imitate, and they want to have a good time. They also do not have the motivation an adult does in participating in physical fitness activities. The following exercises therefore require participation of other children, a parent, older brother or sister or could be used as family activities.

Once the warm-up activities have been completed, a run, jog or swim should follow. Running is a simple as well as beneficial exercise for this age group. Children should run every day and should be encouraged but *not* pressured to run progressively longer distances.

Tortoise and Hare (cardiovascular)
Starting position: Child stands at attention.
Action:
Count 1—Jog slowly in place.
Count 2—On the command, "Hare," the tempo doubles. The knees are lifted high, while arms pump vigorously.
Count 3—On the command, "Tortoise," the tempo slows to an easy jog. Repeat the commands, "Tortoise," "Hare."

Gorilla Walk (flexibility and coordination)
Starting position: Child spreads feet shoulder width, bends at the waist, and grasps ankles, keeping the knees fully extended.
Action: Walk forward holding firmly to the ankles. Keep the knees extended and the legs straight.

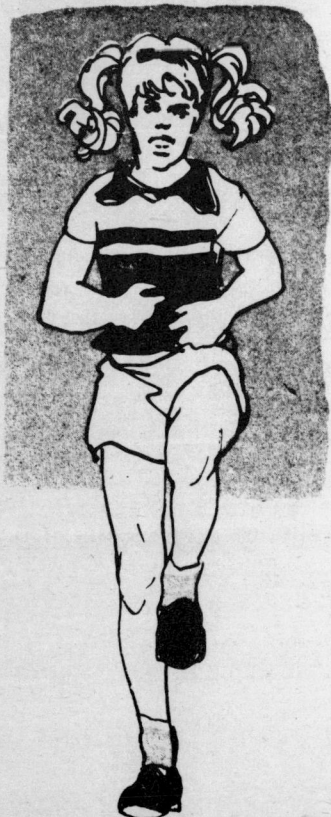

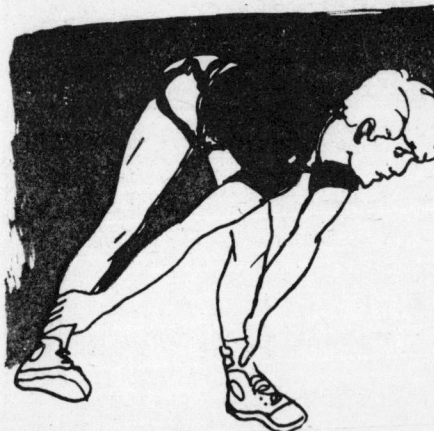

Bear Walk (flexibility—hamstrings)
Starting position: Child stands in position to move around in a circle. Bend from the waist and place hands on the floor.
Action: Child travels around in a circle, moving right arm and right leg simultaneously as one step, then left arm and left leg.

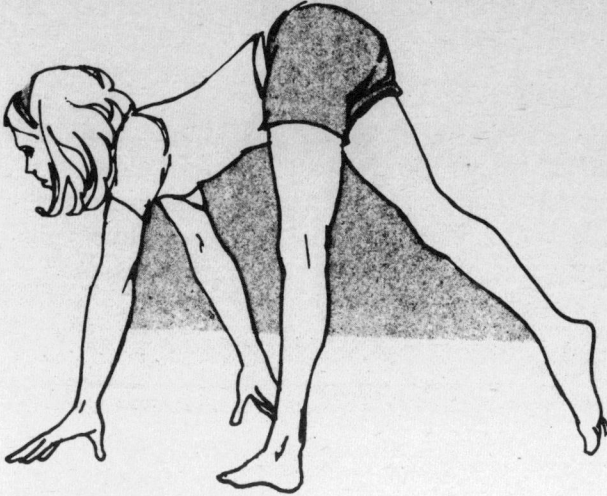

Trees in the Wind (flexibility — lateral trunk)

Starting position: Child stands in position to move around in a circle, with arms raised and extended overhead.

Action: Child runs slowly around in a circle, bending left, right, forward and back as though she or he were swaying in the breeze.

Bunny Hop (leg extensors)

Starting position: Child assumes semi-squat position, with hands behind his or her ears, palms forward, to stimulate rabbit ears.

Action: Child moves around in a circle by hopping with both feet together, landing in the semi-squat position.

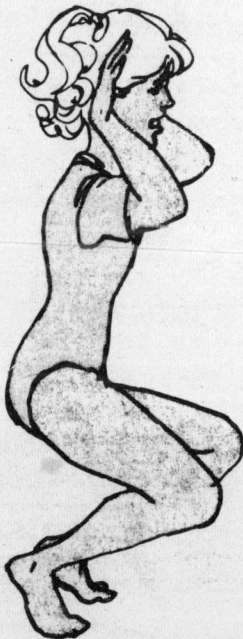

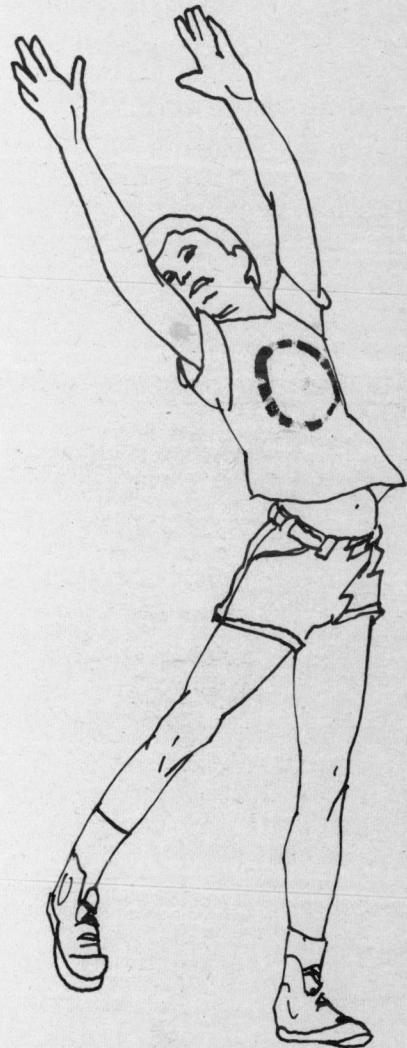

Rabbit Race (cardiovascular and leg extensor)

Starting position: Children stand in a straight line side by side, 3 feet apart. A finish line is designated 60 feet in front of the children.

Action: Children race by hopping with both feet together—first to the right, then to the left, then straight ahead, repeating this pattern until reaching the finish line. The race may be varied by hopping in other ways; e.g., on one leg.

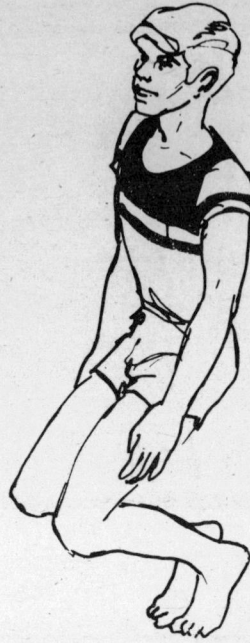

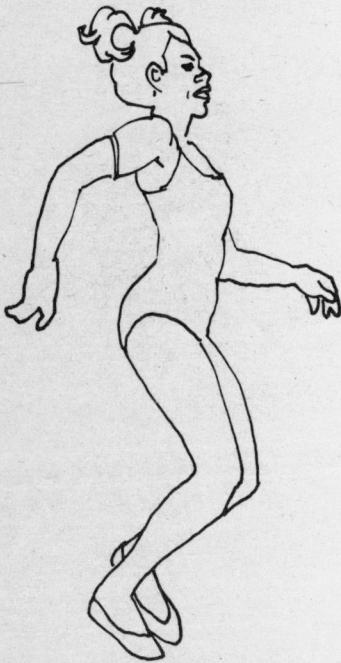

Hop (leg extensors)

Starting position: Child stands in position to move around in a circle.

Action: Child moves forward by hopping on the left foot, taking several long steps.

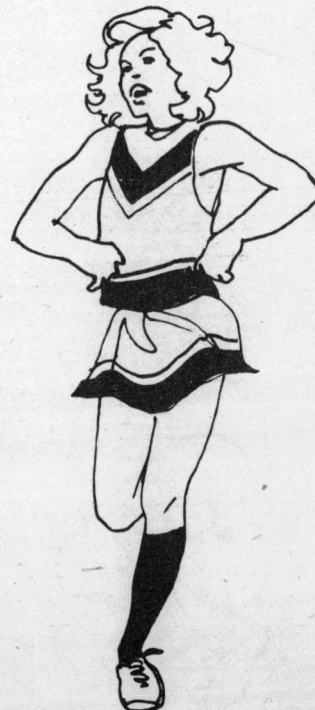

Knee Down (leg extensor strength and balance)

Starting position: Child stands with toes of both feet on a line.

Action: Without using the hands or moving the toes from the line, kneel on both knees. Return to standing position without using hands and keeping toes on the line.

Frog Stand (balance and arm strength)

Starting position: Child assumes squat position, hands on floor, fingers pointing forward. The elbows are inside of, and pressed against, knees.

Action: Lean forward slowly, transferring body weight to hands, raising feet clear of the floor. Maintain balance, keeping head up. Hold for several seconds, then return to starting position. Repeat, maintaining balance for increasingly longer periods.

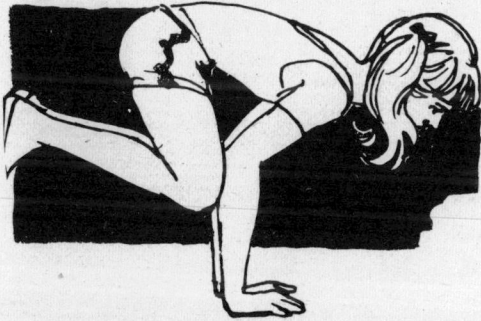

Coffee Grinder (arm, shoulder and lateral trunk strength)

Starting position: Child supports extended body (turned sidewards) on right arm and both feet. Right arm and both legs are fully extended, feet slightly apart.

Action: Move feet and body in a circle using the right arm as a pivot. Repeat, using the left arm.

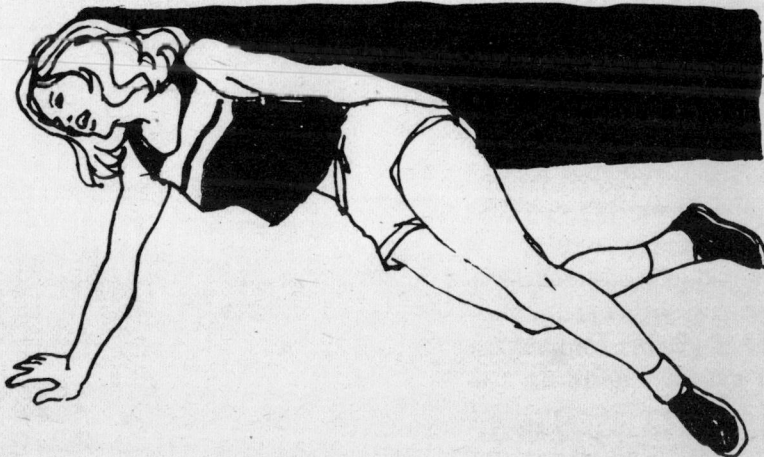

Measuring Worm (flexibility—lower back and hamstrings)

Starting position: Child assumes the pushup position, body extended, face down, arms extended fully, shoulder width apart, hands on floor, fingers spread and pointed forward. The body is supported on hands and toes.

Action: Hold the hands stationary and walk feet up, as close to the hands as possible. Then, keeping the feet stationary, walk hands forward to starting position. Repeat alternate actions.

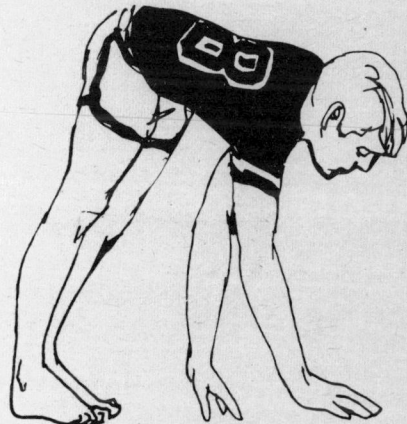

Wheelbarrow (arm, shoulder and abdominal strength)

Starting position: This exercise requires two children. One takes "hands and knees" position. The hands are directly under the shoulders, fingers pointing forward. His partner grasps the kneeling child's ankles, raising his legs.

Action: The first child walks forward on his hands. His feet and legs are supported by partner walking between the outstretched legs.

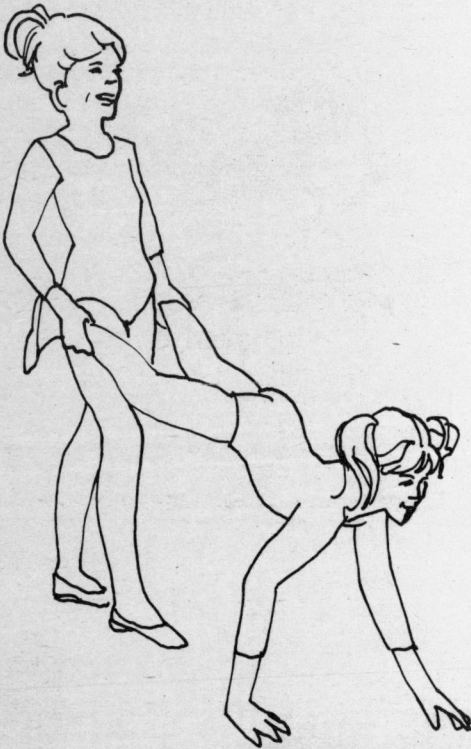

Warm-Up Activities: Ages 10-18

The exercises and activities selected for the 10-18 age group are more formal than those presented for the 6-8 group. The calisthenic exercises have been arranged in a sequence that places the easier warm-up exercises first.

It is not necessary for a child to do all the warm-up exercises prior to engaging in the formal jogging and swimming programs which follow this section, but it is recommended that exercises be selected that affect the strength and flexibility of the major muscles groups of the body. The number of repetitions for each warm-up exercise selected should be 10 and then week by week should be increased in number.

Deep Breather (warm-up—respiratory system)

Starting position: Child stands at attention.

Action:

Count 1—Rise on toes while circling the arms inward and upward slowly, and inhaling deeply. At the end of movement, arms are extended overhead.

Count 2—Continue circling arms backward and downward while lowering the heels and exhaling. This exercise should be done slowly and rhythmically.

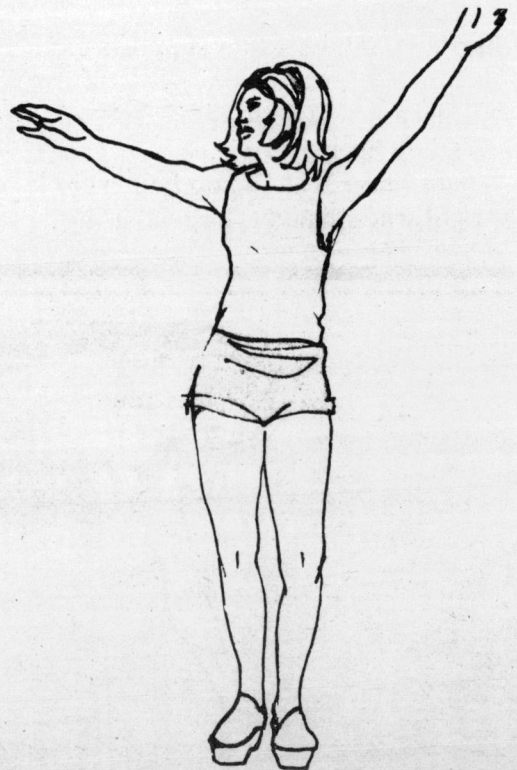

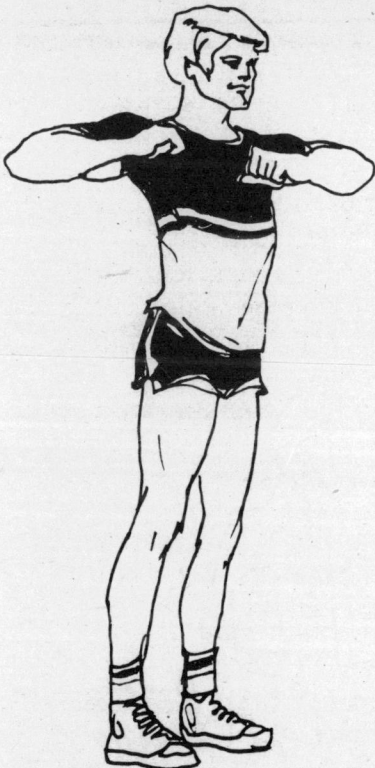

Wing Stretcher (flexibility—back and chest)

Starting position: Stand erect; raise elbows to shoulder height, fists clenched, palms down in front of chest.

Action: Thrust elbows backward vigorously and return. Be sure head remains erect. Keep elbows at shoulder height.

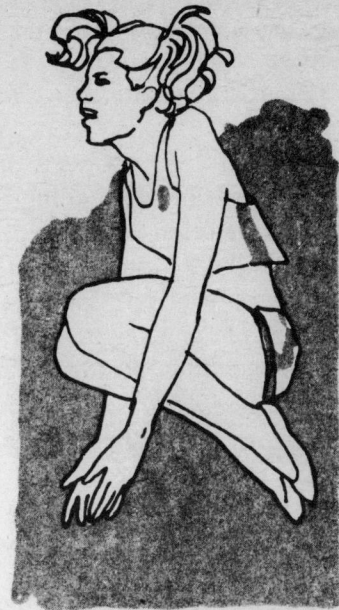

Bear Hug (thighs)

Starting position: Child stands, feet comfortably spread with hands on hips.

Action:

Count 1—Take a long step diagonally right, keeping left foot anchored in place; tackle the right leg around the thigh by encircling the thigh with both arms.

Count 2—Return to the starting position.

Counts 3 and 4—Repeat to the opposite side.

Jump and Touch (legs extensors)

Starting position: Child assumes a half-crouch position, bending from the waist as though about to begin a broad jump. Arms are extended backward.

Action: Spring straight upward, bringing knees to the chest and heels to buttocks, meanwhile swinging the arms downward and around the legs, attempting to touch hands together under the legs. Land in the starting position, ready for the next upward leap.

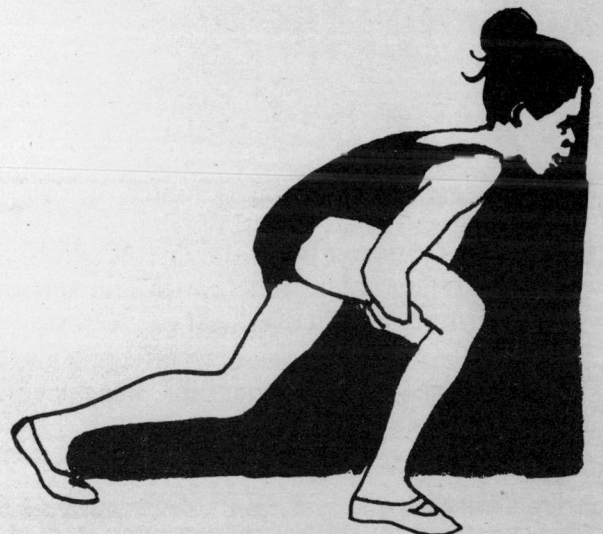

One-Foot Balance (balance)

Starting position: Child stands at attention.

Action:

Count 1—Stretch left leg backward, while bending trunk forward and extending arms sideward until this position is reached: The head is up, trunk parallel to floor; the left leg is fully extended with toes of left foot pointed. The supporting leg is kept straight. Hold this position for 5 to 10 seconds. Return to starting position.

Count 2—Repeat, using the opposite leg for support.

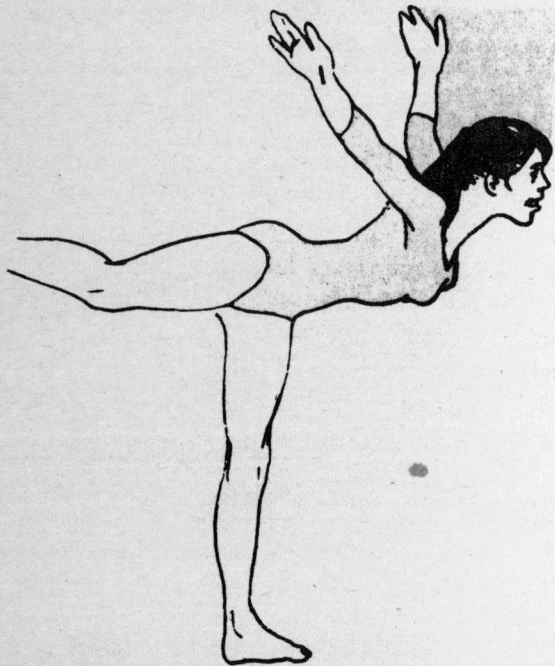

Back Stretcher (lower back—thighs)

Starting position: Child stands with feet spread apart, arms extended overhead.

Action:

Count 1—Bend forward from hips, knees bent. Swing arms downward between legs.

Count 2—Return to starting position.

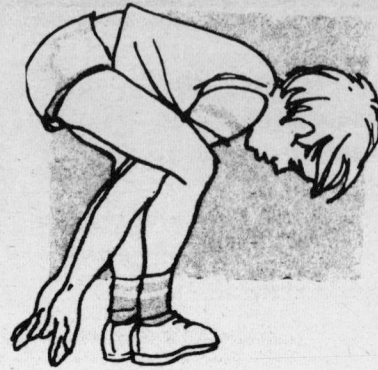

Jumping Jack (coordination—cardiovascular)

Starting position: Pupil stands at attention.

Action:

Count 1—Swing arms sideward and upward, touching hands above head (arms straight) while simultaneously moving feet sideward and apart in a single jumping motion.

Count 2—Spring back to the starting position.

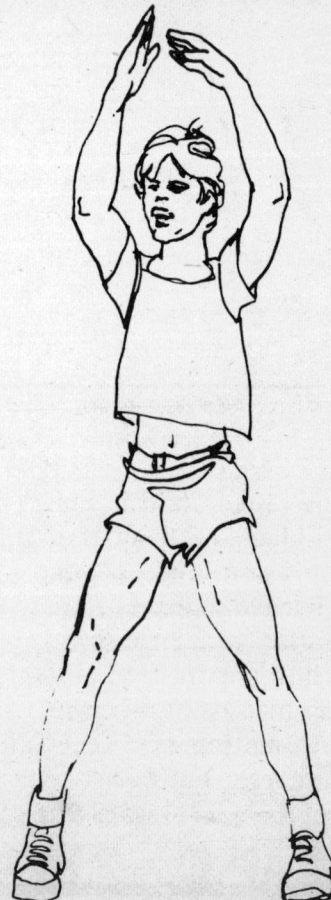

Body Bender (flexibility—lateral trunk)

Starting position: Pupil stands, feet slightly apart, hands clasped behind the head.

Action:

Count 1—Bend sideward at the hips to the left as far as possible. Keep the feet stationary and the toes pointed straight ahead.

Count 2—Return to starting position.

Count 3—Repeat, bending to the right.

Count 4—Return to the starting position.

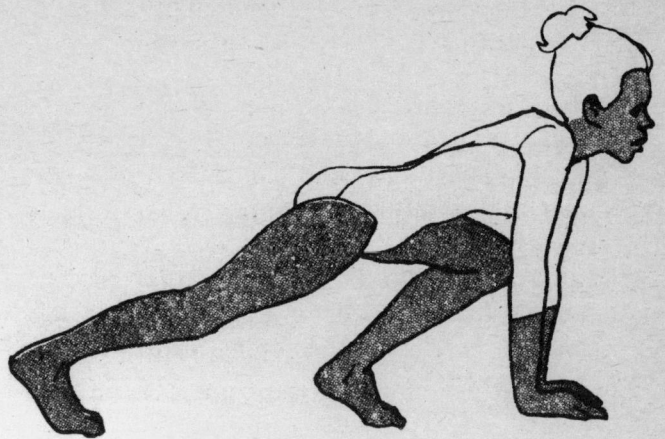

Squat Thrust (cardiovascular—agility)

Starting position: Child stands at attention.

Action:

Count 1—Bend knees and place hands on the floor in front of the feet. Arms may be between, outside of or in front of the bent knees.

Count 2—Thrust the legs back far enough so that the body is perfectly straight from shoulders to feet (the pushup position).

Count 3—Return to squat position.

Count 4—Return to erect position.

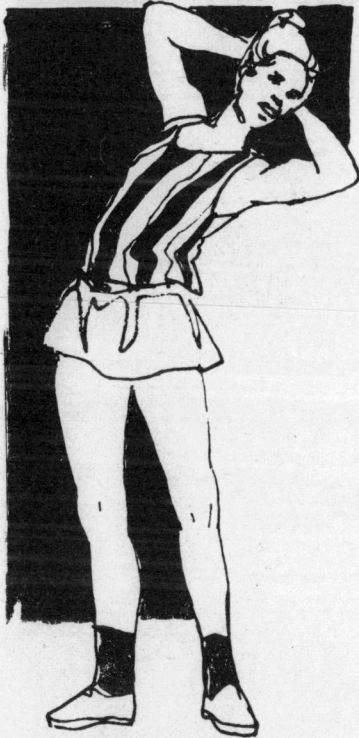

The Sprinter (cardiovascular, arms and legs)

Starting position: Child assumes squatting position, hands on the floor, fingers pointed forward, left leg fully extended to the rear.

Action:

Count 1—Reverse position of the feet by bringing left foot to hands and extending right leg backward, all in one motion.

Count 2—Reverse feet again, returning to starting position. Repeat exercise rhythmically.

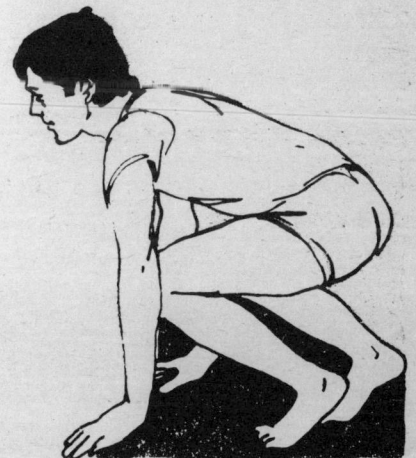

Windmill (flexibility—lower back, hamstrings)

Starting position: Child stands, knees flexed, feet spread shoulder-width apart, arms extended sideward shoulder-high, palms down.

Action:

Count 1—Twist and bend trunk, bringing right hand to the left toe, keeping arms straight, knees flexed.

Count 2—Return to starting position.

Count 3—Twist and bend trunk, bringing left hand to the right toe, keeping arms straight, knees flexed.

Count 4—Return to starting position.

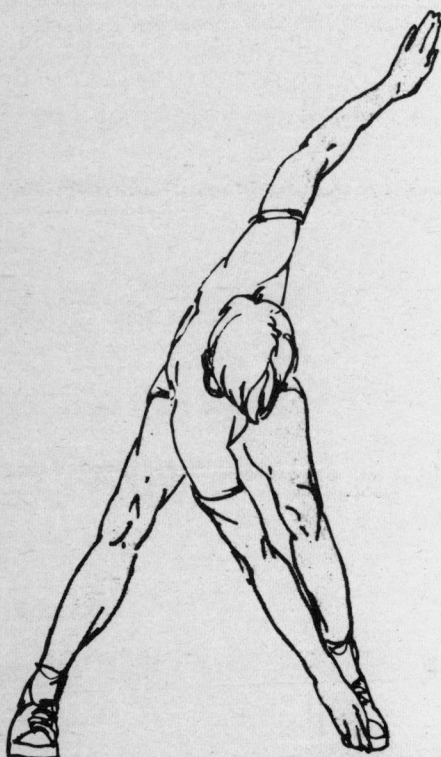

Squat Jump (leg extensor strength)

Starting position: Child assumes semisquat position, hands clasped on top of head, feet 4 to 6 inches apart, heel of left foot on line with toes of the right foot.

Action:

Count 1—Spring upward from the floor, reversing the position of the feet and coming down to the semisquat position. Hands remain on head.

Count 2—Same movement, reversing feet.

Continue, reversing feet on each upward jump.

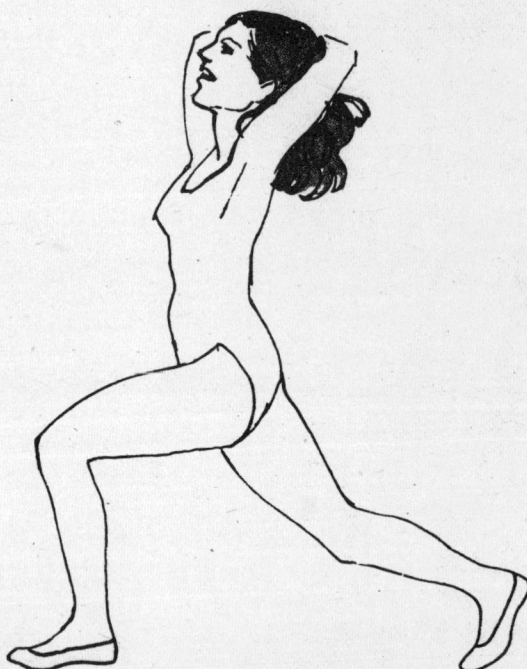

Up Oars (abdominals and hip flexors)

Starting position: Child lies on back with arms extended behind head.

Action:

Count 1—Sit up, reach forward with the extended arms, meanwhile pulling the knees tightly against the chest. Arms outside knees.

Count 2—Return to starting position. The exercise is done rhythmically and without breaks in the movement.

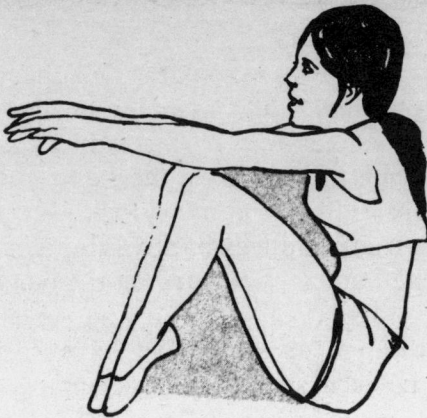

Back Twist (hip flexors and abdominals)

Starting position: Child lies on back, arms at sides, palms on the floor, and legs raised to a vertical position.

Action:

Count 1—Keeping both feet together, swing legs slowly to the left until almost touching the floor. Keep arms, shoulders and head in contact with the floor.

Count 2—Return to starting position.

Count 3—Repeat the movement to the right.

Count 4—Return to starting position.

The Coordinator (coordination—cardiovascular)

Starting position: Child stands at attention.

Action:

Count 1—Hop in place on left foot, swinging right leg forward, touching toe to floor in front of left foot, meanwhile bringing both arms forward to shoulder level, fully extended.

Count 2—Hop again on left foot, swinging right foot to the right side and touching toe to floor, meanwhile flinging arms sideward at shoulder level.

Count 3—Hop again on left foot, returning to position of Count 1.

Count 4—Hop again on left foot, returning to starting position.

Repeat, hopping on right foot. Continue, alternately hopping on each foot. As exercise is mastered, tempo should be increased.

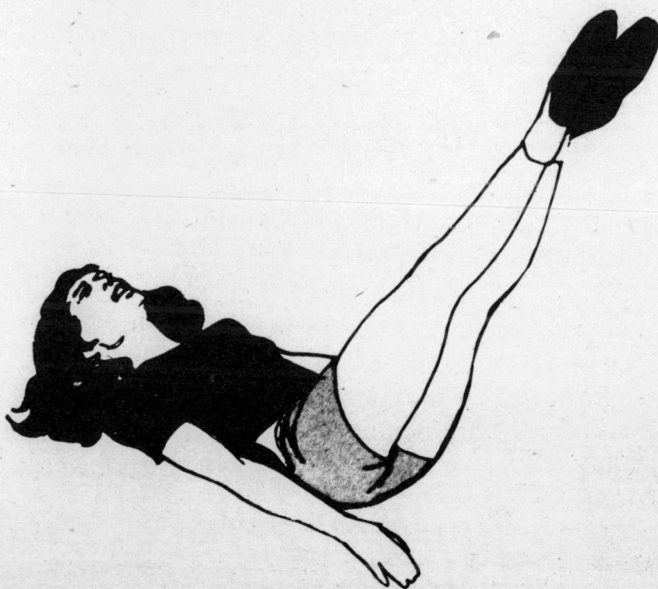

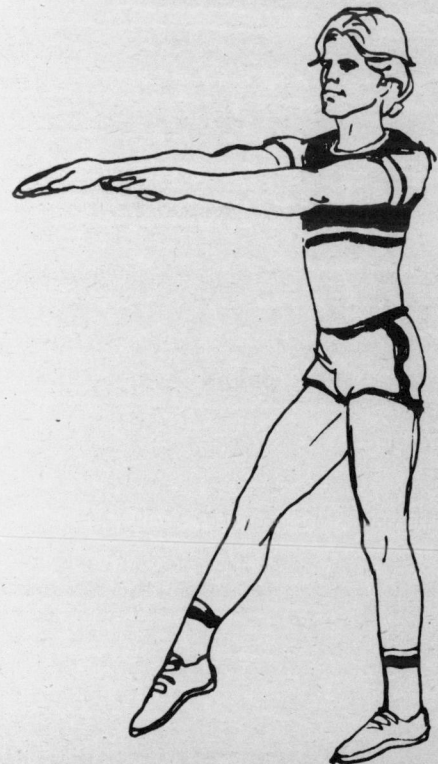

Knee Raise (hip flexors and abdominals)

Starting position: Child lies on back with knees slightly flexed, feet on floor, arms at sides.

Action:

Count 1—Raise one knee up as close as possible to chest.

Count 2—Fully extend the knee so the leg is perpendicular to the floor.

Count 3—Bend knee and return to chest.

Count 4—Straighten leg and return to starting position. Alternate the legs during the exercise. The double knee raise is done in the same manner by moving both legs simultaneously.

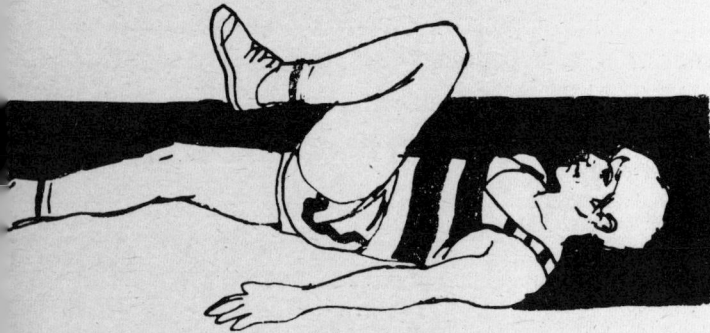

Head and Shoulder Curl (abdominals and hip flexors)

Starting position: Child lies on the back with hands at sides, palms down.

Action:

Count 1—Lift the head and shoulders off the floor. Hold the tense position for four counts.

Count 2—Return to starting position.

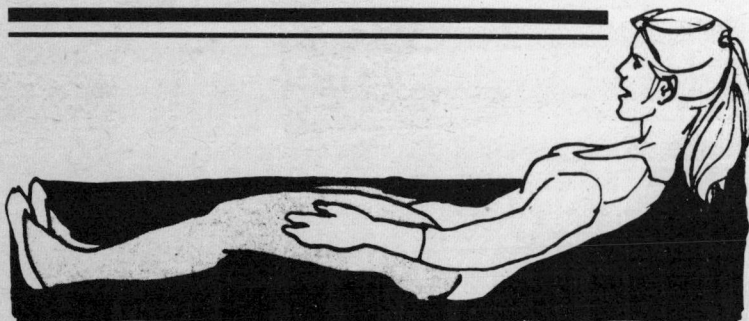

Bouncing Ball (arms, shoulders and chest)

Starting position: Child assumes pushup position, by bending forward extending the arms and placing the hands on the floor, shoulder width apart, fingers pointing forward, and extending trunk and legs backward in a straight line. The body is supported on the hands and toes.

Action: Bounce up and down by a series of short, upward springs. (Try clapping hands together while body is in the air.)

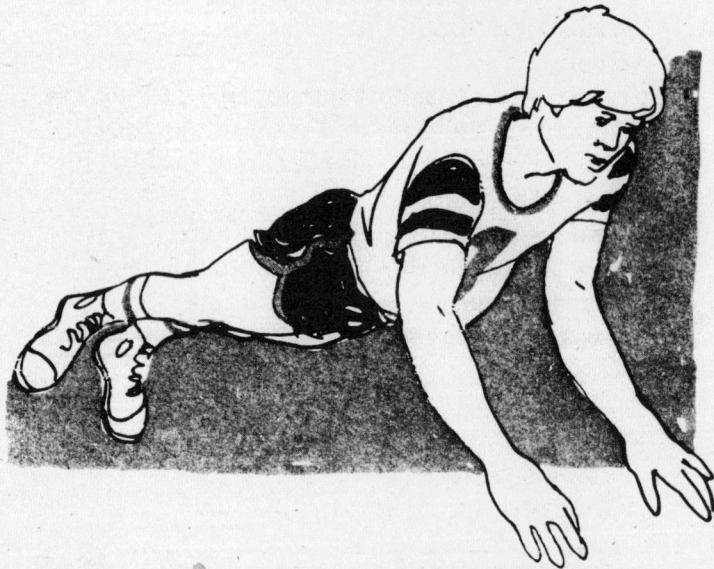

Leg Extension (hip flexors and abdominals)
Starting position: Child sits, legs extended, body erect and hands on hips.
Action:
Count 1—With a quick, vigorous action, raise and flex the knees by dragging feet backward toward the buttocks with the toes lightly touching the ground.
Count 2—Extend the legs back to the starting position.
The head and shoulders should be held high throughout the exercise.

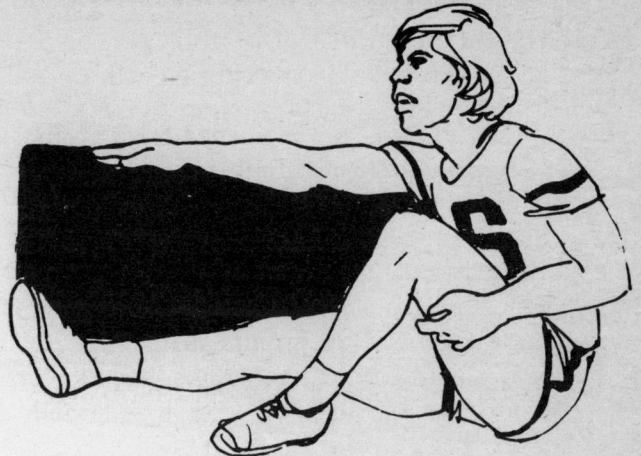

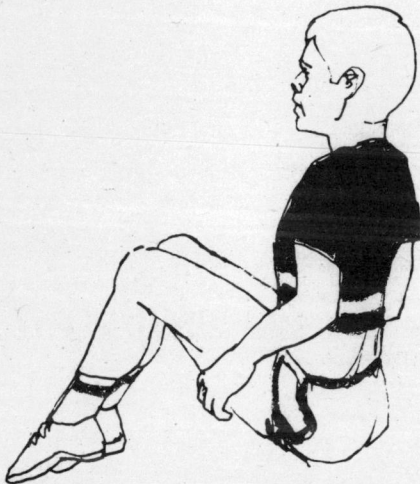

Side Leg Raise (lateral muscles of the leg)
Starting position: Child lies on side, arms extended overhead. The head rests on the lower arm. Legs are extended fully, one on top of the other.
Action:
Count 1—With a brisk action, raise the top leg vertically.
Count 2—Return to starting position. Repeat for specified number of counts and repeat on other side.

Snap and Twist (abdominal and hip flexors)
Starting position: Child lies on back with arms extended beyond head.
Action:
Count 1—With a vigorous action, sit up and bring the left knee to chest while extending right arm forward and the elbow backward. (This is an "explosive" type of movement.)
Count 2—Return to the starting position.
Count 3—Repeat the movement to the opposite side.
Count 4—Return to starting position. The exercise is done rhythmically.

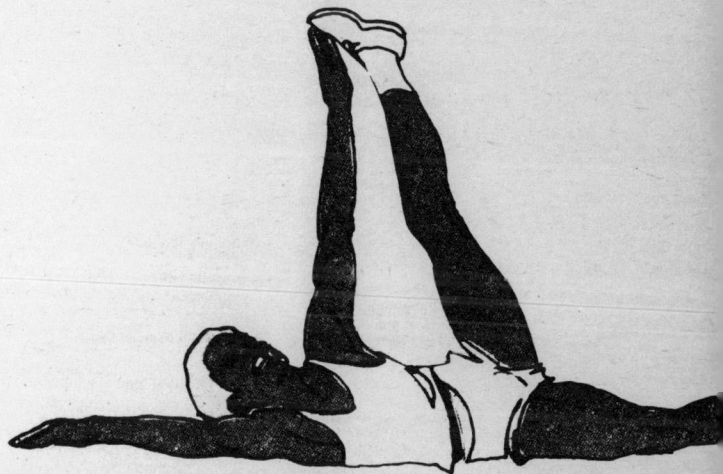

Pushups (arms, shoulders and chest muscles)

Starting position:

Boys—Extend arms and place hands on ground just under and slightly outside of the shoulders, fingers pointing forward. Extend body so that it is perfectly straight. The weight is supported on the hands and toes.

Girls—Extend arms and place hands, fingers pointing forward, on ground just under and slightly outside of the shoulders. Place knees on floor and extend body until it is straight from the head to the knees. Bend knees and raise the feet off the floor. The weight is supported by the hands and knees. (Also for boys who cannot do regular pushups.)

Action:

Count 1—Keeping body tense and straight, bend elbows and touch chest to floor.

Count 2—Return to original position. (The body must be kept perfectly straight. The buttocks must not be raised. The abdomen must not sag.)

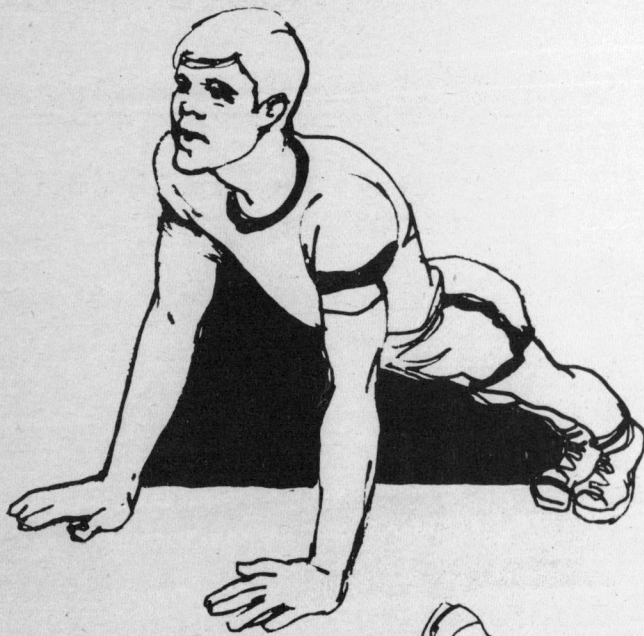

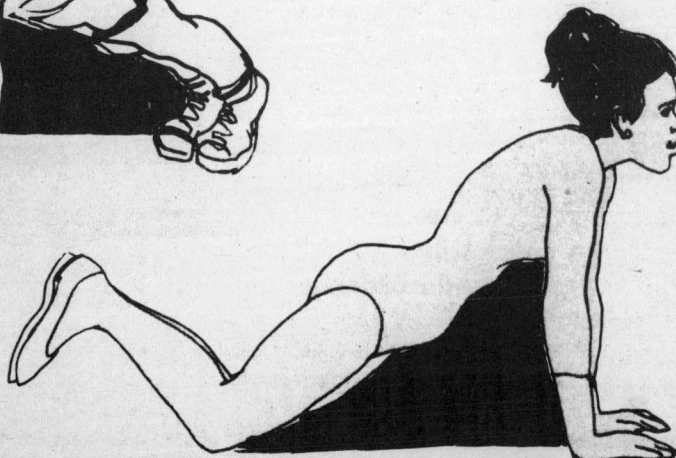

Cardiovascular Endurance Programs: Ages 10-18

Jogging Program

For the following jogging program, each "X" stands for 1 day of the week. For example, in Week 1 of the Girls' 12-Week Schedule, a distance of 440 yards should be run each of the first 2 days of the week and 660 yards should be run each of the next 3 days of the week.

For information on how, when and where to jog, see Chapter 4, page 147.

GIRLS' 12-WEEK JOGGING SCHEDULE

Distance	1	2	3	4	5	6	7	8	9	10	11	12
440 Yards	XX	XX	X	X								
660 Yards	XXX	XX	XX	X	X	X	X					
880 Yards		X	XX	X	XX	X	X	X	X	X	X	X
1100 Yards				XX	X	XX	X	X	XX	X	X	X
1320 Yards					X	X	XX	X	X	XX	X	X
1 Mile								XX	X	X	X	X
1¼ Mile										X	X	X

BOYS' 12-WEEK JOGGING SCHEDULE

Distance	1	2	3	4	5	6	7	8	9	10	11	12
660 Yards	XX	XX	X	X								
880 Yards	XXX	XX	XX	X	X	X	X					
1320 Yards		X	XX	X	XX	X	X	X	X	X	X	X
1 Mile				XX	X	XX	X	X	XX	X	X	X
1¼ Mile					X	X	XX	X	X	XX	X	X
1½ Mile								XX	X	X	X	X
1¾ Mile										X	X	X

Swimming Program

Level 1: 15 minutes aquatic exercise

1. Side Straddle Hop
Standing in waist-to-chest deep water with hands on hips, swimmer:
(1) Jumps sideward to position with feet approximately 2 feet apart.
(2) Recovers. Repeat for 15 seconds.

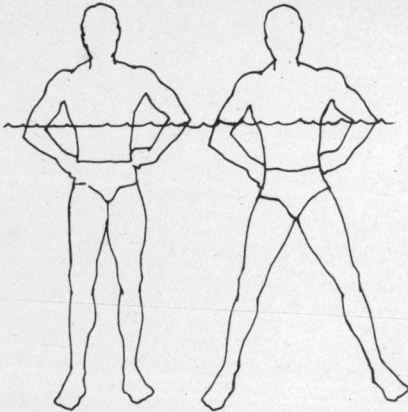

2. Walking Twists
With fingers laced behind neck, swimmer:
(1) Walks forward, bringing up alternate legs, twisting body to touch knee with opposite elbow. Repeat for 15 seconds.

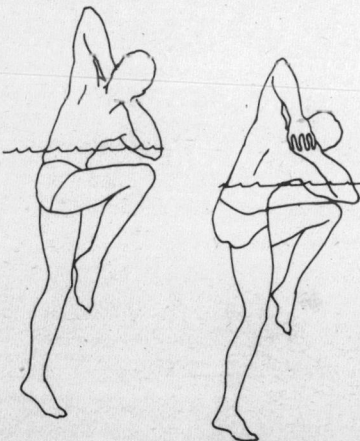

3. Standing Crawl
Standing in waist-to-chest deep water, swimmer:
(1) Simulates the overhand crawl stroke by:
(a) Reaching out with the left hand, getting a grip on the water, pressing downward and pulling, bringing the left hand through to the thigh.
(b) Reaching out with the right hand, etc. Repeat for 30 seconds.

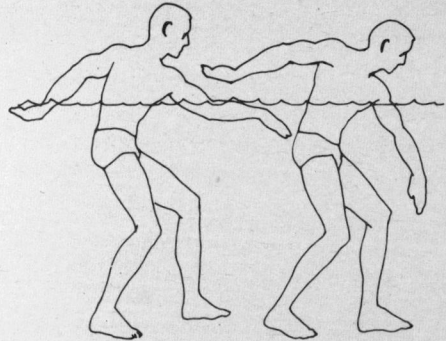

4. Toe Bounce
Standing in waist-to-chest deep water with hands on hips, swimmer:
(1) Jumps high with feet together through a bouncing movement of the feet. Repeat for 15 seconds.

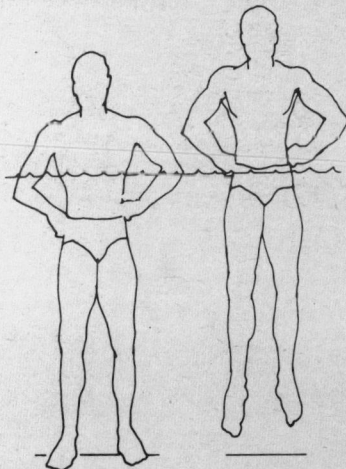

5. Flat Back

Standing at side of pool in waist-to-chest deep water, swimmer:

(1) Presses back against wall, holding for six counts.

(2) Relaxes to starting position. Repeat for 15 seconds.

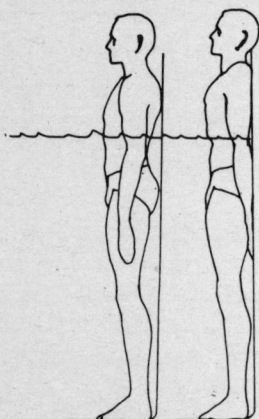

6. Pull and Stretch

At side of pool, back against wall, swimmer:

(1) Raises left leg and clasps shin with both arms pulling leg vigorously to the chest.

(2) Recovers to starting position.

(3) Raises right leg and clasps shin with both arms, pulling leg vigorously to the chest.

(4) Recovers to the starting position. Repeat for 30 seconds.

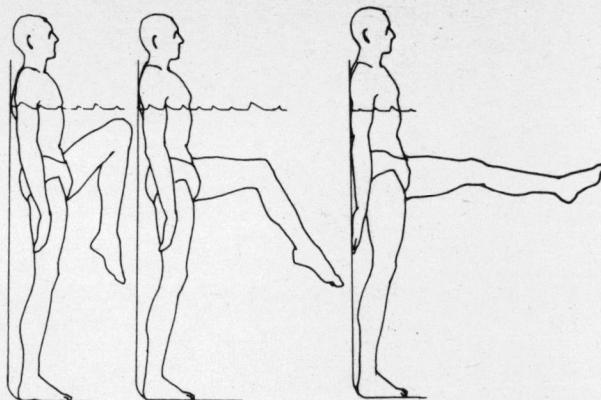

7. Leg Out

Standing at side of pool with back against wall, swimmer:

(1) Raises left knee to chest.

(2) Extends left leg straight out.

(3) Stretches leg.

(4) Drops leg to starting position. Repeat. Reverse to right leg. Repeat for 30 seconds.

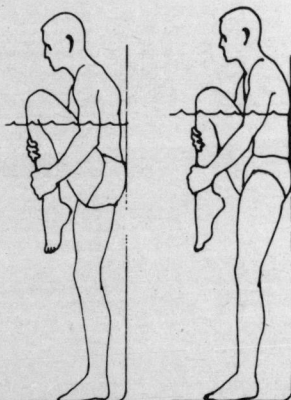

8. Front Flutter Kicking

Lying in a prone position and holding onto side of pool with hand(s), swimmer:

(1) Kicks flutter style in which toes are pointed back, ankles are flexible, knee joint is loose but straight and the whole leg acts as a whip.

(2) Do for 30 seconds.

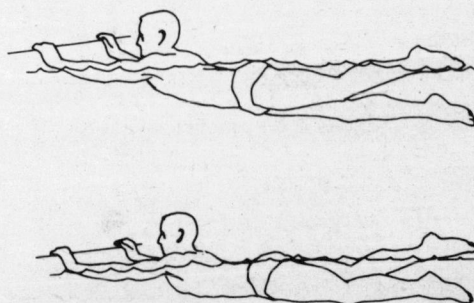

9. *Back Flutter Kicking*

Lying in a supine position and holding onto sides of pool with hand(s), swimmer:

(1) Flutter kicks for 30 seconds.

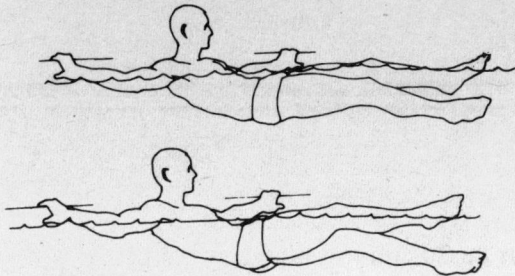

10. *Alternate Leg Rearward Bobbing*

Standing in shallow water, swimmer:

(1) Takes a breath.

(2) Submerges in shallow water with left leg in a squatting position with left foot on the pool bottom and right leg extended rearward. Exhales during (2) and (3).

(3) Shoves up off the bottom reversing the position of the legs, inhaling when the head is out of water.

(4) Submerges with right leg in a squatting position with right foot on pool bottom and left leg extended rearward. Exhales during the action.

(5) Repeat (1), (2), (3) and (4) for 60 seconds.

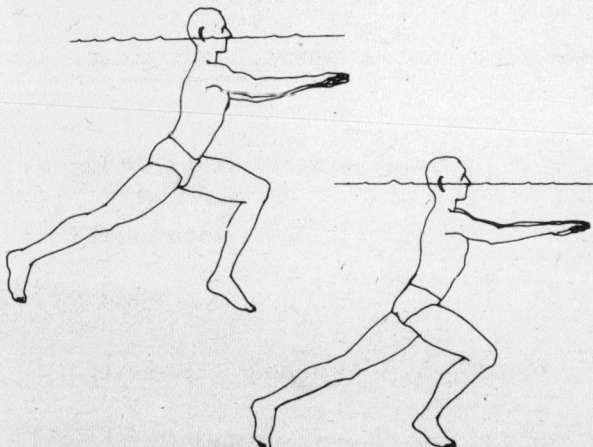

11. *Leg Swing Outward*

Standing with back against poolside, and hands sideward holding gutter, swimmer:

(1) Raises left foot as high as possible with leg straight.

(2) Swings foot and leg to left side.

(3) Recovers to starting position by pulling left leg vigorously to right. Reverses to right leg and repeats. Repeat for 30 seconds.

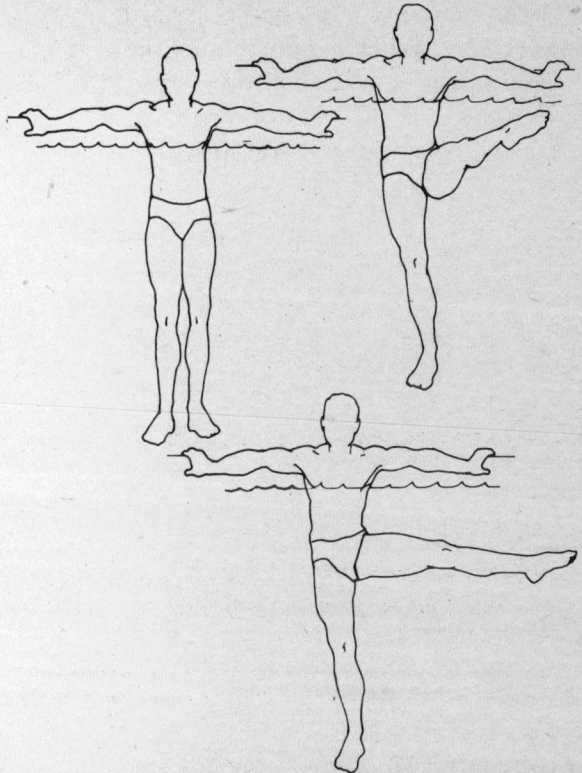

12. Bounding in Place (With Alternate Arm Stretch Forward)

Standing in waist-deep water, swimmer:

(1) Bounds in place with high knee action; right arm outstretched far forward when left knee is high, and the left arm and hand stretched rearward.

(2) When right knee is high, outstretches the left arm and hand forward, with the right arm and hand stretched rearward.

Special Note: When the position of the arm and hand are reversed, pull down and through with hand simulating the propulsion of the crawl stroke. Repeat for 30 seconds.

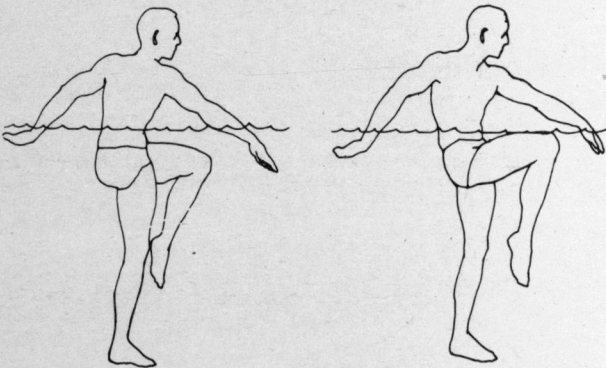

13. Elementary Treading

In water deep enough that toes will not touch bottom, in a perpendicular position, swimmer:

(1) Sculls or fins as he kicks bicycle, scissors, or frog style.

(2) Tread for 30 seconds.

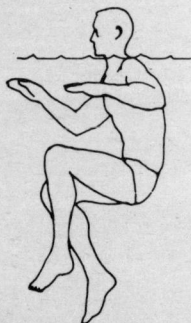

14. Lap Swimming

Use any one of the five basic swimming strokes described in Chapter 4. Using the interval training method, swim one lap, walk back to starting point, swim one lap, etc. Continue this for 9 minutes.

Level 2: 20 minutes aquatic exercise

1. Stride Hop

Standing in waist-to-chest deep water with hands on hips, swimmer:

(1) Jumps, with left leg forward and right leg back.

(2) Jumps, changing to right leg forward and left leg back. Repeat for 15 seconds.

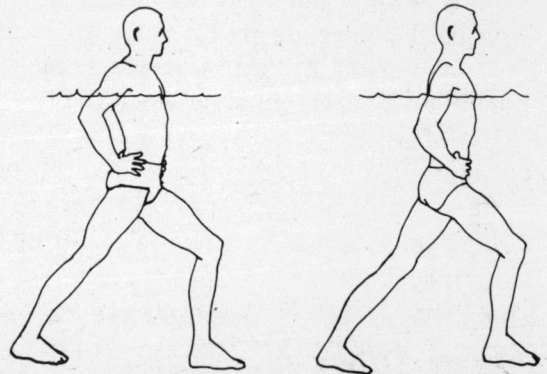

2. Standing Crawl — 30 seconds. (See **Level 1.**)

3. Front Flutter — 1 minute. (See **Level 1.**)

4. Back Flutter — 1 minute. (See **Level 1.**)

5. Front Flutter — 1 minute. (See **Level 1.**)

6. Pull and Stretch — 30 seconds. (See **Level 1.**)

7. Leg Swing Outward — 1 minute. (See **Level 1.**)

8. Advanced Bobbing
Treading in deep water, swimmer:
(1) Assumes a vertical position with hands extended outward from the sides, just under the surface of the water, with palms turned downward. Legs are drawn in a position of readiness for a frog or scissors kick.
(2) Executes kick as hands are pulled sharply to thighs and legs. (As a result of this action, the head and shoulders rise out of the water and a deep breath is taken at the highest point reached.)
(3) As the body sinks, the arms are outstretched overhead and swimmer exhales. Repeats (1), (2) and (3) for 1 minute.

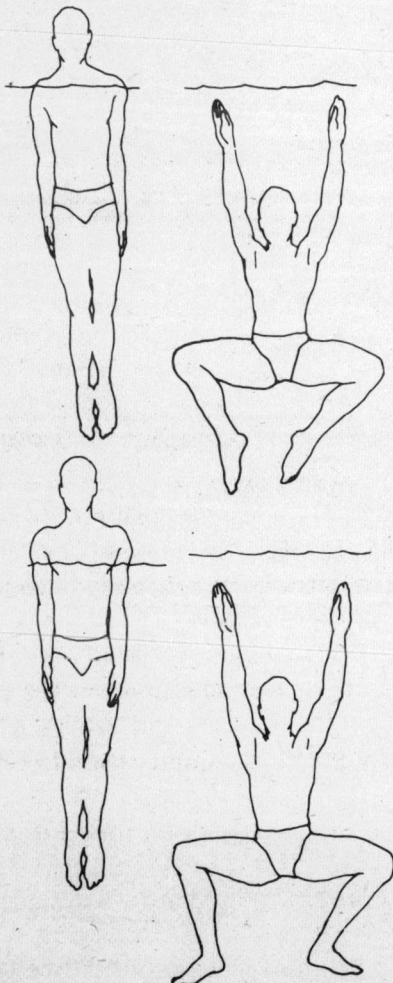

9. Left Knee Up, Back
Assuming a supine position, swimmer:
(1) Sculls, drawing left knee up to chest with right leg extended and toes on the right foot out of water.
(2) Sculls straightening the left leg, thus returning to the starting position. Repeat for 30 seconds.

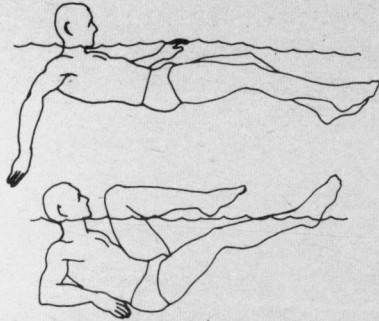

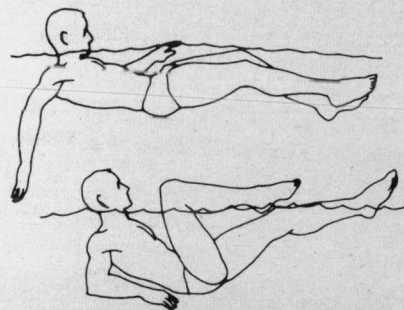

10. Right Knee Up, Back
Assuming a supine position, swimmer:
(1) Sculls, drawing right leg up to chest with left leg extended and toes on the left foot out of water.
(2) Sculls, straightening the right leg, thus returning to the starting position. Repeat for 30 seconds.

11. Alternate Leg Rearward Bobbing — 30 seconds. (See **Level 1.**)

14. Bounding in Place (With Arm Stretch) — 45 seconds. (See **Level 1.**)

---

12. Knees Up, Back
Starting from a back-lying position, swimmer:
(1) Sculls, drawing knees up to chest.
(2) Sculls, shoving legs forward, returning to a back-lying position. Repeat for 30 secs.

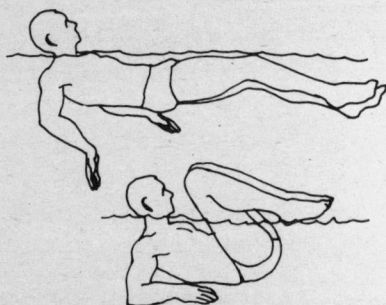

15. Knees Up, Front
Starting from a front-lying position, swimmer:
(1) Sculls, drawing knees up to chest.
(2) Sculls, shoving legs backward, returning to the front-lying position. Repeat for 30 seconds.

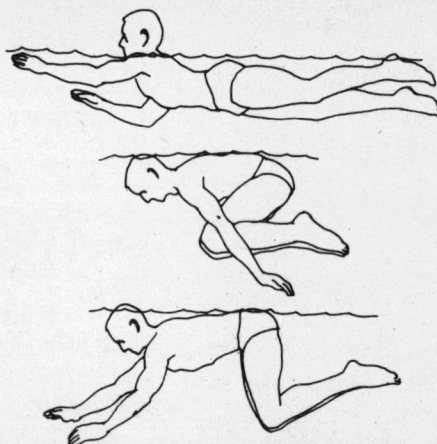

---

13. Alternate Leg Sideward Bobbing
In waist-to-chest deep water, swimmer:
(1) Takes a breath.
(2) Submerges with left leg in a full squatting position, left foot on pool bottom and right leg extended sideward.
(3) Shoves up off bottom, reversing the position of the legs and inhaling when the head is out of water.
(4) Submerges with the right leg in a full squatting position with the right foot on pool bottom and the left leg extended sideward. Repeat for 30 seconds.

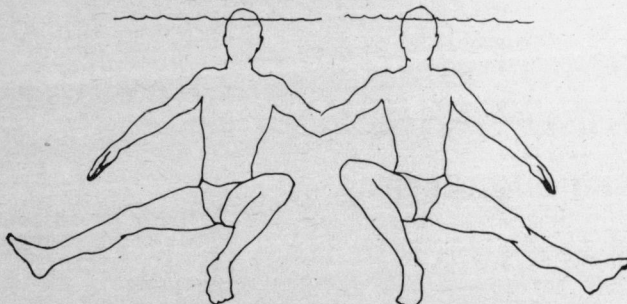

16. Advanced Bobbing — 1 minute. (See Exercise 8 **Level 2.**)

17. Reverse Sides Extension
Starting from a vertical position, swimmer:
(1) Sculls, drawing knees up to chest, shoving legs to left side causing body to be in a right sidestroke position.
(2) Sculls vigorously, drawing knees up to chest and reversing position, shoving legs to the right side, shifting body to a left sidestroke position. Repeat for 30 seconds.

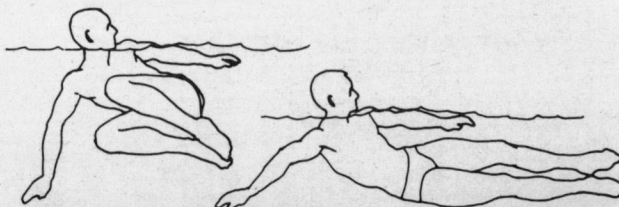

18. Lap Swimming
Use any one of the five basic swimming strokes described in Chapter 4. Using the interval training method, swim one lap, jog back to starting point, swim one lap, etc. Continue this for 6½ minutes.

Level 3 — 30 minutes aquatic exercise

1. Front Flutter — 2 minutes. (See **Level 1.**)

2. Back Flutter — 2 minutes. (See **Level 1.**)

3. Front Flutter — 1 minute (See **Level 1.**)

4. Alternate Leg Rearward Bobbing — 1 minute. (See **Level 1.**)

5. Knees Up, Front — 1 minute. (See **Level 2.**)

6. Knees Up, Back — 1 minute. (See **Level 2.**)

7. Alternate Leg Sideward Bobbing — 1 minute. (See **Level 2.**)

8. Front and Back Extensions
Starting from a vertical position, swimmer:
(1) Sculls, drawing knees up to chest, shoving legs forward coming up to a back-lying position.
(2) Sculls, drawing knees up to chest, shoving legs backward coming to a front-lying position. Repeat for 1 minute.

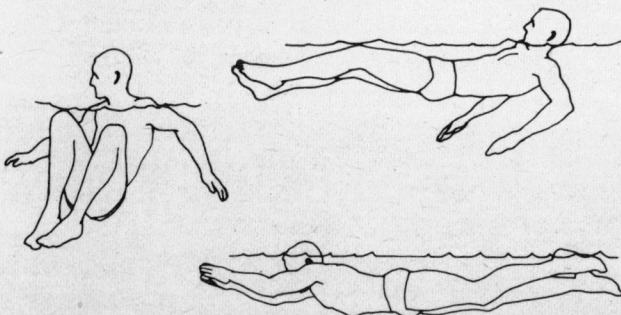

9. High Bobbing
In water approximately 1 to 3 feet over swimmer's head, swimmer:
(1) Takes a vertical position, hands extended outward from the sides with palms turned downward. Legs drawn in for frog kick.
(2) Simultaneously pulls hands sharply to thighs with legs executing frog kick.
(3) Inhales at peak of height.
(4) Drops with thrust of arms downward with palms turned upward until feet reach bottom of the pool and tucks to a squat position. Exhales throughout this action.
(5) Jumps upward with power leg thrust at the same time pulling arms in a breast stroke position downward, causing the head and shoulders to rise high out of water.
(6) Repeats cycles (4) and (5) for 3 minutes.

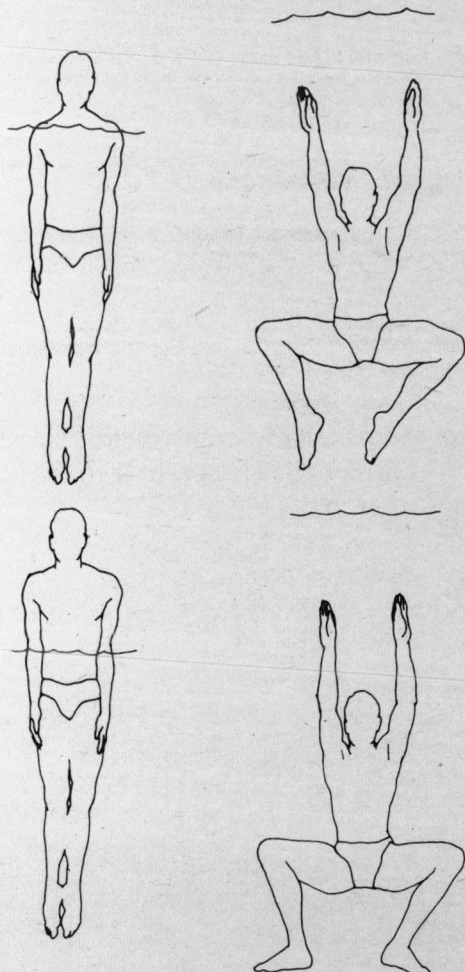

10. Reverse Side Extensions — 1 minute. (See
Level 2.)

11. Progressive "Bunny Hop" Bobbing
Standing, swimmer:
(1) Takes a breath.
(2) Submerges in a tuck or full squatting position with feet on the pool bottom.
(3) Pushes up and forward off bottom of pool,
exhaling during (2) and (3).
(4) Inhales with head out of water.
(5) Repeat for 2 minutes.

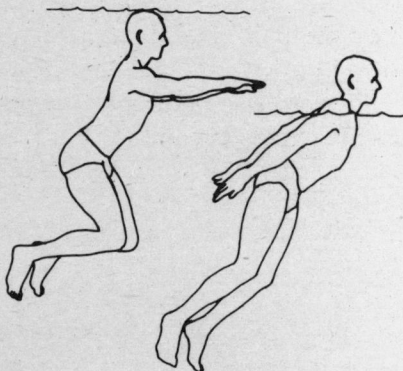

12. Rub-A-Dub-Dub
Starting from a back-lying position in water,
swimmer brings knees to chest with knees and
toes together and:
(1) Spins in a circle by using an opposite scul-
ling motion of hands.
(2) After one full turn, reverses action.

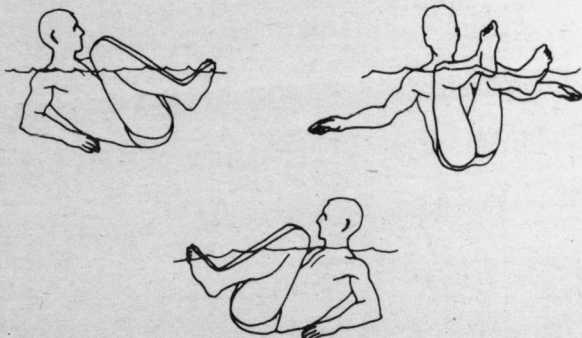

13. Left Leg Raiser
Starting from a back-lying position, swimmer:
(1) Sculls continuously, bringing left knee to
chest until lower leg is nearly parallel to the
surface of the water.
(2) Sculls, straightening the left leg so that the
left leg is perpendicular to the water surface.
(3) Returns to (1), the left knee to chest position.
(4) Returns to back-lying position. Repeat for
15 seconds.

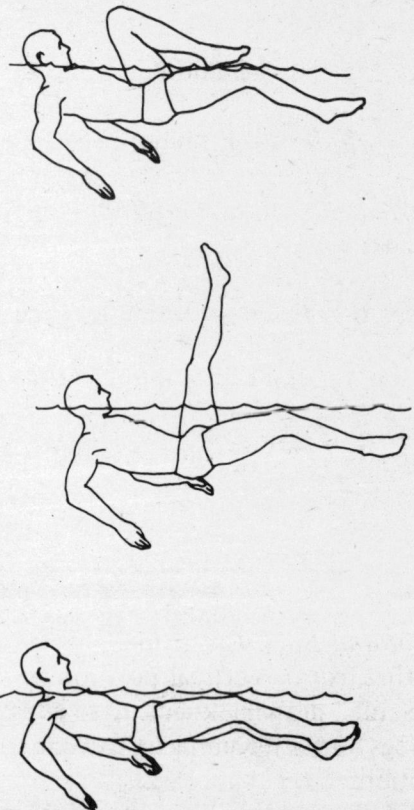

14. *Right Leg Raiser*

Starting from a back-lying position, swimmer:

(1) Sculls continuously, bringing right knee to chest until lower leg is nearly parallel to the surface of the water.

(2) Sculls, straightening the right leg so that the right leg is perpendicular to the water surface.

(3) Returns to (1), the right knee to chest position.

(4) Returns to back-lying position. Repeat for 15 seconds.

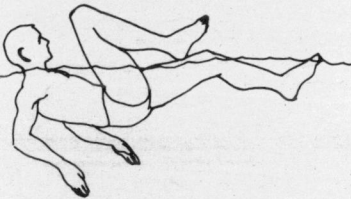

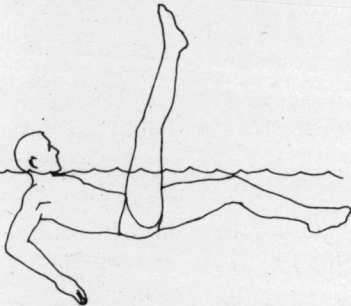

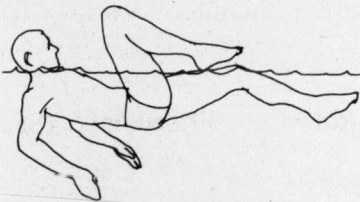

15. *Alternate Leg Raiser*

Starting from a back-lying position, swimmer:

(1) Sculls continuously, bringing left knee to chest until thigh is nearly perpendicular to the surface of the water.

(2) Sculls, straightening the left leg so that the left leg is perpendicular to the water surface.

(3) Returns to (1), the left knee to chest position.

(5) Sculls continuously, bringing right knee to chest until thigh is nearly perpendicular to the surface of the water.

(6) Sculls, straightening the right leg so that the right leg is perpendicular to the water surface.

(7) Returns to (5), the right knee to chest position.

(8) Returns to back-lying position. Continue alternating left and right action for 30 seconds.

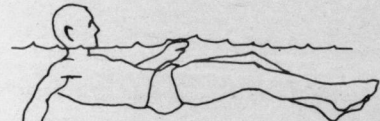

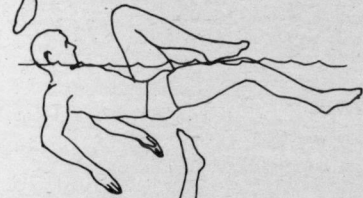

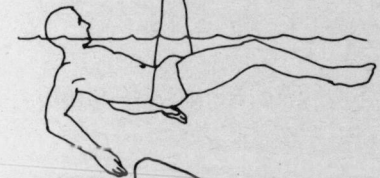

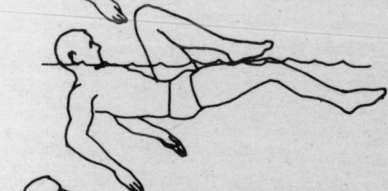

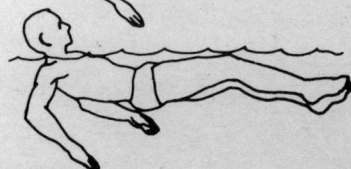

16. High Bobbing — 1 minute. (See Exercise 9, **Level 3**)

17. Lap Swimming
Use any one of the five basic swimming strokes described in Chapter 4. Using the interval training method, swim one lap, jog back to the starting point, swim one lap, etc. Continue this for 10 minutes.

Level 4 — 60 minutes aquatic exercise

1. Front Flutter — 3 minutes. (See **Level 1**.)

2. Back Flutter — 3 minutes. (See **Level 2**.)

3. Advanced Bobbing — 3 minutes. (See **Level 2**.)

4. Left Knee Up, Back — 1 minute. (See **Level 2**.)

5. Right Knee Up, Back — 1 minute. (see **Level 2**.)

6. Knees Up, Back — 1 minute. (See **Level 2**.)

7. High Bobbing — 3 minutes, (See **Level 2**.)

8. Knee Up, Front — 1 minute. (See **Level 2**.)

9. Alternate Leg Rearward Bobbing — 2 minutes. (See **Level 1**.)

10. Front and Back Extensions — 2 minutes. (See **Level 3**.)

11. Alternate Leg Sideward Bobbing — 2 minutes. (See **Level 2**.)

12. Reverse Side Extensions — 2 minutes. (See **Level 2**.)

13. Bounding in Place with Arm Stretch — 3 minutes. (See **Level 1**.)

14. Progressive Alternate Leg Forward Bobbing
Standing, swimmer:
(1) Rearward Bobbing (see **Level 1**), and moves forward the length of the pool for 3 minutes.

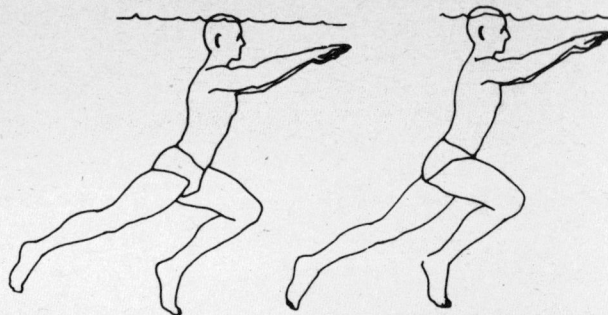

15. Rub-A-Dub-Dub — 3 minutes. (See **Level 3**.)

16. Left Leg Raiser — 30 seconds. (See **Level 3**.)

17. Right Leg Raiser — 30 secs. (See **Level 3**.)

18. Power Bobbing
Power bobbing is similar to "high bobbing" (see Level 3) except that at the top of the upward thrust the hands scull vigorously as the legs flutter kick. In "power bobbing" the swimmer will literally blast out of the water exposing all of body to the hips. Continue for 1 minute.

19. Alternate Leg Raiser — 30 seconds. (See **Level 3**.)

20. Bounding in Place with Arm Stretch — 3 minutes. (See **Level 1**.)

21. Toe Bounce — 90 seconds. (See **Level 1**.)

22. Leg Swing Outward — 2 mins. (See **Level 1**.)

23. Lap Swimming
Use any one of the five basic swimming strokes described in Chapter 4. Using the interval training method, swim one lap, jog back to starting point, swim one lap, etc. Continue this for 18 minutes.

FITNESS PROGRAM FOR THE SENIOR CITIZEN

The years in later life—particularly those of the post-retirement period—should be happy years. But the full promise of this stage of life comes only to those who are healthy, alert, and active. The later years can be truly rewarding if you have the energy and zest to use them well. The purpose of this exercise program is to help older Americans maintain—or regain—a lively way of life.

The way to *keep* lively is to *be* lively; the way to stay active is to move. Energy begets energy, and the only way to develop the capacity to expend more and more energy is to keep increasingly active.

It is nice to come into retirement with a bankroll of physical resources, just as it is comforting to have sufficient financial reserves. Some folks hit their 60's with plenty of bounce, having kept fit and active throughout their adult years. And this is an immense wealth to the older person.

Fortunately, even if you have let too many years slip by when good intentions of keeping fit were sacrificed to other demands of life, you still can pick up at *some level of physical performance* and work yourself up several notches. One of the objectives of this program is to bring you from your present level of fitness up to the point you would like to attain. The move upward will depend on the amount of movement you are willing and able to undertake.

The Importance of Exercise

Why strive in these later years for more "bounce to the ounce?"

Most medical authorities support the belief—and most active people experience the fact—that exercise helps a person look, feel, and work better.

Various organs and systems of the body, particularly the digestive process, are stimulated through activity and as a result work more effectively.

Posture can be improved through proper exercise by increasing the tone of supporting muscles. This not only improves appearance but can decrease the frequency of lower back pain and disability.

Physically active individuals are less likely to experience a heart attack or other forms of cardiovascular disease than sedentary people. And apparently an active person who does suffer a coronary attack will probably have a less severe

A mile a day! At the age of 88 Mrs. Eula Weaver jogs a mile a day, works out at the gym three times a week and pedals 10 miles before dinner on a stationary bicycle at her home.

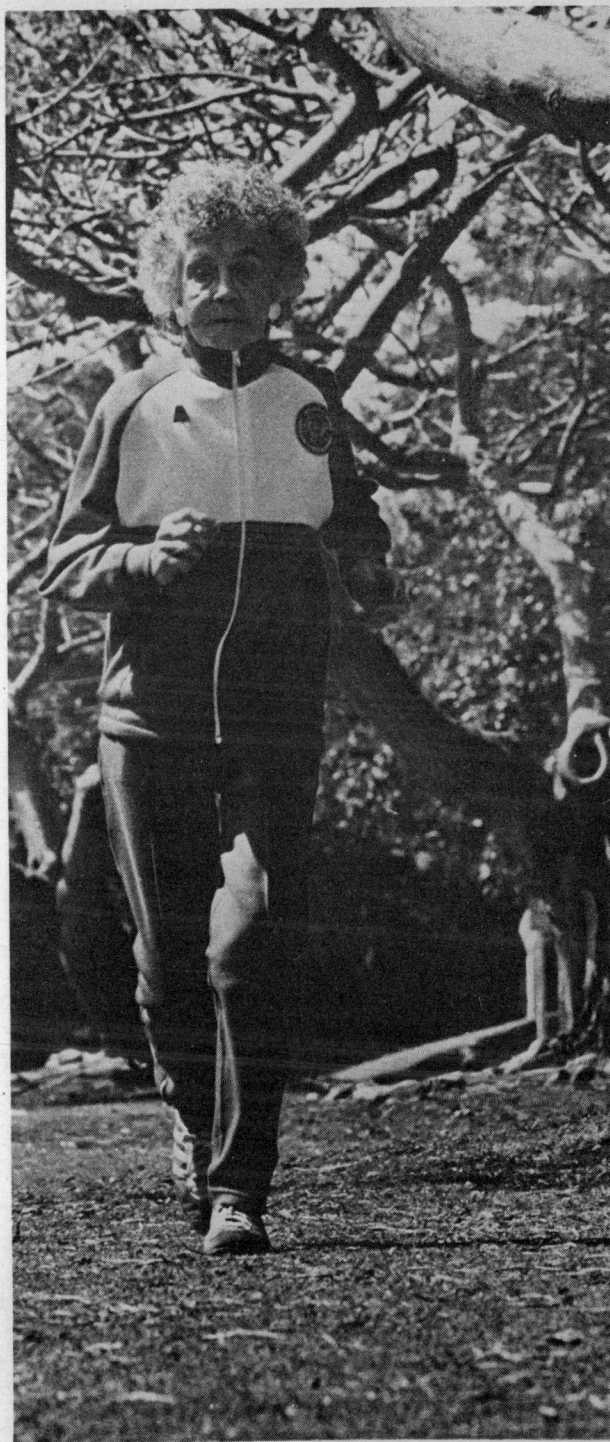

259

form and will be more apt to survive the experience.

Physical activity is as important as diet in maintaining proper weight. And being overweight is more than a matter of individual discomfort. It is related to several chronic diseases, shortened life expectancy and emotional problems. Medical authorities now recommend that weight reduction be accomplished by a reasonable increase in daily physical activity, supplemented, if necessary, by proper dietary controls.

Exercise can't prevent the stresses of life, but it can help you cope with them. For many individuals, frequent involvement in some sort of physical activity helps to reduce mental fatigue, tension, strain or boredom produced by our highly technical and sedentary way of life.

There is an advantage also in keeping fit and maintaining your physical capabilities to meet conditions caused by illness or accident. The person who has good control of his body and physical reserves is much better equipped to cope with such problems and to follow a rehabilitative program if he should have to do so.

The physically active and able person usually has a positive feeling about himself. He also possesses a degree of physical courage that propels him into interesting and stimulating experiences; moves with grace and ease; and generally presents a trim, attractive and self-confident bearing.

Perhaps the greatest benefit of maintaining physical fitness is the degree of independence it affords. This is a quality to be prized in the later years. There is a great psychological and financial advantage in having the ability to plan and do things without depending upon relatives, friends, or hired help. To drive your own car, to succeed with do-it-yourself projects rather than trying to find and pay someone else for the service, to go and come as you please, to be an aid rather than a liability in emergencies—these are forms of personal freedom well worth working for.

How Exercise Promotes Fitness

Efficiency and Endurance of the Heart and Lungs: The proper working of the heart, lungs, and blood vessels is probably the most important aspect of fitness in the adult years. Vital to good fitness are a strong and responsive heart that can

pump the blood needed to nourish billions of body cells, good lungs where gases of cell metabolism are exchanged for life-giving oxygen, and elastic blood vessels free of obstructions. Activities involving leg muscles maintain good circulation by the "squeezing" action of the muscles on the veins. This benefit cannot be achieved by any other means. More and more evidence from scientific research points to the importance of regular physical activity in maintaining good circulation and respiration.

Muscular Strength and Endurance: Muscles grow in size and strength only if they are used. They grow soft and flabby and lose their strength and elasticity if they are not used.

While strength does decrease with advancing years, the rate of decline can be lessened by keeping the muscles toned through regular exercise. Strength and endurance can be promoted by increasing the number of times an exercise is performed, by adding more weight or friction, and by increasing the speed of movement.

Balance: The balance mechanism of the body is commonly neglected and yet is extremely important in the fitness of older people. The balance mechanism is maintained through use and degenerates when not used.

Many older people tend to lose their sense of balance much more quickly than nature intended. The need to use bi-focal or tri-focal glasses increases the hazards for many. A well-maintained sense of balance can help make up for the problems caused by quick changes in vision from one optical focus to another.

Flexibility: The ability to move the joints through their normal range of motion is important, but here again the aging process and disuse cause the tissues surrounding the joints to increase in thickness and lose their elasticity. Moving the joints in a proper exercise program can delay this process. Exercise of the joints also helps slow down the onset or the development of arthritis, one of the most common and painful diseases associated with old age. Proper exercise that stretches the muscles can help keep them supple and prevent them from becoming short and tight.

Traditional "concern" for older people has perhaps done them a disservice. The idea has been to put the pushbuttons in easy reach, to keep the shelves low, to avoid necessity for bending and stretching. Instead, older people should be encouraged to bend, move, and stretch in order to keep joints flexible, muscles springy, and the heart feeling young.

Coordination and Agility: A well-coordinated individual should be able to direct parts of the body in skillful movement, to coordinate different actions with each other and with the eyes, to move and change directions quickly and safely.

Highly refined skills may not be essential in the later years. But for enjoyment of recreation and to keep in condition to move freely and safely, you should exercise regularly in order to maintain reasonably good levels of coordination and agility.

Principles of Exercise and Fitness Programming

Physical fitness can be improved by gradually increasing the amount of work performed, but it is necessary to progress in easy stages. The enthusiast who tackles a keep-fit program too fast soon gives up in discomfort, if not in injury.

While some activity has to be sustained to obtain major benefits, the "cumulative effect" of exercises and activities carried on during a period of time counts. For example, every movement uses calories, so the way to "burn up" calories is to move. And even though certain actions—such as a short walk—may not use many calories at the time, a number of short walks in the course of the day can use up a fair-sized total. Similarly, the benefits of movement to the organs, the joints, the muscles add up little by little.

Therefore, try to step up activity throughout your day, in addition to following specifically planned periods of exercise.

At all ages, but increasingly in later years, it is important to prepare your body for vigorous activity by "warming up." Any individual, and especially an older person, should definitely avoid suddenly undertaking a strenuous activity. A warm-up period should be performed by starting lightly with a continuous rhythmical activity such as walking and gradually increasing the intensity until your pulse rate, breathing, and body temperature are elevated. It is also desirable to do some easy stretching, pulling and rotating exercises during the warm-up period.

Periods of vigorous activity should be alternated with periods of lesser stress. "Put the

pressure on" for a while and then release it. By gradually increasing the stressful interval and reducing the less vigorous interval, you improve your physical condition. This principle of "interval training" is particularly adaptable to walking, jogging, and swimming.

The proper way to advance in strength and physical condition is to put increasing workloads on your system. This is called the "overload principle." Challenge yourself little by little toward improved performance by increasing the amount of exercise performed or the speed at which you perform it. For example, if you repeat an exercise, five times, a certain amount of work has been done and value derived. The next step is to perform the exercise six times, and then gradually increase the count until you can do it, say, 10 times with ease.

Unless the overload principle is employed, only minimal gains will be achieved. This is why it is important to follow a graduated, progressive schedule. This principle applies to the circulatory system as well as to the voluntary muscles. To increase the efficiency of the heart and lungs, the performance of continuous rhythmic exercise for a period long enough to stress the circulatory system is recommended—brisk walking, jogging, bicycling, swimming, rope skipping, or the like. Action should be increased until it can be sustained hard and long enough to keep the pulse rate above 130 for several minutes and to increase the body temperature gradually to the point of perspiration. Programs that promise "fitness" in a minute a day are more than inadequate in their effect on circulation. So, too, are the traditionally recommended activities for the elderly, such as puttering in the garden or taking a leisurely stroll.

Exercise is, of course, only one facet of the active and physically fit life. Medical and dental care, proper diet, sufficient rest, and other good health practices are all important and part of the "balanced life."

However, since this section is concerned with physical activity, it begins with exercise. Other health matters are discussed briefly later on. Now—to work!

Your Exercise Program—Level 1, Level 2, or Level 3?

In this " reasonable" exercise program

planned for you, there are three series of exercises, graded according to their difficulty or the amount of stress involved. They are identified as Level 1, Level 2, and Level 3, with 1 the easiest, 2 next, and 3 the most difficult and sustained. They let you start where you should, and they provide for an easy progression as you improve your physical condition.

Each of these three exercise programs is designed to give you a balanced workout, utilizing all major muscle groups. Performing your program regularly will lead to improvement in the various components of physical fitness, especially in the functioning of the heart and lungs.

As you grow proficient at the exercises in your program, you should increase the number of repetitions of certain exercises, and increase the duration and speed of walking and jogging.

As you become able to increase the number of repetitions and handle more complicated and demanding exercises, you can move up to the next level with new confidence and a growing feeling of well being.

Which Series?

How do you know where to start? Are you at Level 1, Level 2, or Level 3?

First, you should ask your physician for advice. Discuss your plans with your own doctor (or public health clinic physician) and follow his recommendations. Take this book along to show him. Ask him to review the program recommended here and to advise you accordingly. Also give yourself the following simple tests to determine your present condition and your exercise tolerance. In other words, find out just what kind of shape you are in.

The tests will help you select your appropriate exercise level and pace. Keep in mind that there are wide variations in physical performance. Your own individual physical condition must dictate your personal exercise program.

Pre-exercise Tests

Check yourself in easy stages. First, try the walk test below.

Walk Test: The idea behind this walk test is to determine how many minutes, up to 10, you can walk briskly, without undue difficulty or discomfort, on a level surface. Test yourself outdoors preferably, but walking around indoors will do.

If you can finish 3 minutes, but no more, you should begin your daily exercise program with **Level 1.**

If you can go beyond 3 minutes, but not quite to 10 minutes, you can warm-up at **Level 1** for a week or two, and then move up to **Level 2.**

If you can breeze through the whole 10 minutes, you are ready for bigger things. Rest a while, or wait until the next day, and then take "Walk-Jog Test #1."

One note of caution: If at any time during the Walk Test you experience any trembling, nausea, extreme breathlessness, pounding in the head or pain in the chest, STOP immediately. These are signs that you have reached your present level of exercise tolerance. Start your keep-fit program at the corresponding level described in relation to this test. If these symptoms persist beyond a point of temporary discomfort, check with your physician.

Walk-Jog Test #1: This test consists of alternately walking 50 steps and jogging 50 steps for a total of 6 minutes.

Walk at the rate of 120 steps per minute; that is, your left foot strikes the ground once each second. Jog at the rate of 144 steps per minute; your left foot hits the ground 18 times every 15 seconds. Time your walking and jogging intervals for 15 seconds occasionally to check your pace.

If you stop this test before the 6 minutes are up, plan your schedule of exercises at **Level 2.**

If you complete the 6-minute walk-jog test without difficulty, you can probably undertake **Level 3.** It might be well to warm-up for a week or two on the **Level 2** program first, however.

If you can perform this test without difficulty and feel you are capable of a more rigorous trial, rest a day, and then take "Walk-Jog Test #2.."

Walk-Jog Test #2: This test consists of alternately walking 100 steps and jogging 100 steps for a total of 10 minutes. Follow the directions and use the same rates of speed—walking and jogging—as for Walk-Jog Test #1.

If you complete this 10-minute test without difficulty, you can obviously handle the **Level 3** program and might want to consider going beyond it to the Adult Physical Fitness Programs on page 210.

If you do not complete the 10-minute walk-jog, better stay with **Level 3** for awhile, after warming up a few days on the Level 2 program.

Keep an Exercise Schedule

Now that you've tested yourself and determined where to begin, schedule a definite period for your basic exercises every day and stick with it.

This means setting aside 30 minutes to an hour a day for a planned program of physical activity. You should consider your exercises just as important as eating a proper diet or keeping clean.

General Directions—All Levels

The exercises in this program are not graded separately for men and women but are tailored to individuals. A couple can do the exercises together. More than likely, however, a man who has been active can start at a higher level or progress faster than most of the women who undertake the program.

Begin very easily and increase the tempo and number of repetitions very gradually. This will keep stiffness and soreness to a minimum. If you do get a little stiff during the first few days, don't let it slow you down; the stiffness will soon be overcome, and it is an indication that you needed the activity.

Follow the directions for your exercise exactly. If, for example, you are at Level 1 and a particular exercise should be performed only twice as a starter, stop after two repetitions—even though you may feel you can do many more. A warm-up is built into each exercise series. Therefore, the exercises should be performed in the order presented to give best results.

Keep a record of the exercises you perform, and how many times you repeat them. The little extra time required to keep a record of your activities and to set more challenging goals for yourself is well spent. A fitness program should be carefully designed and carefully followed. The best way to keep track of each day's performance is to write it down. The exercise schedules outlined in this section will be more beneficial to you if you keep good records.

One way of adding to the fun of your exercise program is to play music while you are exercising. You can select lively tunes and find music that fits the tempo of the various movements. This is particularly interesting when walking or jogging indoors. Some people also enjoy exercising while watching TV.

You can exercise with family and friends. Many groups get together in each other's homes or at a local center or club.

Wear comfortable clothing. Avoid tight-fitting, restrictive clothes, although, if you feel more comfortable wearing foundation garments, do so. Shorts or slacks, T-shirts or short-sleeved blouses are usually desirable. Wear well-fitting shoes with non-slip soles and low (or no) heels.

Specific Instructions for Individual Programs — Levels 1, 2, 3

Level 1 Program: Try to complete the entire sequence without undue rest periods between exercises, but, of course, rest awhile if you feel overtaxed. One indication of improvement in condition is the ability to go through the workout in less and less time (up to a point), which means doing the exercises at a faster cadence and resting shorter periods between exercises. However, never let the effort to increase speed cause jerky movements or otherwise interfere with correct performance of the exercise.

For the first week at least, perform only the smallest number of repetitions or shortest duration of time shown for each exercise under its illustration. If you find even this amount to be strenuous, or if you feel fatigued at the end of the week, do not increase the repetitions or duration but continue at the same pace for another week.

After the first week—or as you are ready—in each exercise where a range of repetitions is shown, increase the minimum by one. Do this number, but no more, the second week. (If you need to stay at the lowest count, as explained above, don't increase the count at all.) In the following weeks, gradually increase the number of repetitions as you feel you can. Most people should take 3 to 4 weeks to reach the highest counts in the Level 1 program.

After you reach the point where you can do the higher number of repetitions shown for each exercise, continue on Level 1 until you can complete the whole series without resting between exercises.

When you can do this for 3 days in a row, move on to Level 2.

Level 2 Program: When you are ready to undertake Level 2, proceed in a fashion similar to your Level 1 program. That is, start at the lowest frequency of repetitions and gradually work up.

Most people should remain at Level 2 for 3 to 5 weeks before moving to Level 3.

After you pass your "prove-out" test by performing all of the Level 2 exercises at the highest frequency shown without resting in between for three consecutive workouts, move on to Level 3.

Level 3 Program: Follow the same directions as for the Level 1 and 2 programs. Start slowly; step up activity gradually.

When you reach the upper limits of Level 3 exercises and can go through the workout without stopping on 3 straight days, you are ready to tackle bigger things. At this point you can: (1) continue with the exercises in this section, gradually increasing the number and speed of repetitions, the distances walked and jogged, and

also engage in more sports and recreational activities; or (2) proceed to the Adult Physical Fitness Programs for Men and Women on pages 210 to 230, which include more difficult exercises, and advance to its Level 1 without going through the Orientation Program.

Important Note: Most, but NOT ALL, of the exercises illustrated on the next pages are included in all three Exercise Programs; but the same order IS NOT followed in the three programs.

Do only those exercises included in your program level, as indicated.

Perform your exercises in the order indicated for your program.

Order of Exercises (Exercises* to be performed in the following order.)

Level 1 *Program Sequence*
Walk 2 minutes.
Bend and Stretch
Rotate Head
Body Bender
Wall Press
Arm Circles
Wing Stretcher
Walk 2-5 minutes
Lying Leg Bend
Angel Stretch
Walk-a-Straight-Line
Half Knee Bend
Wall Push-Away
Side Leg Raise
Head and Shoulder Curl
Alternate Walk (50 steps) Jog
(10) 1-3 minutes
Walk 1-3 minutes

Level 2 *Program Sequence*
Walk 3 minutes
Bend and Stretch
Rotate Head
Body Bender
Wall Press
Arm Circles
Half Knee Bend
Wing Stretcher
Wall Push-Away
Walk 5 minutes
Lying Leg Bend
Angel Stretch
Walk-the-Beam
(2-inch by 6-inch beam)
Knee Pushup
Side Leg Raise
Head and Shoulder Curl
(arms crossed on chest)
Diver's Stance
Alternate Walk (50) Jog (25) 3-6
minutes
Walk 1-3 minutes

Level 3 *Program Sequence*
Alternate Walk (50) Jog (50)
3 minutes
Bend and Stretch
Rotate Head
Body Bender
Wall Press
Arm Circles
Half Knee Bend
Wing Stretcher
Alternate Walk (50) Jog (50)
3 minutes
Leg Raise and Bend
Angel Stretch
Walk-the-Beam
(2-inch by 4-inch beam)
Hop
Knee Pushup
Side Leg Raise
Head and Shoulder Curl
(hands clasped behind neck)
Stork Stand
Alternate Walk (50) Jog (50)
5 minutes, gradually increasing
to walk 100 steps — jog 100
Walk 3 minutes

---

*Illustrations of each exercise and figures for number of repetitions or length of time to perform it are outlined. Where two figures are given, start at the lower figure; gradually increase the repetitions or duration over a period of days or weeks until you can perform the higher number.

Exercise 1

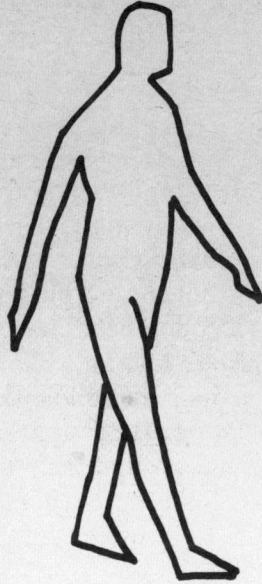

1. Walk
  Level 1: 2 minutes
  Level 2: 3 minutes

Starting position: Stand erect, balanced on balls of feet.

Action: Simply begin walking briskly on a level space, preferably outdoors, but walking around the room will do if necessary.

Value: A good warm-up exercise, loosening muscles, and preparing you for your full exercise schedule.

Exercise 2

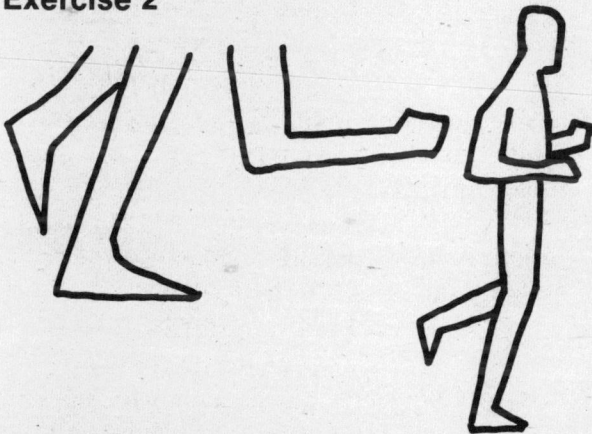

2. Alternate Walk-Jog
  Level 3: Level 3 only at this time. Alternately walk 50 steps and jog 50—for about 3 minutes.

Starting position: As for walking, arms held flexed, forearms generally parallel to the ground.

Action: Jogging is a form of slow running. Begin walking for 50 steps, then shift to a slow run with easy strides, landing lightly each time on the heel of the foot and transfer weight to the whole foot in flatfooted style. (Heel-toe running in contrast to the sprint form of running in which the runner stays on balls of his feet.) Arms should move loosely and freely from the shoulders in opposition to legs. Breathing should be deep but not labored to point of gasping.

Value: Good warm-up for more advanced exercises. Good for legs and circulation.

Exercise 3

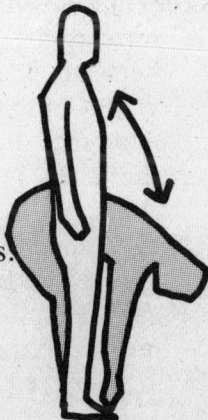

3. Bend and Stretch
  Level 1: Repeat 2 to 10 times.
  Level 2: Repeat 10 times.
  Level 3: Repeat 10 times.

Starting position: Stand erect, feet shoulder-width apart.

Action: Count 1. Bend trunk forward and down, flexing knees. Stretch gently in attempt to touch fingers to toes or floor. Count 2. Return to starting position.

Note: Do slowly, stretch and relax at intervals rather than in rhythm.

Value: Helps loosen and stretch most muscles of body; helps relaxation; aids in "warm-up" for more vigorous exercise.

Exercise 4

4. Rotate Head
 Level 1: Repeat 2 to 10 times each way.
 Level 2: Repeat 10 times each way.
 Level 3: Repeat 10 times each way.

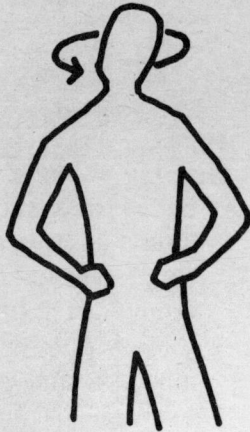

Starting position: Stand erect, feet shoulder-width apart; hands on hips.
Action: Count 1. Slowly rotate the head in a full circle from left to right. Count 2. Slowly rotate head in opposite direction.
Note: Use slow, smooth motion; close eyes to help avoid losing balance or getting dizzy.
Value: Helps loosen and relax muscles of the neck, and firm up throat and chin line.

Exercise 5

5. Body Bender
 Level 1: Repeat 2 to 5 times.
 Level 2: Repeat 5 to 10 times.
 Level 3: Repeat 10 times.

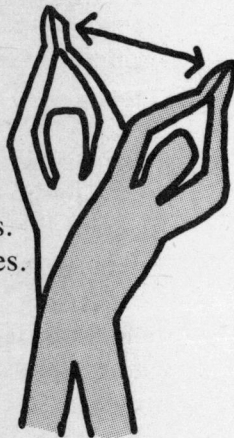

Starting position: Stand with feet shoulder-width apart, hands extended overhead, finger-tips touching.
Action: Count 1. Bend trunk slowly sideward to left as far as possible, keeping hands together and arms straight (don't bend elbows). Count 2. Return to starting position. Counts 3 and 4. Repeat to the right.
Value: Stretches arm, trunk and leg muscles.

Exercise 6

6. Wall Press
 Level 1: Repeat 2 to 5 times.
 Level 2: Repeat 5 times.
 Level 3: Repeat 5 times.

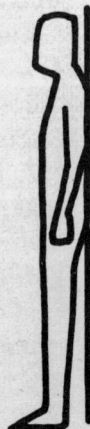

Starting position: Stand erect, head not bent forward or backward, back against wall, heels about 3 inches away from wall.
Action: Count 1. Pull in the abdominal muscles and press the small of the back tight against the wall. Hold for 6 seconds. Count 2. Relax and return to starting position.
Note: Keep entire back in contact with wall on Count 1 and do not tilt the head backward.
Value: Promotes good body alignment and posture. Strengthens abdominal muscles.

Exercise 7

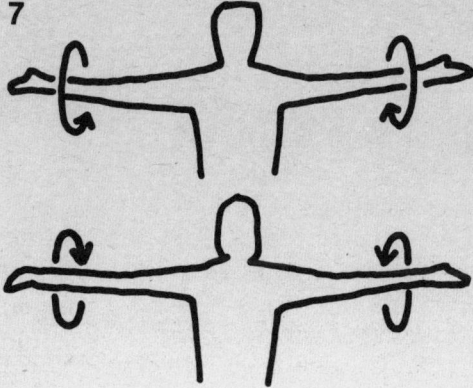

Starting position: Stand erect, arms extended sideward at shoulder height, palms up.

Action: Describe small circles backward with hands. Keep head erect. Reverse, turn palms down and do circles forward.

Value: Helps keep shoulder joint flexible; strengthens muscles of shoulders.

7. Arm Circles
  Level 1: Repeat 5 each way.
  Level 2: Repeat 5 to 10 each way.
  Level 3: Repeat 10 to 15 each way.

Exercise 8

8. Half Knee Bend
Level 1: Skip this exercise at this time.
Level 2: Repeat 5 to 10 times.
Level 3: Repeat 10 to 15 times.

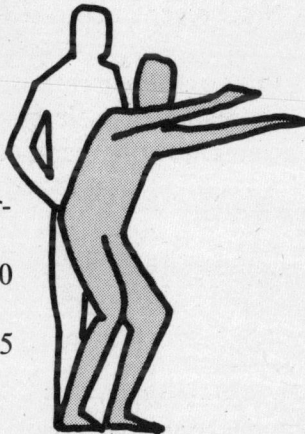

Starting position: Stand erect, hands on hips.

Action: Count 1. Bend knees halfway while extending arms forward, palms down. Keep heels on floor. Count 2. Return to starting position.

Value: Firms up leg muscles and stretches muscles in front of legs. Helps improve balance.

Exercise 9

Starting position: Stand erect, bend arms in front of chest, extended finger tips touching and elbows at shoulder height.

Action: Counts 1,2,3. Pull elbows back as far as possible, keeping arms at shoulder height and returning to starting position each time. Count 4. Swing arms outward and sideward, shoulder height, palms up and return to starting position.

Note: This is a bouncy, rhythmic action, counting "one-and-two-and-three-and-four."

Value: Strengthens muscles of upper back and shoulders; stretches chest muscles. Helps promote good posture and prevent "dowager hump."

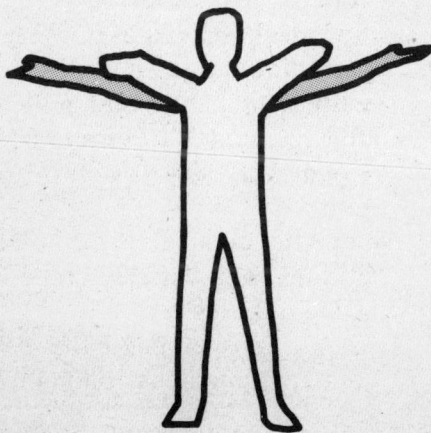

9. Wing Stretcher
  Level 1: Repeat 2 to 5 times.
  Level 2: Repeat 5 to 10 times.
  Level 3: Repeat 10 to 20 times.

NOTE:
Level 1: Now return to WALK (Exercise #1) and walk 2 to 5 minutes.
Level 3: Return to Alternate WALK-JOG (Exercise #2) and walk 50 steps, jog 50 for 3 minutes.

Exercise 10

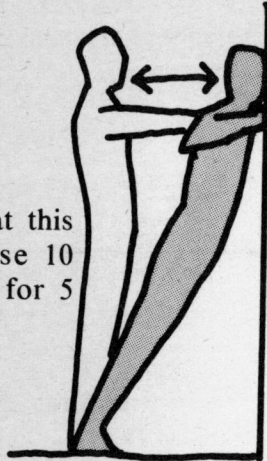

10. Wall Push-Away
Level 2: Level 2 only at this time. Repeat exercise 10 times. Then WALK for 5 minutes.

Starting position: Stand erect, feet about 6 inches apart, facing a wall and arms straight in front, palms on wall, bearing weight slightly.

Action: Count 1. Bend elbows and lower body slowly toward wall, meanwhile turning head to the side, until cheek almost touches the wall. Count 2. Push against wall with the arms and return to the starting position.

Note: Keep heels on floor throughout the exercise.

Value: Increases strength of arm, shoulder, and upper-back muscles. Stretches muscles in chest and back of legs.

Exercise 11

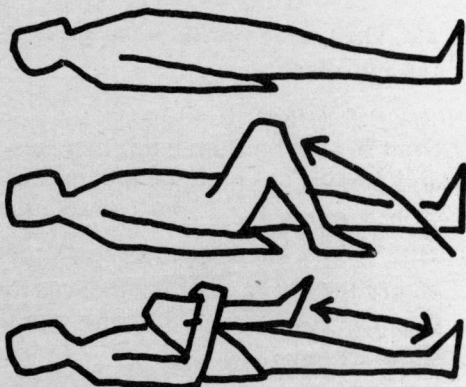

Starting position: Lie on back, legs extended, feet together, arms at sides.

Action: Count 1. Bend left knee and move left foot toward buttocks, keeping foot in light contact with floor. Count 2. Move knee toward chest as far as possible, using abdominal, hip, and leg muscles; then clasp knee with both hands and pull slowly toward chest. Count 3. Return to position at end of Count 1. Count 4. Return to starting position.

Note: After completing desired number of repetitions with left leg, repeat the exercise using right leg.

Value: Improves flexibility of knee and hip joints; strengthens abdominal and hip muscles.

11. Lying Leg Bend
Level 1: Repeat 2 to 5 times, each leg.
Level 2: Repeat 5 to 10 times, each leg.
Level 3: Skip this exercise.

Exercise 12

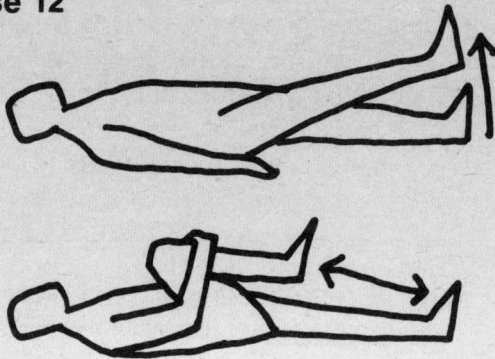

12. Leg Raise and Bend
 Level 3: Level 3 only. Repeat 2 to 5 times. After completing desired number with left leg, do exercise with right leg.

Starting position: Lie on back, legs extended, feet together, arms at sides.
Action: Count 1. Raise extended left leg about 12 inches off the floor. Count 2. Bend knee and move knee toward chest as far as possible, using abdominal, hip, and leg muscles; then clasp knee with both hands and pull slowly toward chest. Count 3. Return to position at end of count 1. Count 4. Return to starting position.
Value: Improves flexibility of knee and hip joints; strengthens abdominal muscles.

Exercise 13

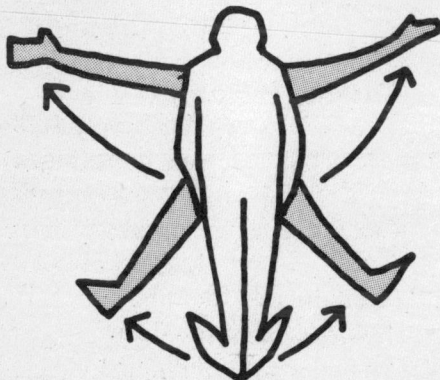

13. Angel Stretch
 Level 1: Repeat 2 to 5 times.
 Level 2: Repeat 5 times.
 Level 3: Repeat 5 times.

Starting position: Lie on back, legs straight, feet together; arms extended at sides.
Action: Count 1. Move arms and legs outward along the floor to a "spread-eagle" position. Slide—do not raise—arms and legs. Count 2. Return to starting position.
Note: Throughout the exercise, try to compress the lower back against the floor by tightening the abdominal muscles. Do not "arch" the lower back.
Value: Stretches muscles of arms, legs, trunk, aids posture; improves strength of abdominal muscles.

Exercise 14

14. Walk a Straight Line
 Level 1: Level 1 only. Walk for 10 feet. Levels 2 and 3 skip this, do Walk-the-Beam (#15) instead.

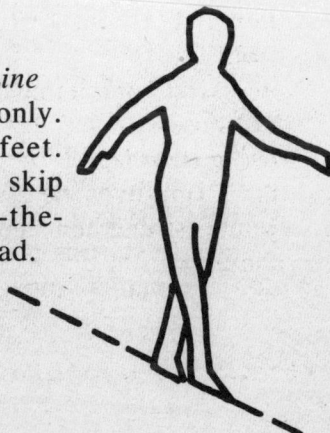

Starting position: Stand erect with left foot along a straight line. Arms held away from body to aid balance.
Action: Count 1. Walk the length of the straight line by putting the right foot in front of the left foot with right heel touching left toe, and then placing the feet alternately one in front of the other, heel-to-toe. Count 2. Return to the starting point by walking backward along the line, alternately placing one foot behind the other, toe-to-heel.
Value: Improves balance; helps posture.

Exercise 15

15. Walk the Beam

Level 2: Walk 10 feet on 2″ x 6″ board.

Level 3: Walk 10 feet on 2″ x 4″ board.

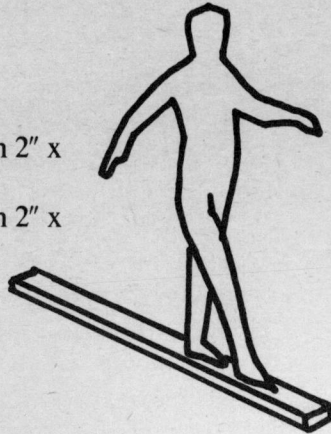

Starting position: Stand erect with left foot on board, long axis of foot in line with board.

Action: Count 1. Walk the length of the board by putting the right foot in front of the left foot with right heel touching left toe, and then placing the feet alternately one in front of the other, heel-to-toe. Count 2. Return to the starting point by walking backward along the length of the board, alternately placing one foot behind the other, toe-to-heel.

Note: The board is placed flat on the floor, not on the 2″ edge.

Value: Improves balance; helps posture.

NOTE: At this point in sequence:
Level 1: Perform Half Knee Bend (#8), repeating it 2 to 5 times; Wall Push-Away (#10), repeating 2 to 10 times; then skip #15, 16 & 17, moving to #18 next.

Exercise 16

16. Hop

Level 3: Level 3 only. Hop 5 times on each foot.

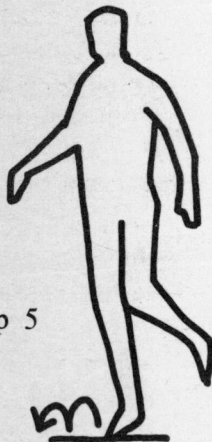

Starting position: Stand erect, weight on right foot, left leg bent slightly at the knee, and left foot held a few inches off the floor; arms held sidewards slightly away from the body to aid balance.

Action: Count 1. Hop on right foot, moving few inches forward each hop.

Note: Perform the desired number of hops on right leg, then change to left leg and hop.

Value: Improves balance, strengthens extensor muscles of leg and foot; increases circulation.

Exercise 17

17. Knee Pushup

Level 2: Repeat 1 to 3 times.
Level 3: Repeat 3 to 6 times.

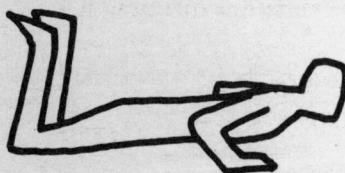

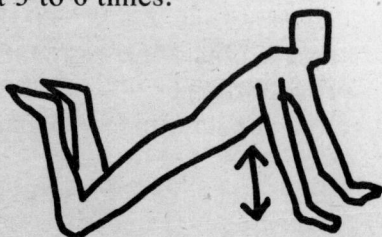

Starting position: Lie on floor, face down, legs together, knees bent with feet raised off floor, hands on floor under shoulders, palms down.

Action: Count 1. Push upper body off floor until arms are fully extended and body is in straight line from head to knees. Count 2. Return to starting position.

Value: Strengthens muscles of arms, shoulders and trunk.

Exercise 18

18. Side Leg Raise
  Level 1: Repeat 2 to 5 times each leg.
  Level 2: Repeat 5 to 10 times.
  Level 3: Repeat 10 times.

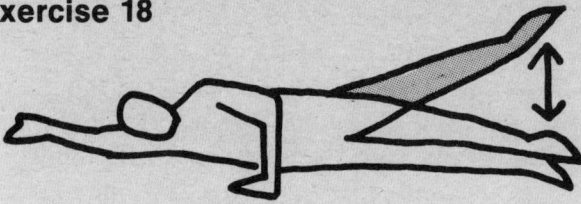

Starting position: Right side of body on floor, head resting on right arm. Count 1. Lift left leg upward about 30 inches off floor. Count 2. Return to starting position.

Note: Do the desired number of repetitions with the left leg and then turn over, lie on left side and exercise the right leg.

Value: Helps improve flexibility of the hip joint and strengthens lateral muscles of trunk and hip.

Exercise 19

19. Head and Shoulder Curl
  Level 1: Repeat 2 to 5 times; hold each for 4 seconds.

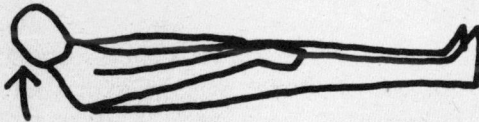

Starting position: Lie on back, legs straight, feet together, arms extended along the front of the legs with palms resting lightly on the thighs.

Action: Count 1. Tighten abdominal muscles and lift head and shoulders so that shoulders are about 10 inches off the floor. Meanwhile slide arms along legs, keeping them extended. Then hold the position for 4 seconds. Count 2. Return slowly to starting position, keeping abdominal muscles tight until shoulders and head rest on floor. Relax.

NOTE: LEVEL 1 skip Exercises #20, 21.

Exercise 19

19. Head and Shoulder Curl
  Level 2: Repeat 5 times; hold for 6 seconds.

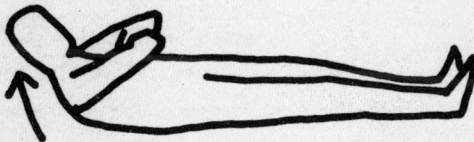

Same as Level 1 except on starting position arms are crossed over chest (kept in that position throughout).

Exercise 19

19. Head and Shoulder Curl
  Level 3: Repeat 5 times; hold for 10 seconds.

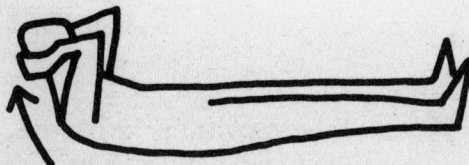

Same as Level 1, except on starting position, hands are clasped behind the neck (held that way throughout).

Note: The head should lead in a "curling" motion, chin tucked to chest, back rounded, not arched.

Value: Excellent for improving abdominal strength and stretching back muscles.

Exercise 20

20. Diver's Stance
   Level 2: Level 2 only; hold position for 10 seconds.

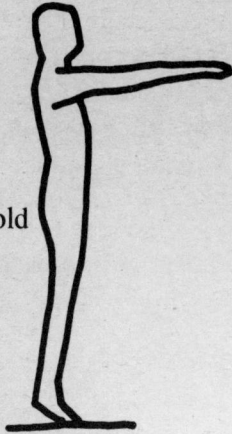

Starting position: Stand erect, feet slightly apart, arms at sides.

Action: Rise on toes and bring arms upward and forward so that they extend parallel with the floor, palms down. When this position is attained, close eyes and hold balance for 10 seconds.

Note: Head should be straight and body should be held firmly throughout.

Value: Improves balance; strengthens extensor muscles of feet and legs; helps maintain good posture.

Exercise 21

21. Stork Stand
   Level 3: Level 3 only; hold position 10 seconds on each leg.

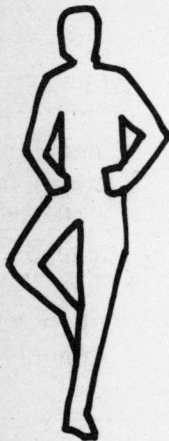

Starting position: Stand erect, feet slightly apart, hands on hips, head straight.

Action: Transfer weight to the left foot and bend right knee, bringing the sole of the right foot to the inner side of the left knee. When this position is reached, close eyes and hold for 10 seconds.

Note: After holding on left leg, change to the right leg and repeat.

Value: Improves balance.

Exercise 22

22. Alternate Walk-Jog (Repeats Exercise #2)
Level 1: Walk 50 steps, jog 10; 1 to 3 minutes.
Level 2: Walk 50 steps, jog 25; 3 to 6 minutes.
Level 3: Begin to walk 50 steps, jog 50, gradually increasing to walk 100 steps, jog 100. Continue for 5 minutes.

Value: Provides an "interval" of exercise for circulatory system, and for strengthening leg muscles.

Exercise 23

23. Walk
   (Repeats Exercise #1)
   Level 1: Walk 1 to 3 minutes.
   Level 2: Walk 1 to 3 minutes.
   Level 3: Walk 3 minutes.

Value: Tapering off, as heart rate, breathing, body heat, and other functions return to normal.

Alternatives to Your Daily Exercise Schedule

If you can enroll in a keep-fit program at the Y, at a school, or the local recreation center, you can skip your home-exercise routine on those meeting days.

If you are able to take part in a sport appropriate for your physical condition, by all means do so. Swimming is an excellent activity if you really swim. Take advantage of any opportunities you may have to swim regularly. Hiking, hunting, bicycling, tennis, or similar sports may sometimes be available to you.

On days when you can participate in such sports, you can substitute the sport for your home-exercise routine, or better still, add it to your day's activity. But make sure, if you substitute it, that the exercise involved in the sport is the equivalent of your regular workout. Incidentally, by doing your home exercises, you can keep in shape for an occasional opportunity to participate in a sport, and also help avoid soreness, stiffness, injury or over-fatigue.

Other active forms of recreation should be worked into your daily life whenever possible. Such activities as gardening, fishing, archery, horseshoes, ping-pong, shuffleboard, a family outing, an evening of social or square dancing are not only fun, but will also help you keep vigorous. Age need not be a barrier to participation. These activities should be added to—not substituted for—your daily exercise.

Stepped Up Daily Activities

To the Daily Exercise Schedule and your supplementary recreation add a little more action. Gradually, day by day, find ways to move more rather than less. Walk to the neighborhood store instead of driving (or being driven). Walk down a flight of stairs instead of taking the elevator; when you're back in shape, walk up the stairs.

In today's sedentary world, particularly the older person's world, you need to look for opportunities to move your body. Many well-meaning friends and relatives try to spare older people from any exertion. It is satisfying to be able to say: "Thank you, but I'd rather do it myself. I can, you know."

It is good to always have some active project underway—putting in a new flower bed, cutting wood, building a fence, painting a room, mowing the lawn, and a thousand other jobs and interests that keep you busy and youthful.

Special Notes on Exercise

Jogging: The fast-growing number of people who are jogging nowadays is good testimony to its value as a fitness-producing activity.

Jogging lends itself very well to the interval method of gradually increasing the stress of the activity. The main idea is to alternate walking and jogging bouts and to gradually increase the proportion of jogging to walking. In addition, the total distance covered can be gradually increased, as well as the speed with which the distance is traversed. However, the speed element is not emphasized beyond the point of getting a good workout within a reasonable time.

The walk-jog intervals outlined in the Level 1, Level 2, and Level 3 exercise schedules provide for easy progressions. If you can handle Level 3 fairly easily and wish to go forward with jogging, by all means do so. First work up both the walking and the jogging intervals simultaneously until you are ultimately walking 100 yards and jogging 100 yards (about the length of a city block). Then hold the walking interval constant at 100 yards, but gradually increase the jogging interval to 200 yards—or more as you feel ready. Also, gradually increase the total distance covered. There are many people around the country in their 60's and 70's who are jogging 2 to 5 miles daily. But don't set your goals this high unless you have gradually raised the distances jogged without experiencing severe reactions or extreme fatigue lasting for several days. Remember to "taper off" by walking the last interval and moving around until your breathing and pulse rate return to near normal.

It is important to wear the correct shoes and clothing while jogging. Clean, thick, well-fitting socks are a "must," and the shoes should also fit well and have soft, nonslip soles, with no heels. If gym shoes are worn, they should have a built-in arch support. Shoes made especially for jogging, having short rippled soles, are now being sold. Other clothing should fit so as not to restrict movement and should be sufficiently warm to protect the jogger on cool days. In cold weather, a cap and ear protectors, as well as gloves are often desirable. It is generally not advisable for older people to jog in midday during the summer.

273

Jogging is great for the circulatory system and the legs but does not provide a complete and balanced workout. Therefore, calisthenics or other conditioning exercises should be added to the jogging session each day. The exercises described in this section will serve this purpose very well.

Swimming and Water Exercises: Swimming is such a good activity it deserves special mention. It involves all the major muscle groups, can be adjusted from very mild to strenuous responses, and can be easily graded for progressive conditioning by gradually increasing the distances.

You can work out your own system of interval training. For example, swim across the pool, get out and walk around to the other side and repeat this procedure until your swimming trips across total a good distance. The next progression might be to swim the length of the pool and walk back, and so on. The workout can be varied by using different strokes to swim the intervals.

The buoyancy of the water makes it easier to do some exercises. Therefore, if your physical condition is such that you cannot do even some of the Level 1 exercises on land, find the ones that you can do in the water and get your workout that way. On the other hand, the water also causes resistance for certain other exercises. Use this medium as a way of increasing the workload.

Exercise Problems Due to Foot Conditions or Leg Pains: Problems with the feet, the legs, and the knee and hip joints are fairly common. Any problem of the lower extremities, be it bunions, arthritic knees, or varicose veins, may interfere with proper performance of some of the exercises outlined in this section, particularly walking and jogging.

If you have such a problem, first make sure that you have done all that you can do to obtain needed medical care.

Next, don't let your ailment sidetrack you in your determination to get fit. The following activities can be substituted for walking and jogging, and can provide healthful exercises.

- Swimming and water exercises.
- "Bicycling" movement, while lying on the floor, hips and legs in the air, supported by the arms and elbows. Do not try this if you think you will have difficulty supporting your weight.

- Riding a bicycle (choose a safe area).
- Exercising on wall pulley-weights or rowing machine.
- Passing a medicine ball with a partner while standing or seated—or bouncing the ball off a wall in continuous rhythmic movement.

Special Notes on Health

A program of physical fitness must, of course, include much more than exercise. It should begin with basic health considerations. Here are a few reminders:

Medical and Dental Supervision and Care: The importance of having continuing supervision by a physician and dentist cannot be overemphasized. Periodic checkups, at least annually, are the best form of preventive maintenance.

If you do not now have a personal physician, check on available health services with your local public health officer or the public health nurse who visits your neighborhood. If you cannot find a local public health person, ask at the closest hospital to you, or call the local medical society. Remember, it is not only important to find the physician and dentist, but it is even more necessary to follow their advice once it is given.

Remember also, your medical "advisor" should know your exercise plans before you start your program. And let him really advise you—follow his recommendations.

Diet and Nutrition: A good basic diet is necessary at all ages and does not change radically when one approaches age 60. Authorities recommend that the older person makes sure he gets the adequate nourishment provided by the four food groups. These groups and recommended daily servings are:

Bread and cereals
(4 or more servings)
Fruits and vegetables
(4 or more servings)
Meat, poultry, fish, eggs
(2 or more servings)
Dairy products
(2 or more cups of milk or its equivalent)

Overweight is a problem with many older persons and, therefore, the total number of calories consumed should be carefully adjusted according to individual needs. Because many persons become less and less active as they increase in years and tend to continue eating the same amounts, it becomes difficult for them to avoid getting heavy.

This is often the case even when they attempt to reduce their diet. Sometimes the energy expenditure is so low that they would have to go hungry most of the time to keep from growing fat. But to do this would be risking the loss of an adequate amount of certain vitamins and minerals necessary to maintain good health. Another reason for increasing your physical activity.

Some older people find that they become uncomfortable after eating a large meal. There is evidence to support the suggestion that it may be better to spread food intake over five or six small meals a day rather than the traditional three hearty meals. The total amount of food, however, should be considered in terms of the individual's daily need for calories and nutrients.

The matter of vitamin supplements or special adjustments in the diet for health conditions is for your physician to decide.

Sleep and Rest: There is some indication that as you grow older, you require more sleep or rest. The day's program should include rest periods. A nap in the afternoon is probably a good idea. Several rest periods or "cat naps" are particularly desirable for the person who usually sleeps less than 8 hours during the night.

Cigarette Smoking: The relationship of cigarette smoking to lung cancer, emphysema (a serious condition of the lung affecting breathing), bronchitis, and heart disease has been well established. The data show that the chances of developing these chronic diseases are related to the number of years a person has been smoking as well as the amount or number of cigarettes smoked. The evidence also indicates that it is possible to overcome some of the harmful effects. That is, the sooner a smoker stops and the longer he stays stopped, the better his chances of improved health.

Detrimental effects of smoking cigars and pipes are not as pronounced as in cigarette smoking—but the risk is greater than for nonsmokers. Also, the incidence of cancer of the lip and oral cavity is greater among those who use cigars and pipes.

The data call out loudly, "If you smoke, stop; if you don't smoke, don't ever start." By increasing the amount of daily exercise, you can help prevent an increase in weight that some people experience when they stop smoking.

Studies show that children are more apt to start smoking if their parents smoke—and probably if their grandparents do, too.

It's Up to You!

The exercises are here—their reasons and promises—goals and scores to keep. Now the rest is up to you. It won't be easy to get going, especially if you haven't been active for a long time. There is no easy way to fitness.

But once you get started, you'll begin to feel the benefits, and before long you will be looking forward to each day's activities. The self-discipline you must employ pays off in two ways—the act of overcoming the tendency toward a sedentary, self-pampering existence gives a psychological boost; and your activity opens the way to a more zestful and worthwhile life.

An eminent physician, commenting on the phenomenon of aging, has said: "Most of us don't wear out, we rust out." Disuse is the mortal enemy of the human body. We know today that how a person lives, not how long he lives, is responsible for many of the physical problems normally associated with advanced age.

This fitness program was prepared to help the elderly take advantage of the added years of life which medical science is making possible. It outlines methods for maintaining youthful health and energy, and it suggests ways of enhancing the enjoyment of leisure.

Advanced age need not mean inactivity or infirmity. For those who are physically and mentally active, it can be a time when long experience of life enriches each passing day.

PERSONALIZED FITNESS PROGRAMS

CIRCUIT TRAINING PROGRAM

Circuit Training was introduced by R. E. Morgan and G. T. Adamson at the University of Leeds in England with the purpose of motivating students to participate in conditioning programs. It utilizes the fact that when about two-thirds of a maximum number of repetitions are performed against a fixed resistance, you develop optimum strength and endurance. Morgan and Adamson start with a series of six to 10 exercises. At the start, the exerciser tries to achieve a maximum number of repetitions for each exercise. After the maximum number of repetitions for each exercise is established, it is cut by one-third.

The object becomes to complete the circuit of all the exercises in a progressively lessened amount of time. Falls, Wallis and Logan, in their book *Foundations of Conditioning,* cite a good example in a biceps curl exercise with 55 pounds of resistance. If the exerciser can perform 21 repetitions, the number of repetitions is decreased by one-third to 14 and the exercise is performed three times during the exercise period. In other words, once during each circuit, 14 repetitions of the biceps curl are performed. To intensify the biceps curl, the number of repetitions and the amount of resistance are increased.

Any assortment of exercises may be included in a circuit, but most authorities recommend eight essential exercises that are picked for all-over body improvement.

Circuit Training is based on the excellent idea of progressive body development. The program is so versatile that it can be fitted to location, exercise facilities, equipment and apparatus. A short circuit can be completed in 10 minutes, while a really comprehensive circuit may call for as much as 25 minutes. The program is flexible enough so that it can be tailor-made to fit any individual. Exercises within the circuit should be and usually are arranged in an order that insures active functioning of different muscle groups.

It's interesting to note that Circuit Training is employed by a great many college and university athletic coaches, the exercises incorporated into their schedules depending upon the sport being coached. Most professional athletic teams participate in Circuit Training for early season training and during the sports season. Theoretically, at least, they have a Circuit Training routine for the entire year, although coaches and trainers complain that their players don't always follow it. It can be said that Circuit Training, which started as a theory, has become practice.

A Circuit Training Exercise Program with Minimum Equipment

1. For circulorespiratory endurance: The Jumping Jack, which starts from the attention position. The exerciser hops with both feet, moving the feet sidewards from 2 to 3 feet. As this is being done, the hands are clapped together overhead, arms fully extended. On the second hop, the exerciser goes back to the starting position.
2. Run in Place: As described in the Adult Physical Fitness Program page 218.
3. Bench Stepping: 30 times in one minute. Step Test, page 14.
4. Scissors: Standing erect, legs in a striding position and hands on hips, the exerciser jumps and exhanges stride positions of the feet by scissoring the legs.
5. Pushups: As described in Chapter 3, page page 97.
6. Rowing: Start from flat on back position, arms extended overhead. Sit up and flex the knees fully. Lean forward and shove arms forward to rowing position. Return to starting position.

The number of repetitions depends on individual differences in physique and health. However, every exerciser should aim for intensity, repetition and duration. This routine benefits flexibility, muscle strength, muscle endurance and cardiovascular endurance and can be done almost anywhere.

Some people add weight-lifting to their Circuit Training programs, doing the power press, squats, two-arm curl, and rowing.

In over-all effectiveness, Circuit Training is superior to interval training, weight training, weight lifting, calisthenics and isometrics. It can contribute to every phase of physical fitness.

Circuit Training Prescription Chart

Instructions

For each of the programs proceed through the circuit, putting down the maximum load and repetitions for each exercise. Rest intervals may be taken after each exercise.

The maximum repetitions for each exercise go on the chart under Maximum Dose.

The Training Dose is two-thirds the Maximum Dose. For example, if the Maximum Dose is 24 repetitions, the Training Dose would be 16 repetitions.

The Target Time is a one-third reduction of the Total Time. The Target Time should be arrived at after the second session. The fitness condition of the exerciser should influence the number of laps.

The exerciser should then follow the program. When a Training Dose is completed in less than the Target Time, one repetition should be added to each exercise.

Cardiovascular Endurance

Exercises	Maximum Dose	Training Dose
1. *Straddle Hop*	_____	_____
2. *Run in Place*	_____	_____
3. *Bench Stepping*	_____	_____
4. *Scissors*	_____	_____
5. *Pushups*	_____	_____
6. *Rowing*	_____	_____

Circuit Laps _____
Total Time _____
Target Time _____

All-Over Fitness

Exercises	Effects	Maximum Dose	Training Dose
1. *Bench Stepping*	Hip and knee flexors	_____	_____
2. *Chinup***	Arm extensors, elbow flexors	_____	_____
3. *Side Twister***	Trunk flexors and extensors	_____	_____
4. *Pushups***	Arm flexors, elbow extensors	_____	_____
5. *Back Lift***	Trunk, head, neck extensors	_____	_____
6. *Heel and Toe** Raises	Calf, foot extensors	_____	_____
7. *Shoulder Curl‡*	Abdomen, endurance	_____	_____
8. *Leg Raiser†*	Thigh abductors	_____	_____

Circuit Laps _____
Total Time _____
Target Time _____

---

* See Chapter 2 for description of each of the exercises.
**See Chapter 3 for description of each of the exercises.
†See Adult Physical Fitness Program for description of the exercises.
‡See Fitness Program for the Senior Citizen for description of the exercises.

Weight Training Program

Exercises	Effects	Maximum Dose	Training Dose
1. *Situp***	Abdominal muscles	_____	_____
2. *Bicep Curl***	Bicep muscles	_____	_____
3. *Bench Press***	Arm and chest muscles	_____	_____
4. *Half-Knee Bend***	Hip, ankle and thigh muscles	_____	_____
5. *Bent Rowing***	Upper back muscles	_____	_____
6. *Triceps Extension***	Triceps	_____	_____
7. *Trunk Raise***	Lower back, hip, thigh muscles	_____	_____
8. *High Pull***	Shoulder muscles	_____	_____

Circuit Laps _____
Total Time _____
Target Time _____

_____

**See Chapter 3 for description of each of the exercises.

A MINIMUM-TIME PHYSICAL FITNESS PROGRAM FOR ADULTS

This program isn't designed to make you a professional athlete. Most programs are more strenuous. Some may get quicker results but will require much more time and effort during the process. It is not intended to build a super musculature that you don't really need.

Spending ½-hour or a little more a week, it goes through three 8-week periods.

Before you start, get approval from your doctor.

Then you begin with a few simple flexibility or "limbering" exercises, spending about a quarter of a minute on each one.

Flexibility Exercises

Exercise 1: Standing flat-footed, reach as close to the ceiling as you can get your right hand to go, so that you feel the stretch all the way down to your feet. Then drop the arm and repeat the exercise with the other arm.

Exercise 2: This is the familiar torso twist, done with the arms out to the sides, parallel to the floor, feet spread comfortably apart. Twist as far as you can go to the right and then reverse it and twist to the left.

Exercise 3: Sitting with knees bent, grip your hands together behind your knees and pull your shoulders as close to the knees as possible in an easy stretch.

Exercise 4: Bend your head forward with chin touching chest and turn your head as far to both sides as you can get it to go. Then reverse the process. Stretch the head backward and twist to either side.

It's not necessary to do these flexibility exercises more than two or three times a session.

Strength Exercises

Exercise 5: Standing a little farther than arms' length away from a wall, lean forward enough to put the palms of the hands against the wall. Then continue to lean forward until your chest is close to the wall. Push slowly away until you're back to starting position. Repeat this one 12 or 15 times a session.

Exercise 6: Reverse situps — this exercise emphasizes stress on the abdominal muscles that situps don't greatly affect. You sit with the knees drawn up to your chest, your feet hooked under a chair or davenport. You move the upper body backward, going back slowly as far as you can. Don't go any farther back than you think you can and still be able to come up to the starting position again. Repeat 12 or 15 times.

Follow this with 5 minutes of running in place, jogging or hopping from one foot to the other.

Each week, increase the intensity of the exercises, stretching more, working harder on the reverse situps and wall push.

Once you've developed some muscular strength, which you should be able to do in 7 or 8 weeks, increase the number of push-aways to at least double the number, but try to do them in the same length of time.

In doing the reverse situps, stop with your back about half-way toward the floor and hold the position for 10 to 12 seconds. Then with your body three-fourths of the way to the floor, stop and hold the position for 10 or 12 seconds again. Try to get so you can hold it a full 30 seconds.

Start jogging, running in place or hopping at the same rate as you were doing it, but maintain that rate for only 30 seconds. In the next 30 seconds, speed up.

In the third 30 seconds, slow down again. Keep alternating fast and slow for a full 6 minutes.

For the third period of progression, go to pushups. Then do a reverse situp with such tension that you can only hold it 5 or 6 seconds. You get that tension by extending your arms above your head as you start going back.

Then for your interval training cardiovascular pulmonary exercise, you alternate 15 seconds at slow speed and 15 seconds fast, for 8 minutes.

After the end of the second period, a maintenance program can consist of a minute of flexibility stretching, one to five wall pushes, one to five reverse situps, and anywhere from 2 to 10 minutes of cardiovascular pulmonary exercise.

A HOME FITNESS MAINTENANCE ROUTINE

As with most exercise routines. It's wise to start with a warm-up consisting of 4 or 5 Neck Rolls* — rolling the head back, around, down and around then reversing the direction. This is followed by Arm Circles, 4 or 5 times in one direction and then in the reverse direction.

This should be followed by Side Benders* and

---

*See Chapter 2 for descriptions of each of these exercises.

Flexed Leg Back Stretches.* These warm-up exercises can be preceded or followed by 1 minute stationary run.

The exercises that follow are intended to improve flexibility, strength and muscular endurance and cover the whole body, starting with the neck.

1. Neck Flexion and Extension: With a head harness that holds a weight, you lie face up on a bench or table, neck above shoulders extending over the edge of the bench. You bend the head up and back down as far as possible, repeating 5 or 6 times. Then you turn over, face down, with head extended over the edge of the bench or table and lift head up and down as far as possible, 5 or 6 times.

2. Lateral Neck Flexion: Standing erect, you bend the head as far as possible, first to the left and then to the right, repeating 5 or 6 times.

3. Do a series of weight-lifting presses and curls, followed by a High Pull, Bench Press and Bent Rowing. (See Chapter 3 for exercise descriptions.)

4. Lateral arm raise with dumbbells. Holding a dumbbell in each hand, hands at sides, lift both arms out to straight overhead position without bending elbows. Repeat 6 or 7 times. Start with 10-pound dumbbells.

5. Double Leg Lift, for abdominal muscles and hip flexors. Face up on floor, hands clasped behind the neck, lift both legs together to straight overhead position and then lower them to within a couple of inches of floor. Hold as long as possible.

6. Situps: Hands clasped behind neck, do 10 to 20 situps.

7. "V" sit: Lying face up on floor, simultaneously sit up and lift both legs, touching the hands to the toes. Only the buttocks are still resting on the floor.

8. Weight lifting exercises for back and legs, as detailed in the weight training exercises in Chapter 3.

9. Stride Stretch (See Chapter 2). Repeat 7 or 8 times with each leg.

10. Scissors. Lying flat on floor with arms perpendicular to sides, touch right toe to left hand, return and then touch left foot to right fingers. Repeat 7 or 8 times.

11. Seated Toe Touch. Repeat 7 or 8 times. (See Chapter 2).

12. Skip rope for 3 or 4 minutes. Rope skipping is the simplest exercise, but bench hopping, 30 repetitions a minute for 5 minutes, is vigorous and effective in building cardiovascular pulmonary endurance.

Running in place, lifting the knees high and swinging the arms vigorously while running as fast as possible in stationary position for 4 or 5 minutes is equally good.

Anyone who follows the above routine, three times a week, will maintain his or her physical fitness.

SIX MINUTES BEFORE BREAKFAST

1. Do 20 pushups, hands flat on floor.
2. Do 20 situps, with hands clasped behind head.
3. With feet together, flat on floor, stand erect, hands extended above head, and try to touch the floor or your toes, 10 times.
4. Chin yourself 10 times or as many times as you can do it.
5. Do any of the barbell exercises described elsewhere in this book. If you don't have barbells, use a heavy skillet, the iron or any other heavy object.
6. Do a minute of stationary running or rope jumping.

This is by no means a good cardiovascular pulmonary endurance exercise program, but it will make you feel better, have a better appetite, start the day more alert and refreshed, and put you miles ahead of the nonexercisers around you. In a few weeks, it should have you at the point where you *want* to do some cardiovascular pulmonary endurance exercise such as running or jogging, cycling, swimming, or jumping rope. Doing the quick program 5 times a week is better than 3 times—but 3 times is better than not at all.

The lasting effectiveness of anything less than 3 times a week is doubtful.

If any part of the program becomes boring or irritating to you, substitute another exercise for the one you don't like.

If you feel that one certain part of your body needs more improvement than the others, stress the exercise that applies to the problem.

Weigh yourself every fifth day to see how well you're controlling your weight. If it goes up, you probably need to exercise closer control over your diet.

FAMILY EXERCISE PROGRAMS

This program is designed to be within the scope of the whole family, with application to children and the elderly, regardless of sex. It should not be done at a speed that would discourage either group.

1. Arms extended straight out from the shoulders, move the hands in circles five times. Then move them in circles five times in the opposite direction. Then try to make the left-hand circles forward while making right-hand circles in reverse motion.

2. A different member of the family is appointed for every session to lead a "Simon Says Thumbs Up" exercise routine, picking from such exercises as pushups, situps, touching toes from an erect stance, etc. The fun of this is to try to change the exercise to a new one while somebody in the group is still doing the previous one.

3. Rope jumping to rhythm, the family keeping time to a recording or music on the radio. Each member tries to keep with the rhythm on one foot, hopping, jumping backward, etc.

4. Situps from face up on floor, arms extended over head. Each member of the family tries to swing the arms as little forward from overhead position as possible. Do 10 times.

5. From face up position on floor, keep legs stiff from foot to hip. Alternate lifting each leg up straight above hips and as far back

toward head as possible. Do it 15 times. On both No. 4 and No. 5, there will be considerable variation in accomplishment. All that matters is that each exerciser extend himself or herself to do the best possible.

6. From standing position, feet together, bend upper body from waist as far down and forward as possible. Repeat 10 times. On this one, the youngsters quite often do better than the adults.

7. With one foot well forward from the other, in standing position, quickly alternate positions of the feet, making a little hopping motion. Do as fast as possible for 2 minutes.

In addition to these floor exercises, there are several great approaches to family exercise that are enjoyable for everyone.

These entail walking to areas where floral, bird life, animal life or woods give an opportunity for observation, with each member of the family pointing out things of interest he or she sees. It may prove surprising how observant the children are. And grandpa and grandma know from long experience what's apt to be found in an area. Often, on weekends, families take picnic lunches along on their nature walks and make a pleasant day's outing of their exercise.

Walking to points of historical or scenic interest that aren't too far for the youngsters can be another fine exercise experience. Fathers and mothers often see things they've heard about but have never gotten around to visiting. State parks offer a wealth of exploratory investigation. If such a park is too far away for hiking, it's possible to drive to the park and then do the family hiking within its confines.

Family cycling is becoming an increasingly popular exercise in the United States and is splendid exercise. In my neighborhood, there's one family—father and mother, two children and a grandfather—that goes cycling past our home early every evening in cycling weather. Every member of the group seems to be having a good time. There are now bicycle paths and bicycle tours in most localities, and there's nothing that would compel a family to go any further than the youngsters can handle. Parents tell me their experience is that the children are so interested and

so like being with their parents that they really extend themselves to keep going. Wisconsin, where our summer home is located, has a reference directory of bike trails, with descriptive information, and some of the trails are terrific. They vary from easy jaunts to those with stiff grades that may be too difficult for young children.

Nearly every indoor swimming pool in YMCAs and similar organizations has family swim periods at least once or twice a week. Some have them early every morning or early in the evening. This is healthful exercise that permits each member of the family to set his or her own pace.

Family Exercise Games

Here are some games that all children enjoy, and adults who participate in them with their youngsters are usually surprised how much strenuous exercise they can get.

The ancient *sack race* can be as strenuous as players want to make it, and the sack in which each participant stands, coming up to his or her neck, is not only an equalizer but often gives children an advantage over adults. If sacks aren't available, the arms can be tied to the sides with a piece of rope and the legs tied together at the knees and ankles.

When my son was a Boy Scout, he talked me into entering a father-and-son *three-legged race* with him. My right leg and my son's left leg were tied together at the thigh, knee and ankle. All of the fathers were physically exhausted at the finish of the 50-yard race, and the boys were sweating profusely.

Keep Away, played with a basketball or beanbag, can be rugged physical exercise if the four players are fairly evenly matched in height.

Hare and Hounds is a great game for a Boy Scout Patrol, with an adult leader getting a 3-minute headstart as the hare. He carries a bag of paper torn up to confetti size and must drop some of it every 15 yards. The ''hound'' who first reaches him is the winner.

The old *Kick the Can* game is always good exercise for children.

Kite Flying may not sound like much exercise, but it offers a lot more of a contribution to physical fitness than sitting and watching television. Youngsters who get interested in the art of kite flying often hold tournaments, and anyone who has watched such an event knows that the participants get a lot of healthful exercise.

Encouraging youngsters to make money from physical labor is certainly commendable. Having a paper delivery route is not only healthful but profitable, and many boys and girls build up quite a nest egg by the time they're out of high school.

When I was a kid, I had a deal mowing five lawns in our neighborhood, at 50¢ each. Today, youngsters get $5 for mowing the same size lawn.

I don't think a boy or girl can possibly mow lawns all summer long without improving his or her condition.

Snow shoveling greatly augments the incomes of four youngsters in the square block where I live. I regret to say that one of the boys uses a gas-powered snow blower, but even *he* gets some exercise from his efforts.

Sometimes it's difficult for parents to tear their children away from TV sets, but they owe their youngsters that much concern.

CORRECTIVE EXERCISE PROGRAMS

"BAD" OR SORE BACK PROBLEMS AND EXERCISE

The medical profession is generally agreed that most back problems—about three-fourths of them—are caused by weak muscles or back inelasticity. Muscles aren't strong enough or flexible enough to stand up to the punishment they must take. A muscle that can't deliver what it's called on to do will temporarily quit functioning.

And the weak muscles aren't always in the back. Weak abdominal muscles are the worst offenders, and aren't able to function properly with stronger back muscles. The back muscles normally use 150 foot-pounds of energy (approximately) to keep a person erect with every step he takes, which keeps those muscles strong.

And the pull of the strong back muscles against weak abdominal muscles rotates the pelvis and consequently strains the back.

The best known way to prevent recurrence of back pain is a regular exercise routine. It's been established that a muscle which isn't used in 10 days has lost a third of its strength. It's also true that exercise calms the nerves, relieving the nervous tension that knots muscles and leads to spasms.

A person shouldn't aggravate the back by starting all-out with a slam-bang exercise program. The demand on the muscles should be increased gradually.

A simple abdominal muscle exercise that can be done anywhere is to squeeze the abdominal muscles, sucking in the belly and holding the position for a brief count. This is followed by relaxing the muscles and pushing the belly out as far as possible, holding the position briefly and then relaxing.

Pushups are also excellent, but you should start with only five or 10 and eventually work up to 50 or 75.

A simple exercise to stretch the back muscles is done from a sitting position in a straight-backed chair. The torso drops forward until the head is between the knees. Then the upper body slowly pulls back up to a normal sitting position. This shouldn't be done more than two or three times at the outset.

Standing properly lessens the strain on the back. If you stand against a wall with your heels, hips, shoulders and head pressed firmly against it and there is space enough between the small of your back and the wall so that you can put your hand into it, your back is arched too much. You need to tilt your pelvis back to get a flat lower back.

Tests for Back and Abdominal Muscle Strength and Flexibility

From a supine position on the floor with legs together and hands clasped behind the nape of the neck, you should be able to lift your feet 10 inches above the floor, holding them there for 10 or 12 seconds. If you can't do it, your hip-flexing muscles need strengthening.

Flexed knee situps with hands behind the neck should be accomplished with the elbows back. If you can't do it, your abdominal muscles need strengthening.

Lying down face-down with feet held anchored

by a chair or davenport, hands clasped behind the neck, you should be able to bend your torso back so that your elbows, chin and chest are off the floor. The position should be held for a count of at least 10. If you can't do it, your upper back muscles need strengthening.

Then, from the same face-down position, try to lift the legs, holding the knees straight and maintaining the position for a count of at least 10. If you can't do it, you have proof that your lower back muscles need strengthening.

If you can't do a straight-knee toe-touch as you bend forward from the waist, then your tight back muscles and shortened hamstrings need to be made more flexible.

Any needs indicated by these tests can be fulfilled by exercise—and in no other way.

A Quick Exercise Routine for a Sore Back

1. From either a doorway or a rod at the proper height for you, grip the rod or the top of the doorway with both hands and hang limply. The feet should hang limply, not touching the ground, and the arms should be fully extended. Hold the position for a full minute.
2. Rest flat on the back for 3 minutes, trying to relax the back muscles as much as possible.
3. Only if the back muscles feel relaxed, do five or six slow situps.
4. Use a Water-Pik or similar massage unit on the back, with water warm but not hot. Move the body around so that every part of the back gets the effect of the shower massage.

Back pains are difficult to diagnose. Some people are stoical about them when they're excruciatingly agonizing, while others scream in agony at a slight back twinge. If a back pain persists for a week, it's a good idea to consult a doctor about it. There are types of back soreness where even mild exercise should be done only with the utmost caution.

Most experts agree that for run-of-the-mill sore backs, a good, firm mattress is an excellent remedy.

At one time, I had occasional sore back muscles just below the waistline. At my doctor's recommendation, I started to wear the Mandate undershorts, and in the 6 or 7 years since I began wearing them, I've never had a twinge in that area. Mandate is a copyrighted brand which is available nearly everywhere.

For a slight sprain, some doctors recommend rubbing the affected area with rubbing alcohol or liniment. It has always seemed to me that the results from both are more psychological than therapeutic. However, I've seen many cases of back soreness where psychology was the most effective treatment.

Massage by a competent masseur will often relieve a sore back almost immediately.

A good piece of advice is not to do *any* violent exercise or engage in any contact sport while a sore back is plaguing you. I've known athletes in competition to use a local anesthetic on their backs before a game—and damage their backs even more—some of them to the point where the back problem became chronic.

A WATER EXERCISE PROGRAM FOR ARTHRITIS SUFFERERS

There is nothing new about water exercise to help arthritis sufferers. When my wife first began to have problems with arthritis in her knees and shoulders, her doctor told her to do a lot of swimming—not hard, competitive-type swimming but the kind of swimming that's done for pleasure. He also gave her some knee and shoulder exercises.

A 65-year-old arthritis sufferer, Dvera Bernson, has put her water exercise routine into a book, *Pain-Free Arthritis*. Written in collaboration with Sander Roy and published by Simon and Schuster in 1978. The book has been accepted with enthusiasm by people with arthritis and if they follow the Bernson exercise routines, they'll be better off.

As with most exercise programs, it is important in this one not to try to do too much at the outset. The slow progressive overload principle is the effective one. And if you overload too much, don't do the exercise for a day or two and then decrease the overload.

Since arthritis is a chronic ailment with most of the people who suffer from it, you don't help it much by exercising a day or two every week. Rather, my wife's orthopedic surgeon told her, it would take a 5-day-a-week routine to accomplish results, and that the exercises wouldn't cure her—that she should make up her mind to continuous exercise to battle the arthritis.

While in some exercises it's recommended that you strain your muscles for short periods of time, arthritis exercises should never do such a thing. The idea is first, to stretch the muscles and second, to gradually strengthen them. Slow and easy does it. In the water is the ideal place to stretch and strengthen without pain or strain. Everyone who has ever done much swimming knows that exercising in the water is considerably easier than exercising out of it.

Arthritis strikes some people first in the hands and fingers, and some people never have a great deal of trouble with it anywhere else. Other arthritics tell me that trouble with the hands is an advance warning of trouble in other parts of the body.

For this exercise, you should be in a part of the pool where the water isn't above your waist. With your hands hanging naturally at the sides, under water, of course, move your fingers back and forth as far as they'll go without forcing them. Don't move them simultaneously side by side but independently of each other. An easy way to do it is to start moving the little finger in toward the palm. As it begins to move, the third finger follows it, and then the second finger, followed by the first finger. The last finger to move is the thumb, which moves out to the side of the hand instead of into the palm, which is the natural way for it to go. The routine might be described as a finger flourish.

You should get the feeling that each finger is gently but firmly pushing the water away from it.

After you have done this a few times, you stand with the hands in the same position, palms toward the body. Then close your fist over the thumb. Next, move the thumb and fingers back and out, stretching the digits as much as you can without straining.

This can be followed by an exercise for the wrist joints, standing in the same depth and position. Without moving your arm, you raise your wrist as far as possible and then lower it, slowly and gently with a pushing motion. After doing this a few times, revolve the wrists of the open hands in circles, reversing the rotation after a few times clockwise to a counterclockwise rotation.

To exercise the elbow joints, stand in water up to your neck. With the palm open, lift the arm below the elbow from the side to a point where the finger tips are above water. As you reach that point, reverse the motion, lowering the arm below the elbow to the starting position. After doing this a few times with the right arm and elbow, do it with the left.

Then, as you did with the wrists, rotate the forearm in a circle, first to the right for a few times and then to the left.

Follow this with an exercise to stretch and strengthen the shoulder muscles. The water should be up to your chin. Keep your arms straight, unbent at the elbow, and raise and lower your arms while pushing your palms against the water. The palms should be open, in a straight line from the arm and wrist, so that you push the water gently as you make the movements. As with the wrists and elbows, then move the shoulder first a few times in a circular motion clockwise, then in a counter-clockwise rotation. Follow that by shrugging your shoulders, up and down. Then lift your shoulders and rotate them back and down to their starting position.

Follow this by standing with arms at the sides, bring them up and forward straight out in front of you and cross the arms at the elbows without bending the elbows. Now bring them back down to the sides and behind you, doing the whole movement slowly and smoothly, pushing the water with your arms.

Follow this by standing in water up to your waist. Raise your leg in front of you, without bending your knee and then swing it back behind you, in what amounts to a pendulum motion, pushing the water away with the leg throughout the movement.

After you've done these gentle exercises for a few weeks, add to them by doing a flutter kick while floating on your back. While you're doing it, raise and lower your arms 7 or 8 inches, alternately.

Next, floating on your back, spread your legs as far apart as possible while moving your arms out from the sides. Repeat this exercise movement, pushing the water gently away from your arms and legs as you make the motions.

After you've done this routine for a few weeks, you should be able to swim the backstroke. When an arthritic does the backstroke and treads water, there should be an effort to move every part of the body that has an arthritic tendency, even if the part isn't directly involved in swimming the backstroke or treading water.

That and treading water are about as far as you should go. When you can do those two things readily, five times a week, your battle against arthritis will have come a long way.

Some people advance to this point but can't do the backstroke and treading water satisfactorily.

They should not give up. A life belt around the waist will make the backstroke much easier and a pair of waterwings put at the back of the neck will simplify treading water.

For those whose arthritis isn't yet so painful as to prevent it, the flexibility exercises in Chapter 2 are excellent for stretching the muscles. The arthritic should use the flexibility exercises that apply to the troubled joints and muscles.

After these have been done for about 3 weeks, exercise to strengthen the affected parts can be started, but on a very gentle basis.

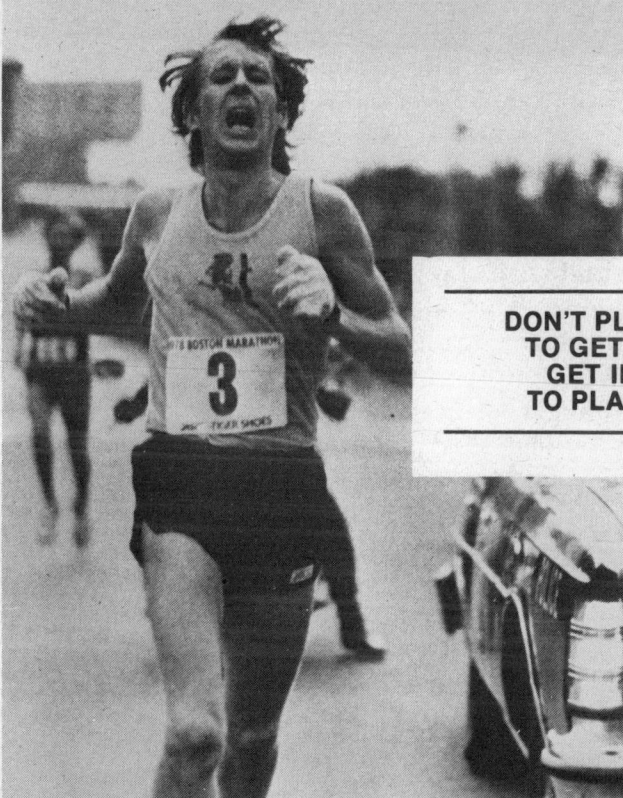

**DON'T PLAY SPORTS
TO GET IN SHAPE
GET IN SHAPE
TO PLAY SPORTS**

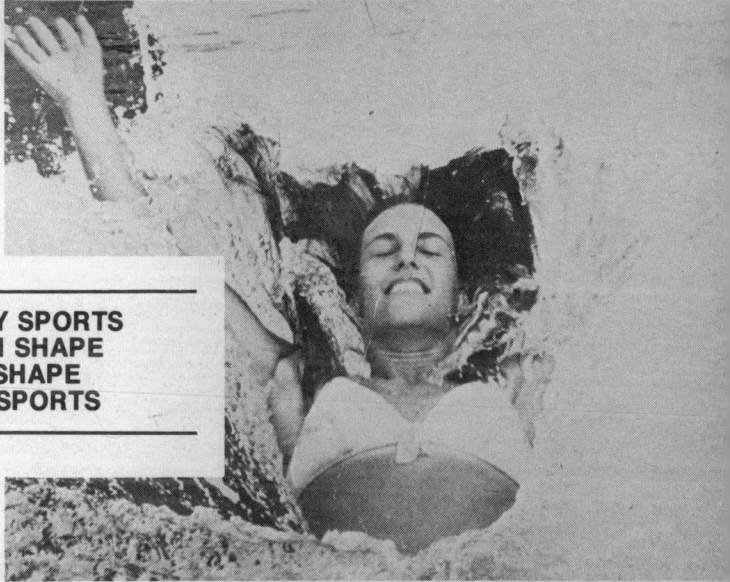

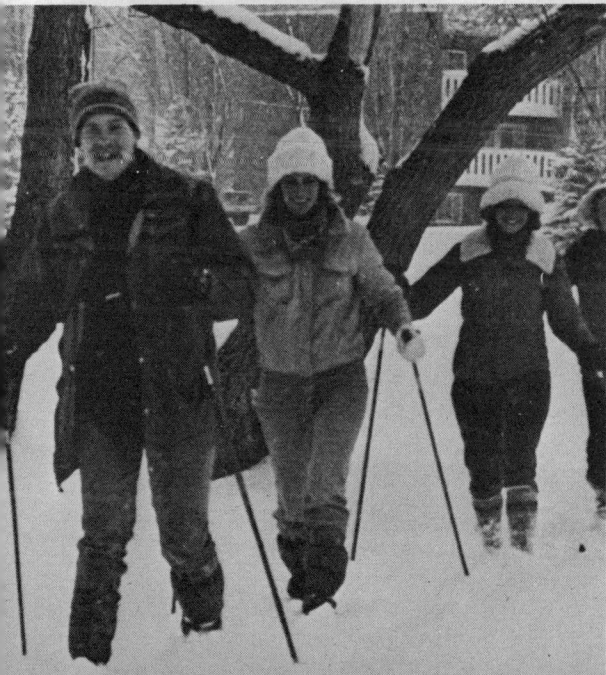

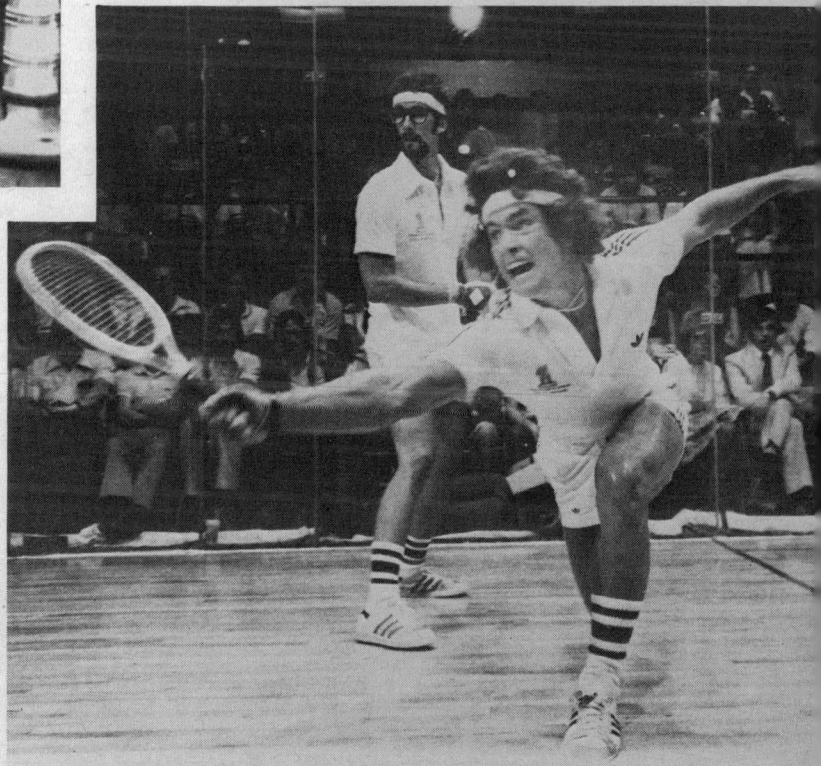

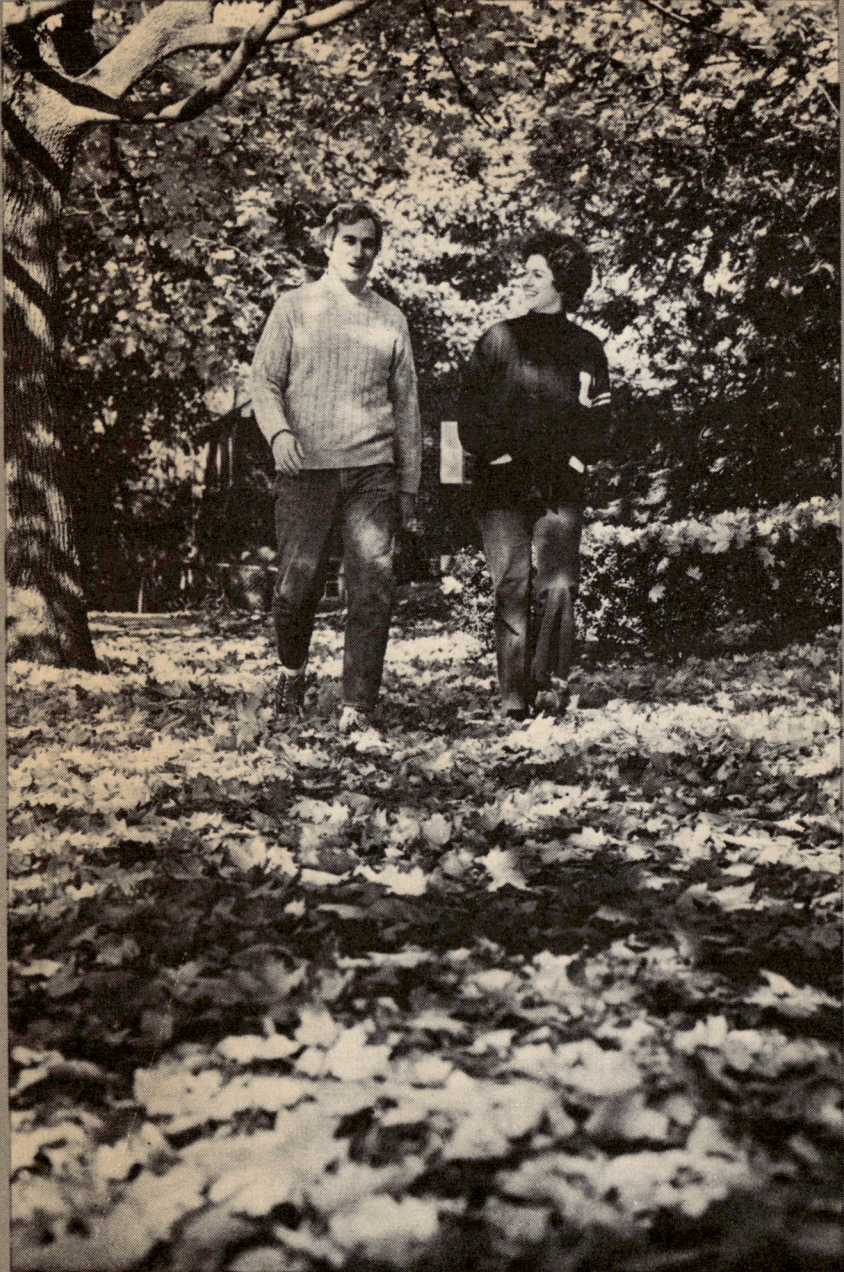

chapter 7

Now It's Up To You

THE WAY TO physical fitness and good health has been charted. You've been given a wide choice and by this time should have elected to follow one specific exercise or fitness program.

But remember that you were told early in the book—that there's no ending to any successful physical fitness routine. It has to be a *continuing* way of life for lasting benefits.

By now, results should be so dramatic and so pleasing that you'd never *want* to revert to sedentary existence. You should be *enjoying* your exercise, regardless of what form it takes.

Any tendency to return to a life of physical inactivity will inevitably result in a deterioration of what you've built up.

Young athletes in particular have a tendency after graduation from college to discontinue exercise, and they soon go to pot, both literally and figuratively.

Getting the glow of good health in your grasp doesn't mean that it's permanent. It can soon disappear if you don't keep it alive and flourishing.

Some basic minimal exercise routines for the maintenance of physical fitness are included in this book, but they *are* minimal. They're better than nothing, but not nearly as good as the vigorous, all-out programs are.

Regardless of your age, your program should be for keeps.

Youngsters who have finally gotten into good shape can quickly revert to unhealthy weaklings if they don't make a habit of proper and sufficient exercise.

Young married couples and middle-aged people are often guilty of letting other interests interfere with getting sufficient exercise.

The elderly are fighting what may be considered the toughest battle of all. Unless they continue a vigorous exercise regimen, they can quickly deteriorate—and once organs and muscles have deteriorated, bringing them back to life at a late age is an almost hopeless cause.

Some readers may ask at this point, "Is an exercise program that continues for the rest of my life worth the effort?"

I'll answer that question with a few counter-questions.

Is staying healthy worth an effort?

Is being vitally alive and vigorous instead of having a dormant existence worth the effort?

Is not being tired all the time worth the effort?

Is being mentally alert and fresh worth the effort?

If the reader's answer to any one of these questions is "Yes," the proper procedure is obvious.

I'm thinking of an elderly man who made a great deal of money as a top professional athlete. When he retired from athletic competition, he had no financial worries and announced to his friends, "Thank goodness, from now on, I can take it easy. No more training. No more watching my diet. No more jogging. No more sprinting, no more nursing bumps and bruises.''

Today, he's a pitiful sight. It's my opinion that he's dying by inches. He complains constantly about his health, and the complaints aren't imaginary. His old friends avoid him and, worse yet, pity him.

I talked to him awhile back and asked, "Why don't you get back into decent shape?"

He shrugged his shoulders. "I'd like to," he admitted, "but I'm afraid it's too late. I'm run down and worn out to the point where there's not much left to rebuild. About a month ago, I decided to start jogging again. I couldn't do it. By the time I'd gone three blocks, I was all in, puffing like a steam engine, and my heart was giving me trouble. Oh, I suppose I could take it a little step at a time, but the hell of it is, the steps would have to be so small that I don't think I'll be alive long enough to get back into shape. I made a bad mistake, and I guess I have to be resigned to paying for it."

I know men 10 years older than this fellow who never went through the rigorous routines he did who are exercising every day and are in excellent health. They've *maintained* their physical fitness to the best of their ability.

Your body is not a steel and concrete skyscraper that, once built, needs little or no maintenance. Some physical education experts say that a normally healthy person who's maintained moderately good physical condition begins to decline after reaching a peak, usually somewhere in the 30s. Unless he fights that regression with vigorous exercise, the decline will gain momentum as he ages.

Wishful thinking won't stop the process. Nothing combats it successfully except adequate exercise and proper diet. Some day, there may be a magic potion that will stop the deterioration of the human body and freeze good health permanently, but that time has not yet arrived. Until it does, we have to exercise or become physically unfit.

There are a few people who *look* fit but who never seem to do enough exercise to raise a mild sweat. I was baffled by one such person until he confided that he had a bad case of ameobic dysentery that doctors had been unable to cure. Actually, he was in bad physical shape.

Another man who used to joke that whenever he felt like exercising, he took a nap until the urge

wore off, died at his desk about a year ago. I don't know about the few others I've run across, but I'd be willing to bet a few bob that their appearance belies their physical condition.

In contrast, I know a professional football guard who looks like a big, fat slob. His size makes it seem that he would *have* to be slow.

His coach told me, "At first, opponents got the same impression you've arrived at. But they revised their thinking in a hurry. That's not fat on his body. It's muscle. He's hard as a rock. And he can get from one side of the line to the other before an opponent can stop him. I wish every man on our squad was in such good condition."

A YMCA gym instructor told me he'd had quite a time deciding what to do about a more lucrative job that had been offered him in business. He said, "On this job, I'm exercising almost eight hours a day, with a lot of variety in the routines. I think my physical condition's about as good as it can get. The new job would have me on the road as a salesman for the first year after a 3-month instruction course. I'd be shuttling from airports to hotel rooms, with the working day spent in showing our line.

"The more I thought about it, the more I was convinced that taking the job would be a good way to go down hill physically. I enjoy the Y job, I'm good at it, I like the people I'm working with and I'm keeping in great condition. I decided that money's nice but isn't everything, and I stayed on the Y job."

A friend of mine protested to his doctor that he didn't have the time to exercise as much as the doctor wanted him to. And the doctor told him, "You can't beat the rap. Either you'll take the time to exercise or you'll spend much *more* time in a hospital or nursing home. Take your choice."

I was amused by a man in his mid-60s who was telling me about his plans for the expansion of his business. And he'd thought of every contingency. "If I should die," he said, "the business wouldn't suffer much, thanks to the way I have it organized."

"If he should die." What does he mean, *if* he should die? He's *going* to die, some time, sooner or later. That's guaranteed.

That's true for all of us. But in the meantime, as far as I'm concerned, I'm going to enjoy good health to the fullest. I hope you do, too.